Psychological Insights for Understanding COVID-19 and Society

In the *Psychological Insights for Understanding COVID-19* series, international experts introduce important themes in psychological science that engage with people's unprecedented experience of the pandemic, drawing together chapters as they originally appeared before COVID-19 descended on the world.

This book explores how COVID-19 has impacted society, and chapters examine a range of societal issues including leadership and politics, community, social status, welfare, social exclusion and accountability. Addressing the social and psychological processes that structure, and are structured by, our social contexts, it shows not only how groups and individuals can come together to manage global crises, but also how these crises can expose weaknesses in our society. The volume also reflects on how we can work together to rebuild society in the aftermath of the pandemic, by cultivating a shared sense of responsibility through social integration and responsible leadership.

Showcasing theory and research on key topics germane to the global pandemic, the *Psychological Insights for Understanding COVID-19* series offers thought-provoking reading for professionals, students, academics and policy makers concerned with the psychological consequences of COVID-19 for individuals, families and societies.

S. Alexander Haslam is Professor of Psychology and Australian Laureate Fellow at the University of Queensland. Alex's research focuses on the study of group and identity processes in social, organisational and health contexts. Together with over 250 co-authors around the world, he has written and edited 15 books and published over 250 peer-reviewed articles on these topics. He is a former editor of the *European Journal of Social Psychology* and currently Associate Editor of *The Leadership Quarterly*.

Psychological Insights for Understanding COVID-19

The *Psychological Insights for Understanding COVID-19* series aims to highlight important themes in psychological science that engage with people's unprecedented experience of the COVID-19 pandemic. These short, accessible volumes draw together chapters as they originally appeared before COVID-19 descended on the world but demonstrate how researchers and professionals in psychological science had developed theory and research on key topics germane to the global pandemic. Each volume includes a specially commissioned, expert introduction that contextualises the chapters in relation to the crisis, reflects on the relevance of psychological research during this significant global event, and proposes future research and vital interventions that elucidate understanding and coping with COVID-19. With individual volumes exploring society, health, family, work and media, the *Psychological Insights for Understanding COVID-19* series offers thought-provoking reading for professionals, students, academics and policy makers concerned with psychological consequences of the pandemic for individuals, families and society.

Titles in the series:

Psychological Insights for Understanding COVID-19 and Families, Parents, and Children
Marc H. Bornstein

Psychological Insights for Understanding COVID-19 and Media and Technology
Ciarán Mc Mahon

Psychological Insights for Understanding COVID-19 and Society
S. Alexander Haslam

Psychological Insights for Understanding COVID-19 and Work
Cary L. Cooper

Psychological Insights for Understanding COVID-19 and Health
Dominika Kwasnicka and Robbert Sanderman

For more information about this series, please visit: https://www.routledge.com/Psychological-Insights-for-Understanding-COVID-19/book-series/COVID

Psychological Insights for Understanding COVID-19 and Society

Edited by S. Alexander Haslam

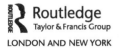

Routledge
Taylor & Francis Group

LONDON AND NEW YORK

First published 2021
by Routledge
2 Park Square, Milton Park, Abingdon, Oxon OX14 4RN

and by Routledge
52 Vanderbilt Avenue, New York, NY 10017

Routledge is an imprint of the Taylor & Francis Group, an informa business

British Library Cataloguing-in-Publication Data
A catalogue record for this book is available from the British Library

Library of Congress Cataloging-in-Publication Data
A catalog record for this book has been requested

ISBN: 978-0-367-64760-5 (hbk)
ISBN: 978-0-367-64759-9 (pbk)
ISBN: 978-1-003-12612-6 (ebk)

Typeset in Times New Roman
by Apex CoVantage, LLC

Selected chapters are taken from the following original Routledge publications

Selma Rudert, Rainer Greifeneder, Kipling Williams, *Current Directions in Ostracism, Social Exclusion and Rejection Research*, ISBN: 978-0-8153-6813-7 (hbk) ISBN: 978-1-351-25591-2 (ebk)

Ken J. Rotenberg, *The Psychology of Trust*, ISBN: 978-1-138-67848-4 (hbk) 978-1-315-55891-2 (ebk)

Barry Richards, *The Psychology of Politics*, 978-1-138-55167-1 (hbk) ISBN: 978-1-315-14769-7 (ebk)

Wendy Stainton Rogers, *Perspectives on Social Psychology: A Psychology of Human Being*, ISBN: 978-1-138-50132-4 (hbk) ISBN: 978-1-315-14427-6 (ebk)

Catherine Haslam, Jolanda Jetten, Tegan Cruwys, Genevieve Dingle, S. Alexander Haslam, *The New Psychology of Health: Unlocking the Social Cure*, ISBN: 978-1-138-12387-8 (hbk) ISBN: 978-1-315-64856-9 (ebk)

Carolyn Kagan, Mark Burton, Paul Duckett, Rebecca Lawthom, Asiya Siddiquee, *Critical Community Psychology: Critical Action and Social Change*, ISBN: 978-1-138-36405-9 (hbk) ISBN: 978-0-429-43150-0 (ebk)

Polli Hagenaars, Marlena Plavšić, Nora Sveaass, Ulrich Wagner, Tony Wainwright, *Human Rights Education for Psychologists*, ISBN: 978-0-367-22287-1 (hbk) ISBN: 978-0-429-27431-2 (ebk)

Contents

Contributors

Mark Burton, Manchester Metropolitan University, UK (visiting position)

Tegan Cruwys, Research School of Psychology, The Australian National University, Australia

Genevieve Dingle, The University of Queensland, Australia

Paul Duckett, Victoria University, Australia

S. Alexander Haslam, The University of Queensland, Australia

Catherine Haslam, The University of Queensland, Australia c.haslam@uq.edu.au

Jolanda Jetten, The University of Queensland, Australia

Carolyn Kagan, Manchester Metropolitan University, UK C.Kagan@mmu.ac.uk

Rebecca Lawthom, Manchester Metropolitan University, UK

Elizabeth Lira, Alberto Hurtado University, Chile elira@uahurtado.cl

Maria Paola Paladino, University of Trento, Italy

Barry Richards, Department of Humanities and Law, Bournemouth University, UK BRichards@bournemouth.ac.uk

Paolo Riva, University of Milano-Bicocca, Italy

Ken J. Rottenberg, University of Keele, UK k.j.rotenberg@keele.ac.uk

Asiya Siddiquee, Manchester Metropolitan University, UK

Wendy Stainton Rogers, Faculty of Health and Social Care, The Open University, UK w.stainton.rogers@icloud.com

Susanna Timeo, University of Trento, Italy susanna.timeo@unipd.it

Introduction

COVID-19 and society

S. Alexander Haslam

An obvious point about the COVID-19 pandemic is that it has created a huge amount of uncertainty that we are unable to resolve on our own. Much of that uncertainty centres on the nature of the virus itself and questions of biology and epidemiology. How does it spread? What are its effects? How can we find a vaccine? But many others relate to the social and psychological dimensions of the pandemic. Indeed, all of these questions have answers that are social as much as medical. This is particularly true when we reflect on the impact of the virus as it is clear that, after the pandemic, society as a whole will be profoundly altered (Solnit, 2020). For example, previously unquestioned assumptions about work, travel, social interaction and health will have to be substantially revised – in ways that we would have struggled to envisage just a year ago (Jetten et al., 2020a; Pfefferbaum, & North, 2020; Wind et al., 2020).

And, yet, for all this uncertainty, there are two important sets of constants. The first relates to the social and psychological processes that will play out in the context of this change. Certainly, these processes will be operating under a different set of conditions and in a different set of circumstances; nevertheless the processes themselves will be the same. For example, prior to COVID-19 we knew that social interaction and social integration were key determinants of health (Haslam et al., 2018; Holt-Lunstad et al., 2010) and this is no less true today. What has changed, though, is that many forms of interaction (e.g., with colleagues, with those in care; Bentley, 2020; Haslam, 2020) are now a lot more problematic and harder to take for granted than they were a year ago. Likewise, prior to the pandemic it was the case that social inequality created a health gradient which compromised the health and well-being not just of the disadvantaged but also of the advantaged (Marmot, 2014; Wilkinson & Pickett, 2012). This will still be true tomorrow, but what will have changed is that the pandemic will have exposed and accentuated pre-existing inequalities in ways that seem likely to place even greater strain on societies, their citizens and their institutions (Jetten, 2020; Smith & Gibson, 2020; Weible et al., 2020).

Related to this, the second set of constants relates to the knowledge that we have acquired about these various social and psychological processes. Faced with the unprecedented scale and nature of the pandemic, it is easy to imagine that social psychological science would be poorly prepared for the task of understanding the dynamics that would play out in its wake. Indeed, along these lines, several commentators argued that psychology (and social psychology in particular) was not 'crisis ready' – especially in comparison to medical and biological sciences whose understanding of the realities of epidemics and their impact was believed to be in a much more advanced state (Dupuis, 2020; Ijzerman et al., 2020; Ritchie, 2020; Yates, 2020).

There are a range of problems with this argument, but two stand out. The first is that, as events have shown, the novelty of the SARS-CoV-2 virus has meant that medical and biological scientists have themselves often struggled to make sense of, and respond to, the unfolding realities of virus transmission (Krause et al., 2020; Sahu et al., 2020). As a result, their models are imperfect and are constantly being updated and revised (Kuznia & Griffin, 2020; O'Brian, 2020). Nevertheless, alongside the new knowledge that is acquired as the pandemic advances, the main source of guidance has been the body of scientific knowledge that scientists painstakingly built up in the decades leading up to the current crisis. The same is true of social psychological science, and indeed in this respect the scientific fields are no different. Moreover, in this context, a second problem with the idea that psychological scientists are poorly positioned to inform responses to COVID-19 is that since start of the pandemic not only has there been more demand for social psychological knowledge than ever before, but so too that knowledge has proved far more useful than ever before.

As testament to this, a major review article by Van Bavel and colleagues (2020) that was published early on in the pandemic was accessed over 130,000 times in the first three months after appearing in *Nature Human Behaviour*. More importantly, over that time, most of its observations (e.g., about such things as threat perception, leadership, science communication, stress and coping) appeared to have been borne out by developments. For example, the observation that the pandemic would unleash a wave of prejudice and racism – particularly against Asians – proved correct (Huo, 2020) as did the claim that countries' ability to secure compliance with health directives would be linked to leadership that communicated a sense that 'we are all in this together' (rather than that 'we are divided'; e.g., along party political lines; Haslam et al., in press; Steffens, 2020).

It is in this context, then, demands have increased for social psychologists to harvest knowledge from their discipline in ways that would support responses to the pandemic. Prior to the outbreak of COVID-19, very few social psychologists had been explicitly interested in pandemics (although a body of research on public health emergencies and disaster management certainly anticipated some of its key features; e.g., Carter et al., 2015; Drury, 2012, Drury et al., 2020; Williams & Drury, 2009). Accordingly, as the pandemic took hold, researchers scurried to assemble and curate relevant theoretical, empirical and practical insights in ways they thought would be helpful to policy makers, practitioners and other researchers. Here, then, as Abrams (2020) has observed, researchers worked together

> not to find the one truth or "the science", but to deploy [their] different academic insights to best effect under the circumstances . . . [thereby getting] multiple experts to work together to identify how we can get things less wrong.

The review by Van Bavel et al. (2020) was one such effort, but the pandemic has inspired many other reviews (e.g., Holmes et al., 2020; O'Connor et al., 2020), journal special issues (e.g., Jonas & Cesario, 2020; Smith & Gibson, 2020) and books (including our own: *Together Apart: The Psychology of COVID-19*; Jetten et al., 2020a).

The present volume is part of this same orchestrated response and is an attempt to bring together contributions from key researchers and practitioners that speak to issues of leadership, trust, community, human welfare, human rights, social exclusion and disadvantage which are proving to have profound relevance in the context of COVID-19. What follows provides a short introduction to these contributions and goes on to abstract some of the key themes whose importance they explore and underline.

The present volume

The contributions

Our coverage starts in Chapter 1 with a discussion by Barry Richards of the nature of leadership taken from his 2018 book *The Psychology of Politics*. As we noted at the start of this chapter, the COVID-19 pandemic has created demand for effective leadership both to resolve uncertainly about the nature of the threat that the virus poses and to motivate people to work together to minimise that threat. In this context, effective leadership helps people understand what they should be thinking and doing, and inspires them to contribute to a concerted societal response. Effective leadership thus serves the dual function of (a) holding groups together through a crisis and (b) constructively channelling the energies of group members. In this context too, leaders themselves should ideally serve as a model of "the best of us" and in a crisis their first responsibility should be to set aside – and to be seen to set aside – divisive personal or partisan interests (Haslam et al., in press). And yet, as Richards observes, around the world in recent years we have witnessed the ascendancy of populist leaders (generally men) with turbocharged superegos who come to power with a narcissistic interest in pursuing polarising agendas – often underpinned by a narrative in which they cast themselves as representatives of the downtrodden who are fighting back against an all-too-cosy political elite. Think Donald Trump, Jair Bolsonaro, Rodrigo Duterte. Richards explores many of the deficiencies of this model of leadership – not least its authoritarian requirement that followers are excluded from the democratic process of defining and shaping the group that the leader leads. As he observes, this skews agency in the leader–follower relationship in ways that ultimately make groups themselves weak and ineffective (see also Haslam et al., 2011).

Along these lines, prior to the pandemic, a range of scholars and commentators had identified and decried the deficiencies of this model of leadership (e.g., Fitzduff, 2016). Yet Richards makes the point that it takes a crisis to fully expose their shortcomings. He does so with reference to terrorist attacks and international conflicts, but clearly COVID-19 was just such a crisis and here an ego-focused approach to leadership has indeed exposed groups to the full force of the existential threat that the SARS-CoV-2 poses. Going forward, a key question is therefore how to loosen the grip of such models and develop alternatives which are more democratic and inclusive – and safer. Unfortunately, as Richards notes, this goal has been made more challenging because populist leaders have themselves sought – with some success – to erode trust in the political process and in the people and institutions that embody it.

These questions of trust are even more central to Chapter 2. Taken from Ken J. Rotenberg's 2018 volume on *The Psychology of Trust*, this underlines the point that in recent years the rise of populism has transformed healthy political scepticism into rampant cynicism. In the process, he notes that a key form of social capital has itself been eroded – capital which binds citizens to each other and to their communities and institutions. Importantly, this capital is a key resource in efforts both to mitigate against the effects of various forms of disaster and to manage post-disaster recovery (Helliwell et al, 2014; Jovita et al., 2015; Masud-All-Kamal & Monirul Hassan, 2018; Nakagawa, & Shaw, 2004). Accordingly, it should come as no surprise that the countries in which this capital is highest (e.g., in Australasia and Scandinavia) have generally fared better in responding to COVID-19 than those in which it is lower. Not least, this is because social capital is associated with a sense of ties to, and obligation towards, one's fellow citizens in ways that encourage co-operation and compliance with health directives (Borgonovi, & Andrieu, 2020).

At the same time, precisely because the pandemic has underscored the need for sound governance and good leadership, where this has been forthcoming, it has tended to increase trust in government and thereby (re)build social capital. This is true in Australia, for example, where, as Rotenberg notes, prior to the pandemic only 43% of the public agreed that government could 'usually' or 'sometimes' be trusted to do the right thing, but by April 2020 this had risen to 53% and only 13% of Australians said that they had 'no trust' in government (Lewis, 2020). One reason for this is that the pandemic has created a sense of common fate and shared identity, such that rather than snipe at their political opponents, many leaders have been motivated to collaborate with them (Ntontis & Rocha, 2020). Again, though, for some political leaders the pill of solidarity has proved too bitter to swallow. Accordingly, while this upswell in solidarity has been found to have a range of benefits (of a form that Rotenberg's analysis anticipates) it has not been a universal phenomenon.

Issues of community are explored in Chapter 3 in a contribution from Carolyn Kagan, Mark Burton, Paul Duckett, Rebecca Lawthom and Asiya Siddiquee that is taken from their 2011 text on *Critical Community Psychology*. The focus here is on the ways that different types of social ties – those based on affection, interdependence and coercion – contribute to a sense of community and in turn have a role in defining behaviour within that community. A key theme here is that ties are multifaceted and nuanced and create a complex network of forces. For example, the social ties that bind people into a social group and that support positive relations within it can also engender antagonism toward those outside the group who appear to threaten it (Tajfel & Turner, 1979). Similarly, social boundaries can have impacts that are both benign and malign: helping to define a community of 'us' but sometimes also creating a pariah of 'them'. Again, these are dynamics that have played out forcefully in the context of COVID-19 – where international tensions have been inflamed by leaders seeking to build ties with and within their ingroup by tuning its members into various sources of outgroup threat (e.g., as seen in Donald Trump's insistence on referring to SARS-CoV-2 as "the Chinese virus"; Huo, 2020).

As in Rotenberg's chapter, these considerations again feed into reflections on the way that different types of social ties serve to build social capital of a form that not only sustains civic life and polity, but also forms an important resource for communities to sustain themselves in the face of various challenges (Puttnam, 2000). Importantly, though, the authors observe that communities' capacity to do this is conditioned by the degree of inequality within them – so that social capital is harder to build (and hence its benefits harder to access) in communities that have high levels of inequality (Wilkinson & Picket, 2009). As they note, this is a point that is often overlooked by theorists and commentators – in part because they have been insensitive to the political and ideological forces that erode social capital (e.g., those informed by neoliberalism and individualism; Sennett, 1998). Yet the importance of this point has also been forcefully brought home by the COVID-19 pandemic. Here, then, it has become clear that inequality is a major determinant of SARS-CoV-2's impact – so that not only is the virus disproportionately harmful to the poor and disadvantaged, but so too general levels of harm are higher in communities with higher inequality (Farmer et al., 2020).

The mechanisms of such health disparities are the focus of Chapter 4. Taken from their 2018 text, *The New Psychology of Health: Unlocking the Social Cure*, here Catherine Haslam, Jolanda Jetten, Tegan Cruwys, Genevieve Dingle and S. Alexander Haslam provide an analysis of the impact of social status and disadvantage on health. Importantly, this provides a social psychological framework that explains how the health impacts of inequality flow in large part from levels of shared social identity within a given community or society. A key point here is that, on their own, sociological and economic factors do not fully account for the impact of social disadvantage on health. Instead, the authors argue that social psychological processes moderate this relationship such that health (particularly of those who are disadvantaged) will vary as a function of the degree to which members of particular groups perceive themselves, and act, *as a group* (in terms of shared social identity) rather than as individuals. The authors argue that where people act in terms of social identity, this provides them with access to a range of social psychological resources – notably a sense of control, purpose and support – that then help them cope better with various forms of adversity, especially those that are associated with life (and identity) change.

A large body of empirical evidence supports these claims, much of it gleaned from studies of people's capacity to adjust successfully to such things as serious illness, retirement and trauma (Haslam et al., 2020). The latter work is particularly relevant in the context of the COVID-19 pandemic as it provides evidence of the capacity for social identity not only to increase resilience but also to open up pathways to post-traumatic growth (Muldoon et al., 2019). In line with a range of points that we have already made, it thus seems likely that social identity will prove to be an equally critical resource in efforts to tackle, and recover from, the pandemic. Indeed, consistent with this claim, there is already evidence that in the face of COVID-19 people's social identification with a given community – and leadership which helps to build and support this identification (Steffens et al., 2014; Van Dick et al., 2019) – is a key predictor not only of compliance and citizenship but also of solidarity, health and well-being (Haslam et al., in press; Jetten et al., 2020a; Templeton et al., 2020).

These considerations of health provide a segue into broader questions of human welfare upon which Wendy Stainton Rogers reflects in Chapter 5. Taken from her 2019 book *Perspectives on Social Psychology*, this chapter offers a wide-ranging critical perspective on matters of health and well-being, and begins by noting how these constructs have become increasingly personalised, commercialised and medicalised over time (trends which lead her to prefer to talk of 'welfare' rather than of 'health'). In particular, she draws attention to the way in which health – and the task of being healthy – has come to be construed as a matter of personal responsibility. Relatedly, another important contribution of this chapter is to observe how prevailing models of health focus attention on the individual – rather than on the social context in which they are embedded – in ways that lead us to see any illness that a person suffers as 'their problem'. Not only does this draw attention away from structural factors (such as inequality) that drive health outcomes, but so too it stigmatises those who suffer from particular conditions and skews attention away from the role and responsibility of collectives (not least governments) in this process and also overlooks the capacity for collectives (not least thriving communities) to promote resilience.

Again, there is abundant evidence of the problematic implications of such skewing in the trajectory of COVID-19. To start with, the defunding of public health agencies (e.g., the Centre for Disease Control and Prevention in the US) meant that they were poorly prepared to deal with the pandemic and that the burden of care then fell on victims whose capacity to cope was understandably limited (Haeder, 2020; Scott, 2020). As the pandemic has spread, it is apparent too that those who have contracted the virus are often targets of opprobrium and discrimination rather than of empathy and support. As the World Health Organization (2020) notes, "the current COVID-19 outbreak has provoked social stigma and discriminatory behaviours against people of certain ethnic backgrounds as well as anyone perceived to have been in contact with the virus". Not only, then, are those who are disadvantaged more likely to fall prey to the virus, but they are also more likely to be blamed and victimised if they do. At the same time, though, in line with Stainton Rogers' emphasis on the importance of social connection for welfare (which was also a focus of the previous chapter), we see that strong communities have played a vital role in pushing back against the virus – in particular, helping people to resolve local problems (e.g., surrounding access to resources and services) and protecting the vulnerable (Jetten et al., 2020b; Walker, 2020). As Herron (2020) observed on the ground in New Zealand, it takes a village to beat a virus.

Yet if it is true that a sense of shared social identity and community can support adjustment and recovery, then, as a corollary, it should equally be true that social division and social exclusion will tend to work against these things. This is a point that is explored in Chapter 6 by Susanna Timeo, Paolo Riva and Maria Paola Paladino in an analysis of the dynamics of social exclusion taken from Selma Rudert, Rainer

Greifeneder and Kipling Williams's (2019 edited volume, *Current Directions in Ostracism*. As they point out, social exclusion has a range of negative consequences for people's emotional and cognitive states and for their mental and physical health. A primary way it does this is by threatening basic needs – for belonging, self-esteem, control and purpose (Williams, 2009; precisely those needs which group-based inclusion satisfies; Greenaway et al., 2017; Haslam et al., 2018). The authors discuss a range of cognitive strategies for coping with this threat (e.g., re-appraisal, self-distancing, distraction), as well as reaffirmation strategies for restoring threatened needs. In line with observations in the preceding two chapters, many of the latter centre on efforts to reconnect (psychologically and/or physically) with valued groups in ways that (re)create the social bonds that are damaged by exclusion.

The significance of these issues in a world torn asunder by COVID-19 is all too clear. Indeed, even where people have not contracted the virus and been excluded on that basis (e.g., by having to self-isolate or being placed in quarantine), the process of protecting oneself against it (e.g., by practicing physical distancing) can itself be exclusionary (Bentley, 2020; Van Bavel et al., 2020). Thus at a time when, as we have noted, there is a particular need for people to come together to support each other and work on challenges collectively, there are forces driving them apart. This puts health policy makers on the horns of a serious dilemma, and presents as a particular challenge for members of vulnerable populations (e.g., older adults, or those in care; Haslam, 2020; Seifert et al., 2020). Going forward, it is clear too that developing workable solutions to this dilemma will be critical to ensuring that a viral disaster does not pave the way to a mental health catastrophe.

Panning out to reflect on broader challenges of policy making, the volume is brought to a close in Chapter 7 with an analysis of social accountability and action orientation by Elizabeth Lira Kornfield that appeared in a volume edited by Polli Hagenaars, Marlena Plavšić, Nora Sveaass, Ulrich Wagner, and Tony Wainwright (2020) on *Human Rights Education for Psychologists*. This chapter takes as its focus the challenges researchers faced when trying to support victims of the human rights violations that were committed by the military regime in Chile between 1973 and 1990. Under the dictatorship of Pinochet-led government, these violations were rife and centred on the abuse, torture, 'disappearance' and murder of many thousands of the regime's opponents. However, alongside this oppression, there also developed a network of agencies that emerged to provide social, psychological and medical support to those who had been brutalised by the regime. As documented by Kornfield, the problems that these agencies had to deal with were profound and traumatic, and she describes a range of processes designed to help victims work through their experiences and the psychological scarring these had created, and to recover something of their dignity and sense of self-worth. As she describes it, this journey starts with the creation of a therapeutic bond that then creates a platform for victims to regain confidence in their ability to trust and have meaningful relationships with others. Necessarily too, intervention also needs to be social not just personal, as in order for the journey to progress, victims "need[] to know that their society, as a whole, acknowledge[s] what had happened to them".

While many of the harrowing features of Kornfield's analysis are specific to the atrocities that victims of the Pinochet regime had to deal with, there are important lessons here for recovery from all trauma. Moreover, these will undoubtedly be important to take on board in efforts to recover from the trauma caused by COVID-19 (Muldoon et al., in press). Principal among these is the importance of intervention being built around a therapeutic alliance between those who give and receive support (Haslam et al., 2018). Support from the wider society (material as well as psychological) will also be important not only as manifestation of solidarity but also to help repair the enormous damage that COVID has done to social, economic and community infrastructure. Whether or not this will be forthcoming remains to be seen, but if it is not then the traumatic scarring of COVID-19 is likely to be much profound and much prolonged.

Conclusion: key messages for a COVID-stricken society

These, then, are the specific analyses that this volume brings together. No doubt too, as you read the chapters yourself you will discover a wealth of points that are germane to contemporary debates about how we should respond to the COVID-19 pandemic, and how we should work to rebuild our societies in its wake. Indeed, the diversity of these chapters is testimony to the breadth and richness of a wealth of theoretical and empirical research that has investigated the social and psychological foundations of society over the course of many decades (and in some case centuries).

Yet while the chapters that follow are a source of variegated insights, for a reader who is coming to this literature for the first time, the wood here may be hard to see for the trees. So what are the core messages that these contributions (and the broader corpus of work of which they are representative) carry for researchers, practitioners, policy makers and the general public in a time of COVID-19? There are many of these. But in bringing these introductory reflections to a conclusion, there are three inter-related messages that the chapters bring home that seem to be particularly worthy of emphasis.

1. *We are political beings who look to others to help us formulate collective responses to uncertainty and complexity.* As we have already noted, a defining feature of COVID-19 has been the complexity of the pandemic and of its impact on societies around the world. Scarcely a day goes by without some new revelation, some new twist or some new complication. Most of these centre on the implications of the virus for our health, our economies and our communities. In this context our quest for definitive answers to a catalogue of high-stakes questions is insatiable. More particularly, as several chapters in this volume anticipate (notably Chapters 1 and 2), the pandemic has fuelled demand for *leadership* – not just in politics but in multiple spheres including those that centre on matters of health, education, business and community. Importantly too, there is evidence that despite numerous examples of leadership failure, a great many leaders and a great many institutions have risen to this challenge. Importantly, though, they have not done this alone or through the assertion of 'I-ness' or ego. On the contrary, where they have been most successful, this is because they have mobilised

the latent power of communities through efforts to unite them around a shared sense of 'we-ness' and the common cause of fighting the virus.

2. *We are communal beings and our health and welfare is compromised by the erosion of communal ties.* This is a message that is shot through most of the chapters but which is underscored in different ways by Chapters 3, 4, 5 and 6. Each of these contributions points to the importance of community-based social connections for health, but each also identifies ways in which this sense of community can be eroded – by social division, by inequality, by social exclusion. The truth and relevance of this observation in the time of COVID-19 is plain to see and aligns with the general observation that, to date, countries and communities have generally been better placed to weather the viral storm where they have presented a united front against it. At the same time, it needs to be recognised that the virus itself exploits division and disunity, and so its capacity to do this needs always to be actively countered – not least through leadership that focuses on social integration rather than division.

3. *The processes that shape and sustain society are social, participatory and fluid.* In many different ways, one of the big lessons of the COVID-19 pandemic is that nothing in society is set in stone. Indeed, stark testimony to this is provided by the fact that the pandemic has required a radical rethinking of the functionality of the skyscrapers that adorn our city skylines, of the stadia in which sporting and cultural festivals are enacted, and even of our large lecture halls. In the process, much of the social psychological infrastructure that sustains society – and that hitherto we had taken largely for granted – has also been thrown into sharp relief too (Solnit, 2020). For example, the importance of mundane social interaction, of social integration and of compassionate leadership has been brought home in ways that could scarcely have been more dramatic.

As we work together on the challenging tasks of rebuilding society in the pandemic's aftermath, now, then, is the time to take stock of the core lessons of social psychological science and to reflect on their implications for action. The chapters that follow are broadly representative of that science, and, for all their manifold differences, they actually speak with a remarkably clear voice. Never has it been more important for that voice to be heard.

References

Abrams, D. (2020). To solve the problems of this pandemic, we need more than just 'the science'. *The Guardian* (April 29) Retrieved from www.theguardian.com/education/2020/apr/29/to-solve-the-problems-of-this-pandemic-we-need-more-than-just-the-science

Bartscher, A. K., Seitz, S., Slotwinski, M., Siegloch, S., & Wehrhöfer, N. (2020). *Social capital and the spread of COVID-19: Insights from European countries.* Unpublished manuscript: University of Bonn.

Bentley, S. (2020). Social isolation. In J. Jetten, S. D. Reicher, S. A. Haslam & T. Cruwys. *Together apart: The psychology of COVID-19* (pp.59–63). Sage.

Borgonovi, F., & Andrieu, E. (2020). Bowling together by bowling alone: Social capital and COVID-19. *COVID Economics, 17,* 73–96.

Drury, J. (2012). Collective resilience in mass emergencies and disasters. In J. Jetten, C. Haslam, & S. A. Haslam (Eds.), *The social cure: Identity, health and well-being* (pp.195–215). Hove, UK: Psychology Press.

Drury, J., Cocking, C., & Reicher, S. D. (2009b). Everyone for themselves? A comparative study of crowd solidarity among emergency survivors. *British Journal of Social Psychology*, *48*, 487–506.

Dupuis, D. R. (2020). The debate over psychology's COVID-19 response. *Areo* (June 15). Retrieved from: https://areomagazine.com/2020/06/15/the-debate-over-psychologys-COVID-19-response/

Farmer, N., Wallen, G. R., Baumer, Y., & Powell-Wiley, T. M. (2020). COVID-19: Growing health disparity gaps and an opportunity for health behavior discovery?. *Health Equity*, *4*, 316–319.

Fitzduff, M. (Ed.) (2017). *The myth of rational politics: Understanding the allure of Trumpism* (pp.25–39). Praeger.

Greenaway, K. H., Cruwys, T., Haslam, S. A., & Jetten, J. (2016). Social identities promote well-being because they satisfy global psychological needs. *European Journal of Social Psychology*, *46*, 294–307.

Haslam, C. (2020). Ageing and connectedness. In J. Jetten, S. D. Reicher, S. A. Haslam & T. Cruwys. *Together apart: The psychology of COVID-19* (pp.64–68). Sage.

Haslam, C., Haslam, S. A., Jetten, J., Cruwys, T., & Steffens, N. K. (2020a). Life change, social identity and health. *Annual Review of Psychology*.

Haslam, C., Jetten, J., Cruwys, T., Dingle, G. A., & Haslam, S. A. (2018). *The new psychology of health: Unlocking the social cure*. Abingdon, UK: Routledge.

Haslam, S. A., Reicher, S. D., & Platow, M. J. (2011). *The new psychology of leadership: Identity, influence and power.* Psychology Press.

Haslam, S. A., Steffens, N. K., & Peters, K. (2019). The importance of creating and harnessing a sense of 'us': Social identity as the missing link between leadership and health. In R. Williams, V. Kemp, S. A. Haslam, C. Haslam, K. S. Bhui, & S. Bailey (Eds), *Social scaffolding: Applying the lessons of contemporary social science to health, public mental health and healthcare* (pp.302–311). Cambridge: Cambridge University Press.

Haslam, S. A., Steffens, N. K. & Reicher, S. D. (in press). Leadership in a pandemic: Ten lessons from responses to COVID-19. *Social Issues and Policy Review*.

Helliwell, J., Huang, H. & Wang, S. (2014). Social capital and well-being in times of crisis. *Journal of Happiness Studies*, *15*, 10.1007/s10902–013–9441-z.

Herron, J. (2020). It takes a village to beat a virus. *Newsroom* (April 5). Retrieved from: www.newsroom.co.nz/it-takes-a-village-to-beat-a-virus

Holt-Lunstad, J., Smith, T. B., & Layton, J. B. (2010). Social relationships and mortality risk: A meta-analytic review. *PLoS Medicine*, *7*(7), e1000316.

Holmes, E. A., O'Connor, R. C., Perry, V. H., Tracey, I., Wessely, S., Arseneault, L., . . . & Ford, T. (2020). Multidisciplinary research priorities for the COVID-19 pandemic: A call for action for mental health science. *The Lancet Psychiatry*, *7*, 547–560.

Huo, Y. (2020). Prejudice and discrimination. In J. Jetten, S. D. Reicher, S. A. Haslam & T. Cruwys. *Together apart: The psychology of COVID-19* (pp.113–118). Sage.

Ijzerman, H., Lewis Jr, N., Weinstein, N., DeBruine, L., Ritchie, S. J., Vazire, S., . . . & Przybylski, A. K. (2020). *Psychological science is not yet a crisis-ready discipline*. Unpublished manuscript. Retrieved from: https://psyarxiv.com/whds4/

Jetten, J. (2020). Inequality. In J. Jetten, S. D. Reicher, S. A. Haslam & T. Cruwys. *Together apart: The psychology of COVID-19* (pp.101–106). Sage.

Jetten, J., Reicher, S. D., Haslam, S. A., & Cruwys, T. (2020a). *Together apart: The Psychology of COVID-19*. Sage.

Jetten, J., Reicher, S. D., Haslam, S. A., & Cruwys, T. (2020b). 10 lessons for dealing with a pandemic. *The Psychologist, 33* (7–8), 30–32.

Jonas, K., & Cesario, J. (2020). Social psychological contributions to understanding the coronavirus crisis. *Comprehensive Results in Social Psychology, 7* (1).

Jovita, H. D., Nashir, H., Mutiarin, D., Moner, Y. & Nurmandi, A. (2019) Social capital and disasters: How does social capital shape post-disaster conditions in the Philippines? *Journal of Human Behavior in the Social Environment, 29*, 519–534.

Krause, N. M., Freiling, I., Beets, B., & Brossard, D. (2020). Fact-checking as risk communication: the multi-layered risk of misinformation in times of COVID-19. *Journal of Risk Research*, 1–8.

Kuznia, R., & Griffin, D (2020). How did coronavirus break out? Theories abound as researchers race to solve genetic detective story. *CNN.com* (April 6). Accessed 10 April 2020. www.cnn.com/2020/04/06/us/coronavirus-scientists-debate-origin-theories-invs/index.html.

Lewis, P. (2020). Trust in the government is rising – but will Australians accept the coronavirus tracing app? *The Guardian* (April 21). Retrieved from: www.theguardian.com/australia-news/commentisfree/2020/apr/20/trust-in-the-government-is-rising-but-will-australians-accept-the-coronavirus-tracing-app

Marmot, M. (2015). *The health gap: The challenge of an unequal world*. London, UK: Bloomsbury.

Masud-All-Kamal, M., & Monirul Hassan, S. M. (2018). The link between social capital and disaster recovery: evidence from coastal communities in Bangladesh. *Natural Hazards, 93*, 1547–1564.

Morris, C. (2020). Trump administration budget cuts could become a major problem as coronavirus spreads. Fortune (February 27). Retrieved from: https://fortune.com/2020/02/26/coronavirus-COVID-19-cdc-budget-cuts-us-trump/

Muldoon, O., Haslam, S. A., Haslam, C., Cruwys, C., Kearns, M., & Jetten, J. (2019). The social psychology of responses to trauma: Social identity pathways associated with divergent traumatic responses. *European Review of Social Psychology, 30*, 311–348.

Muldoon, O., Lowe, R. D., Jetten, J., Cruwys, C., & Haslam, S. A. (in press). Personal and political: Post-traumatic stress through the lens of social identity, power and politics. *Advances in Political Psychology.*

Nakagawa, Y., & Shaw, R. (2004). Social capital: A missing link to disaster recovery. *International Journal of Mass Emergencies and Disasters, 22*, 5–34.

O'Brian, M. R. (2020). Retractions and controversies over coronavirus research show that the process of science is working as it should be. *The Conversation* (July 6). Retrieved from: https://theconversation.com/retractions-and-controversies-over-coronavirus-research-show-that-the-process-of-science-is-working-as-it-should-140326

O'Connor, D. B., Aggleton, J. P., Chakrabarti, B., Cooper, C. L., Creswell, C., Dunsmuir, S., . . . & Jones, M. V. (2020). Research priorities for the COVID-19 pandemic and beyond: A call to action for psychological science. *British Journal of Psychology*, e12468.

Pfefferbaum, B., & North, C. S. (2020). Mental health and the COVID-19 pandemic. *New England Journal of Medicine*.

Putnam, R. D. (2000). *Bowling alone: The collapse and revival of American community*. Simon & Schuster.

Ritchie, S. (2020) Don't trust the psychologists on coronavirus: Many of the responses to COVID-19 come from a deeply-flawed discipline. *Unherd* (March 31). Retrieved from: https://unherd.com/2020/03/dont-trust-the-psychologists-on-coronavirus/

Sahu, K. K., Mishra, A. K., & Lal, A. (2020). Trajectory of the COVID-19 pandemic: Chasing a moving target. *Annals of Translational Medicine, 8*(11).

Scott, D. (2020). Coronavirus is exposing all of the weaknesses in the US health system. *Vox* (March 16). Retrieved from: www.vox.com/policy-and-politics/2020/3/16/21173766/coronavirus-COVID-19-us-cases-health-care-system

Seifert, A., Cotten, S. R., & Xie, B. (2020) A double burden of exclusion? Digital and social exclusion of older adults in times of COVID-19. *The Journals of Gerontology: Series B*, gbaa098.

Sennett, R. (1998). *The corrosion of character: The personal consequences of work in the new capitalism*. WW Norton & Company.

Smith, L. G., & Gibson, S. (2020). Social psychological theory and research on the novel coronavirus disease (COVID-19) pandemic: Introduction to the rapid response special section. *The British Journal of Social Psychology*, *59*, 571–583.

Solnit, R. (2020) "The impossible has already happened": What coronavirus can teach us about hope. *The Guardian* (April 7). www.theguardian.com/world/2020/apr/07/what-coronavirus-can-teach-us-about-hope-rebecca-solnit

Steffens, N. K., Haslam, S. A., Reicher, S. D., Platow, M. J., Fransen, K., Yang, J., . . . Boen, F. (2014). Leadership as social identity management: Introducing the Identity Leadership Inventory (ILI) to assess and validate a four-dimensional model. *Leadership Quarterly*, *25*, 1001–1024.

Tajfel, H., & Turner, J. C. (1979). An integrative theory of intergroup conflict. In W. G. Austin & S. Worchel (Eds.), *The social psychology of intergroup relations* (pp. 33–47). Monterey, CA: Brooks/Cole.

Templeton, A., Guven, S. T., Hoerst, C., Vestergren, S., Davidson, L., Ballentyne, S., . . . & Choudhury, S. (2020). Inequalities and identity processes in crises: Recommendations for facilitating safe response to the COVID-19 pandemic. *British Journal of Social Psychology*, *59*, 674–685.

Van Bavel, J. J., Baicker, K., Boggio, P. S., Capraro, V., Cichocka, A., Cikara, M., . . . & Willer, R. (2020). Using social and behavioural science to support COVID-19 pandemic response. *Nature Human Behaviour*, *4*, 460–471.

van Dick, R., Lemoine, J. E., Steffens, N. K., Kerschreiter, R., Akfirat, S. A., Avanzi, L. . . ., & Haslam, S. A. (2018). Identity Leadership going global: Validation of the Identity Leadership Inventory (ILI) across 20 countries. *Journal of Occupational and Organizational Psychology*, *91*, 697–728.

Walker, C. (2020). What is remarkable about what we've achieved is that it's unremarkable. *The Psychologist*, *33* (7–8), 50–53.

Weible, C. M., Nohrstedt, D., Cairney, P., Carter, D. P., Crow, D. A., Durnová, A. P., . . . & Stone, D. (2020). COVID-19 and the policy sciences: initial reactions and perspectives. *Policy Sciences*, *53*, 225–241.

Wilkinson, R., & Pickett, K. (2009). *The spirit level: Why more equal societies almost always do better*. London, UK: Allen Lane.

Williams, K. D. (2009). Ostracism: A temporal need-threat model. In M. P. Zanna (Ed.), *Advances in experimental social psychology* (Vol. 41, pp. 275–314). Elsevier Academic Press.

Williams, R., & Drury, J. (2009). Psychosocial resilience and its influence on managing mass emergencies and disasters. *Psychiatry*, *8*, 293–296.

Wind, T. R., Rijkeboer, M., Andersson, G., & Riper, H. (2020). The COVID-19 pandemic: The 'black swan' for mental health care and a turning point for e-health. *Internet interventions*, *20*,100317.

World Health Organization (2020). *Guide to preventing and addressing social stigma associated with COVID-19*. Retrieved from: www.who.int/publications/m/item/a-guide-to-preventing-and-addressing-social-stigma-associated-with-COVID-19

Yates, T. (2020). Why is the government relying on Nudge theory to fight coronavirus? *The Guardian* (March 13). www.theguardian.com/commentisfree/2020/mar/13/why-is-the-government-relying-on-nudge-theory-to-tackle-coronavirus

1

LEADERS

Barry Richards

RAGE AND RETRIBUTION

> You bleed for those sons of a bitch. How many? Three thousand? I will kill more if only to get rid of drugs.[1]

> When I say, 'I will kill you if you destroy my country', and 'I will kill you if you destroy the young of my country', I am asking everybody to find me a fault in those two statements.[2]

> If I make it to the presidential palace I will do just what I did as mayor. You drug pushers, holdup men, and do-nothings, you better get out because I'll kill you.[3]

These are statements made during a successful campaign in 2016 by a candidate for election to the presidency of a country of more than 100 million people. Rodrigo Duterte is a middle-class, university-educated career politician, currently president of the Philippines, who was explaining his strategy for tackling the country's major drugs problem. He is an extreme example of a politician, well-known for the violence and misogyny of his language, but is head of state in one of the world's largest democracies. Later in this chapter we will discuss what responsibility leaders have for the climate of feeling in their countries – in this example, why is the rage about drug trafficking so focussed on savage retribution? But first we must walk through some more general ideas about, and analyses of, the dynamics of leadership.

AUTHORITY AND THE SUPEREGO

Leadership is a central issue in most aspects of human society, perhaps most obviously so in areas such as organisational life and politics. Yet it is one aspect of a wider and perhaps even deeper topic, that of authority. Authority is at the centre of all human relationships, including personal and intimate ones, because it is intrinsic to the questions of how we conduct ourselves, and how we make decisions; what rules we choose to follow, or to break; what standards we seek to achieve, or to subvert; what we expect of people, including ourselves. All such moral questions are at one level about authority, because they are about which or whose rules and standards we relate to, and about how we experience ourselves as moral agents able to act on our own authority.

These are not only questions about which people we respect and which codes we try to adhere to. They are also about a more subterranean area of human life, in which forms of pre-verbal relating to the world hold sway. These are laid down early in our psychological development, when we learn who or what to trust, and what we have to do to keep safe and to fit in with the world. In the technical language of psychoanalysis, it is the area of early superego development. The superego is that part of the mind in which the restraints and rules of the culture are embedded, transferred from one generation of superegos to the next (though with modifications along the way), and which is therefore core to our development as civilised beings. Out of the 'parental matrix', which was described in Chapter 1, there emerges a constellation of feelings and capacities in the developing person which we can call their 'superego', and which define that person's relationships with authority. This includes their own sense of personal authority, the capacity to make judgments and to act independently. So the superego is deeply linked to the individual's experience of both safety and dignity.

In the over-simplified versions of psychoanalysis sometimes found in general psychology textbooks, the term 'superego' can mean much the same as 'conscience'. It is usually painted in severe terms, as a punitive enforcer causing much painful guilt. Undoubtedly, guilt is a major source of pain, and the superego can in some persons be capable of great cruelty. However it is important to see it as a much broader and more complex region of the self, including not only fearful images of a forbidding censor, but also impressions of authority as caring and supportive. Indeed the capacity to feel guilt and remorse will not develop authentically if driven by fear alone, and needs a trusting and loving connection with whoever is doing the prohibiting or commanding.

What does all this early psychology have to do with the psychology of politics? The superego is a core part of the self which is not only an internal regulator but is also a set of powerful templates, deeply embedded in the adult mind and able to shape our experience throughout life of people and organisations we encounter which in one way or another represent authority to us. Our experiences of these authorities will carry the stamp of that early parental matrix, and any social institution or person carrying some meaning as a source of authority will occupy a quasi-parental place in the life of the adult citizen. Of course, that doesn't necessarily mean it will be trusted or followed. As we saw in Chapter 1, there is much ambivalence to be overcome in relationships with parents.

THE EXTERNALISED SUPEREGO

One of the earliest psychological theories of leadership is still a rich source of understanding its dynamics. It was set out by Sigmund Freud in his 1921 essay on group psychology. He noted that when individuals inhabit a collective identity, they merge a part of themselves into that identity. The part in question is what Freud a little later came to call the 'superego'. His crucial observation was that group members were often prepared to hand over their superego functions, at least in part, to the leader of the group, and so were prepared to act in ways that as individuals they would probably not allow themselves. Group membership is therefore a reversal of the process of emotional maturation. Having spent the years of growing up in efforts to internalise restraint, and to build our own internal capacity for self-regulation, we project that back out there, to some-one (or something) in the external world, when we commit to a group which is emotionally significant to us. In return for this loss of full selfhood, of psychic autonomy, the individual can gain the safety and the dignity of belonging to a group, under the protection and blessing of its leader. This experience may however be illusory, and so be a long-term threat to the well-being of the individual. Moreover, there is another more obviously dangerous consequence of this dynamic of group membership, in that group members may find themselves acting on feelings or impulses which are destructive or self-damaging.

There are many ways in which this dynamic can play out, with very different consequences, depending on what feelings the group leader is giving permission to group members to release, or what actions the leader is demanding of the group. In criminal gang cultures, the permission or demand may often be for violent behaviour. In bohe-mian communes, it may be for promiscuity and other hedonistic activities. In political parties or movements, it is a demand for belief in what the organisation stands for, and for action to promote its aims. The content of that demand will vary according to the ideology involved. The demands may conceal permissions as well – to engage in antagonistic behaviour, for example, perhaps even violence, or to take yourself away from your relationships with family or friends.

As was noted in Chapter 1, we are more familiar with the nega-tive versions of this phenomenon. Freud's model of group dynam-ics has influenced many attempts to explain the rise of Nazism and the Holocaust. Indeed, a general implication of the model is that group membership is intrinsically a form of diminished selfhood, a condition into which people with less integrated superegos (i.e. less psychic maturity) are more likely to fall. Freud was influenced by the rise of totalitarianism, in response to which he and many other intellectuals held a suspicion of the collective and an idealisation of the autonomous, fully self-possessed individual who would be less vulnerable to the seductions of leaders.

However, developments in psychoanalytic thinking since Freud about the superego and about groups enable us to expand his model such that we can see leader-follower or leader-public relationships in terms of a wide range of possibilities. Our perceptions of and feelings about leaders may be the result of various aspects of the self being projected onto them, with different elements in leaders' personalities acting as the hook or target for those projections. So to an important degree, we create our leaders through projection. But a leader must be willing and able to inhabit and to own the projected feelings and identities.

What about the leaders themselves? The choice to become a political leader may, in the person's internal unconscious, be an attempt to inhabit a superego role in the external world. At its worst, this might mean gaining the power to inflict on others whatever punishments the person feels they have been threatened with by their own superego. (Our discussion of terrorism in Chapter 4 will explore that scenario.) At its best, it might mean the leader becoming a benign and protective authority, thereby either reproducing their own good developmental experiences of superego figures, or filling a gap in their personal development. Justin Frank's (2012) psychoanalytic study of Barack Obama links both merits and flaws in his leadership style to – amongst other factors – his early loss of a father. His parents separated when he was one, and his father moved away. In later life, including in his role as president, Obama sought to *be* the father he had missed while also being very ambivalent in his relationship with his internal image of father.

There are a number of 'psychobiographies' of leaders which try to trace their emotional development and its shaping of their adult characters, and to examine the fit (or sometimes the lack of fit) between the person and the office occupied, with its political demands and opportunities to respond to the emotional profile of the public. Some recent American presidents have been the subject of interesting psychobiographies; as well as Frank's study of Obama, and an earlier one by him of George W. Bush, there is also one by Vamik Volkan on Richard Nixon's very difficult childhood and his subsequent narcissism and self-destructiveness (Volkan et al., 1997).

In the rest of this chapter we will however focus more on the 'followership' side of leadership. We will consider how broad changes in society have affected leadership styles, by modifying what we want and need to see in leaders. These changes bring the psychological dimensions of leader-follower relations more into focus. We will discuss the question of whether leaders are made in the image of their followers, or vice versa. Then we will look at some examples of how leaders respond to their public's needs for safety and dignity, and of what containment they can offer of the anxieties around those needs.

AMBIVALENCE TOWARDS AUTHORITY

Perhaps the most obvious form of authority in everyday life is that of the law. The law is easily pictured both as an external superego in both a patriarchal, punitive mode, as something designed to oppress rather than protect us, and also as a fundamentally benign source of collective strength and rectitude. There may be many specific situations in external reality which fit one or the other of these dichotomised images of a 'good' law and a 'bad' one. We may consume, in rapid succession, media reports about the heroism of some police officers and the corruption of others. An 'official' and widely shared rhetoric about the goodness of the law and those employed to enforce it exists alongside many narratives that assume the opposite. This cultural ambivalence towards the law reflects the mixed nature of reality, but also echoes the ambivalence towards parental authority which is especially noticeable in adolescence and its oscillations between needy dependence and resentful hostility.

The psychological basis of ambivalence towards authority, in the process of development from infancy through adolescence, is present in us all, though as individuals we are able to resolve it to varying degrees, and express either or both sides of it in endlessly varying ways. These will be strongly influenced by our social environments. It seems that social media have hugely expanded the scope for public expression of negative feelings about politicians, sometimes testing the legal proscription of hate speech. However there is reason to think that expression of the negative side of the ambivalence was gaining strength some decades before social media, due to a number of factors but in particular the broad cultural trend over at least the last half century of falling levels of trust in traditional institutions and professions, and growing scepticism about some types of expertise. Politicians have been especially affected by the weakening of deferential trust in their integrity and competence. They are the least trusted profession in the UK, according to IpsosMORI's annual Veracity Index of 2017,[4] which reports that only 17% of the public trust them to tell the truth.

Globally, the overall picture of trust in politics is complex. Trust in politicians is not quite the same as trust in government, and both differ from trust in political institutions, so recorded levels of trust in politics will depend on the questions asked. And as the 2018 Edelman Trust Barometer shows,[5] there are international year-by-year variations, with some countries such as Argentina, France and Germany showing surprising increases in trust in government since 2012, with fluctuations in between. So some positive attitudes towards authorities remain, but negative ones towards politicians are probably on a long-term rising trend, with some people becoming relentlessly disparaging of them. To be cynical about politics ('I don't trust any of them') seems to have become for many people a criterion of basic worldliness. Amongst other people, positive attitudes may be inflated to the point of idealisation, in denial of a disappointing reality. If we try to understand all this psychologically, we can see it as regressive splitting, a difficulty in holding on to a complex, mixed view of vital social institutions, instead retreating to the simplicities of a black-and-white world. This may suggest that some erosion of our general capacity to trust has occurred, a diminution of emotional capital in society as a whole. In representative democracies, there is obviously risk to the democratic process when attitudes towards elected politicians are dominated by splitting and the negative side of the ambivalence is becoming stronger, a situation facilitating the rise of 'populist' leaders.

THE CHANGING STYLES OF LEADERSHIP: INFORMAL, EMOTIONAL, PERSONAL

Another cultural trend of relevance to understanding the changing dynamics of leader-follower relations has been called the *informalisation* of everyday life (the sociologist Cas Wouters [2007] has led the way in defining this trend). This refers to the fact that social formalities and conventions, including those related to differences in status and authority, no longer regulate social exchanges to the extent that they used to. For example, dress codes are much more relaxed than they were, and less indicative of rank. First name address is common even across wide gaps in age and status. This trend may sometimes mislead by obscuring the hierarchies that continue to exist, but overall must surely be a positive development: it signals that respect should flow 'down' as well as 'up', it may reduce the timidity of younger or more junior people, and it facilitates inclusiveness. It can reduce the distance between politicians and the people, though politicians must be careful in this area, since as they know, affecting an informality which does not come naturally can make for bad publicity.

Informalisation is linked to two other broad cultural changes which are impacting on political leadership: personalisation and emotionalisation. *Emotionalisation* is a complex cultural phenomenon which is linked to the rise of psychology we noted earlier. At its core is an increase in emotional expressivity in everyday life, but amongst many other things it also involves an increased popular interest in emotional experience, and in the intimate lives of celebrities and public figures. Leaders are now permitted a much wider range of emotional expression than previously – in fact, this is now desired of them. The changing leadership styles in a more emotionalised culture have been explored in Candida Yates' study of British political culture from the late 1990s to 2015. The public's interest is partly served by, and partly generates, media content in which politicians are presented as emotional persons as well as, or even rather than, the bearers of policies.

The trend to *personalisation* is therefore closely linked to emotionalisation. There has been a tendency amongst politicians and commentators in the more stable democracies to underplay the importance of leaders. What matters, we have often been told, is policies not personalities. It is as if an attraction to individual leaders sets us on a dangerous path which could lead again to the horrors of twentieth-century fascism. Yet this fear sits in a cultural environment in which there are endless invitations in our media to experience and consider politicians as persons, and to focus on the personalities of our leaders. Two developments have facilitated this personalisation of politics.

One is the process of 'dealignment' – the dissolution of the links between socio-economic position and political affiliation. While in the past the industrial working class could have been expected to vote *en masse* for parties of the left, the dissolution of clear and stable class structures has led to much more complex and unpredictable patters of voting. Ideologies grounded in class identity have much weaker influence, and the 'Left-Right' distinction can no longer organise the diversity of political opinion. In this context, more space is available for the personal qualities of candidates to become important in electoral choice.

The second is to be found in socio-technical developments in media. The arrival of television in the 1950s and 1960s brought the personal presence of politicians into everyday experience. The first televised debate between presidential candidates in the US, between John Kennedy and Richard Nixon in 1960, was seen as a turning point in the campaign. Kennedy subsequently won the election by a narrow margin, with many commentators and polls suggesting this was due at least in part to his much more telegenic presence and performance in the debate. The later rise of the web and of social media, and of the global 24-hour news environment, have afforded deeper audience involvement in many aspects of politics, with the domain of emotional responses to politicians expanding and being of focal interest for many people. There some negative sides to this. The intensive visual presentation of leaders on television and online can have distracting or trivialising effects on political debate, and it may negatively affect the leadership prospects of very capable people who do not have distinctive screen appeal.

However, while this is clearly a mixed development, we might welcome it as being more positive than sinister. It can help to sustain public interest in politics, in times when the sterile ritualism of party competition and the remoteness of political elites has turned large numbers of people away from it. What interests many people most is other people, and what matters most are our relationships with other people. Passionately focussed though some people are on issues like the environment or human rights, productive emotional engagement with politics is for many most likely to develop when it is somehow personalised. This may come about through an issue being dramatised by the case of an individual (say, stories of an individual migrant, CEO or terrorist coming to represent the broad issues of migration, business governance or terror), or through the media presence of an appealing leader (or perhaps through an aversive response to an unappealing one).

Many members of the public have perhaps always ignored the advice to stick to policies, and have instead been heavily influenced by how they relate to leaders and aspiring leaders as people, even though they mostly have only 'para-social' contact with them (i.e. via the media) so that relating is based on impressions gained from media content alone. Certainly, before the age of television some leaders were acutely aware of their emotional impact on their followers, and of how their personal character and its presentation was crucial to their political support. Reflecting this, in the classic sociological theory of charisma, academics have also registered the power of the emotional tie between leader and follower. For the sociologist Max Weber in 1919,[6] the appeal of the charismatic leader rested on personal qualities, distinguishing that style of leadership from 'traditional' and 'bureaucratic' types, which were based on respect for roles defined by custom and by law respectively (say, tribal elder or high court judge) not on the emotional appeal of a person. Perhaps academic theory, which across the social sciences this century has been undergoing a 'turn to affect', is only now just returning to Weber and catching up with reality. Yet reality is also moving, and political leadership is becoming more explicitly personalised and emotionalised, as is culture as a whole.

THE LEADERS WE DESERVE?

This focus on the emotional dynamics of leadership points to a way of answering the old and fundamental question of whether – for better or worse – we get the leaders we deserve. In societies with some degree of functioning democracy it is hard to avoid the conclusion that yes, we do – though in a limited sense, as we will see. While the capacity of wealthy and influential elites to manipulate elections through propaganda and other forms of influence, if not outright corruption, should not be underestimated, voters usually have some choice, and exercise it. On this view, leaders may articulate public opinion, but do not radically shape it.

Insofar as we do exercise choice, it is not in the simple way that rationalist models of democracy would have it. Rational and evidence-based comparative analysis of policy alternatives on offer may play a part amongst some voters, but 'voter competence' levels (how much electorates know about the issues and can make rational, informed judgments about them) are not high even in the most educated societies. So recourse to an intuitive summary judgment of candidates is common, and is likely to be heavily influenced by a voter's emotional responses to the candidates. As we've observed, their judgments may be based on what voters project of themselves onto the public personae of candidates, and therefore on how much they can identify or feel a bond with one candidate more than others, or on how much they are repulsed by a candidate onto whom they have projected some very negative qualities. Or voters may be searching out the candidate who they feel can best meet their needs to feel, say, more safe or more respected. In these circumstances, the successful candidate may likely be the one who, irrespective of competence and even of ideology, has a public persona which best fits the emotional needs of a crucial segment of the public.[7] So we the public are choosing, albeit for what may be largely unconscious reasons, the candidate whom we have ourselves largely constructed. Some would see the role of the media as crucial in that process of construction, although again there is a debate to be had about whether we get the media we deserve. Do the media simply articulate public emotion, or shape it?

LEADING BY EXAMPLE

Let's continue to test the view that neither the media nor leaders actually create their publics, but simply reflect them. Is this true at moments of crisis, when there may be clear choices available to leaders about how to lead? There are always different structures of feeling[8] present in the pool of public emotion, and at times of acute disturbance and uncertainty when leaders are looked to for guidance they may be able to choose which of these to express and support. After a major terrorist attack, for example, there is grief, fear, rage and resolve, and leaders' choice of language in the aftermath shapes and modulates some of these feelings more than others, with differing consequences on a number of fronts, especially in relation to social cohesion and to support for counter-terrorism policies. Two days after 77 terrorist murders in Oslo and on the island of Utoya in Norway in July 2011, the then Norwegian Prime Minister Jens Stoltenberg in a national memorial address spoke powerfully about the victims, and then struck a remarkably positive note of optimistic resolve.

> Amidst all this tragedy, I am proud to live in a country that has managed to hold its head up high at a critical time. I have been impressed by the dignity, compassion and resolve I have met. We are a small country, but a proud people. We are still shocked by what has happened, but we will never give up our values. Our response is more democracy, more openness, and more humanity. But never naïvety. No one has said it better than the Labour Youth League girl who was interviewed by CNN: 'If one man can create that much hate, you can only imagine how much love we as a togetherness can create'.[9]

We can compare this with the quotations at the start of this chapter, a few of the many statements made by the Rodrigo Duterte about the ongoing crisis of massive drug use in his country, the Philippines. The contrast between these two leaders demonstrates the fundamental role of public emotion in shaping leadership. Neither set of statements could conceivably have been made by a national leader in the other country. So something about Norwegian culture and its shaping of the psychology of the Norwegian public produced the Stoltenberg statement, while making it impossible for the Duterte statements to have been uttered in Norway. Nor could Duterte's violence have been released amongst the Philippino public without their substantial collusion. In fact, with his reputation and style as a political leader already established from years as a mayor, he received 16.6 million votes, 39% of the votes cast, in his victory in the presidential election of 2016.

However these examples also indicate the role of individual leaders in giving voice to reserves of particular feeling at particular times. There are politicians in Norway who after Utoya would have spoken in a different tone from that adopted by Stoltenberg. While subscribing to the general horror at this atrocity, the anti-immigration Norwegian Progress Party had a different version of the resolution not to be led into losing its values: it affirmed the importance of retaining its policy priorities. And of course there are many in the Philippines who speak differently from Duterte on how to deal with the drug problem, including Benigno Aquino III, who lost the presidency to Duterte.

Stoltenberg's speech had a strong effect on the Norwegian public, who rallied around his words, and his approval ratings improved considerably. This was not a long-term effect, but the speech seemed to play a major role in containing public feeling during a critical period. However, the difficulty for national leaders is that national publics are emotionally diverse, and finding an appropriate response for *all* the feelings that may be present in the public at the time is an impossible task. Still, good emotional governance requires as wide a containing response as possible. The speech did not address the fear and the rage which many Norwegians must have been feeling, even if they did so against their better judgment. The Oslo/Utoya attack was a major assault on the sense of safety, and on the dignity of Norway as peaceable and cohesive country. The prime minister's speech tended to idealise the Norwegian public as extraordinarily resolute, leaving little space for anything more complicated or ambivalent to be expressed. It followed a claim that this was not naïve with a statement that could be seen as naïve. All this may explain why its unifying effect was short-lived. Most people urgently wanted to regain the experience of safety and dignity, and Stoltenberg's words offered a noble way towards that. As such they offered some containment of the shock and anxiety, in modelling a composed and resilient response. To speak at all at such a time must be extremely hard, and this was a deeply felt and eloquent speech. It would be unrealistic to expect one speech to give voice to all reactions to the killings. In the longer run, however, a more variegated picture of the Norwegian public would need to be presented if the polarising forces which had given rise to the attacks were to be more comprehensively managed and contained.

Duterte also must have 'struck a chord', though in the opposite of a containing way. How can a national presidential candidate brag of murdering people, and then be elected? The Philippines does not only have a drug problem; it also has a major terrorism problem. In the year before Duterte's election as president, several groups with allegiance to or similar aims as ISIS were involved in bombings, burning of villages, extortion, kidnappings and beheadings. The police have been unable to deal with the problem, so the army was continuously deployed against the terrorist paramilitaries, who were especially strong in the region Duterte came from. Later, in 2017, Islamist fighters actually took control of a city in the south of the country, and a military battle involving nearly a thousand deaths was necessary to reclaim it. The country's politics for most of its history have been turbulent and bloody, and the thousands of extra-judicial killings in Duterte's war on drugs are integral to its violent history. This is the kind of situation where one would expect emotional capital to be at very low levels, with the sense of safety seriously depleted, and dignity minimal except in privileged strata of the population. In that context, it is plausible that a population habituated to violence, yet also desperate to escape it, might turn to a violent leader promising to demolish one key part of the ruin that is their society. Potentials for (often sexualised) violence therefore awaited the arrival of a Duterte, though his particular character was perhaps also necessary to break the taboo on a president openly glorifying and promising violence.

At the moments of potential flux occasioned by an election, it is very possible for an incumbent to be replaced by a very different leader, perhaps quite suddenly. This reminds us that a public is never monolithic – there are bodies of feeling present in it other than that expressed in the current regime, such that given the availability of a potential leader with a different emotional appeal and an effective way of communicating it, one of these other structures of feeling may take hold of government. So while leaders must work within the psychological limits of their publics, they can play crucial roles in the complex processes which bring about switches of government from one emotional base to another, by mobilising a particular constituency of feeling, a particular segment of the emotional public. As was suggested in the previous chapter, the 'leave' campaigners in the UK's 2016 'Brexit' referendum were able to do this, by an articulation of anxieties about the loss of British identity or its dignity, and thus overturning a long-standing (if narrow) majority of public sentiment in favour of remaining in Europe.

So we should not overlook the active role of the leader in making history. Leaders are not only chosen by the public to act out the collective will, and it would be misleading for us to rest with a simple assertion that therefore we get the leaders we deserve. A national public is a hugely complex phenomenon, psychologically, so much so that to speak of a 'national psyche' is bound to be a major simplification. Many different structures of feeling within it are available for mobilisation, and through their words, images and deeds some political leaders will, deliberately or not, be working to identify and bring some of those structures to the surface and to foreground or amplify some feelings rather than others. So we have come to the overall conclusion that publics and leaders make each other; there are endless complex interactions involving expressed feelings and unconscious phantasies amongst the public, their representations in mainstream and social media, the internal worlds (the motives and perceptions) of political leaders at all levels, and the external world demands of economic life, diplomacy, and so on. While the default position in psychoanalysis is more towards seeing people as responsible for managing their own feelings, perhaps in the political context we should give a little more emphasis to the opportunities that leaders have to influence how their publics do this, and to help build up emotional capital.

LEADING INTO BATTLE

This influence of leadership may be most clear, and most consequential, in some conflict situations, especially those of potential violence, military or other. Alongside the classical non-psychological causes of inter- and intranational conflicts (such as who governs a territory and its people, or has access to its resources), there are the psychosocial processes by which our internal needs and anxieties fasten themselves onto some aspects of the conflict and rigidify the minds of those involved. The Israeli psychologist Daniel Bar-Tal (2013) has developed the concept of 'conflictive ethos' to describe a situation in which, whatever is objectively at stake in the conflict, the parties involved have come to experience it in certain ways. For example, they see it as fundamental to their identity, and as a zero-sum affair, such that any benefit to their enemy must be a loss to themselves. Those and other related perceptions lock them into pursuit of the conflict, and paradoxically enable them to bear it carrying on, so that it then becomes intractable. In a different theoretical language, Vamik Volkan, through many studies of conflicts around the world, and the roles of leaders within them, has written about how a process of 'large group regression' can take place, involving the majority of people in a society and resulting in the intractability which Bar-Tal describes.

This is most likely to happen when a leader emerges whose own personality is dominated by a malignant narcissism, and who encourages large sections of the public into regressed states of mind in which the world is grossly simplified. The large group's identity (typically that of a 'nation') is idealised, and the process of splitting, on which that idealisation depends, also produces demonised enemies, and a number of other adverse effects. A large group is vulnerable to this process, says Volkan, when it is unable to process and tolerate the level of anxiety to which its members are subject. In terms of the ideas which are outlined in this book, this would mean that an insufficient experience of safety and/or dignity has raised levels of anxiety to a point at which the group will seek a defensive response. This is offered by a leader who promises safety and dignity, linked in more toxic cases to an image of a purified national community, of which more below.

THE 'POPULIST' PHENOMENON

Much discussion of political leadership around the world in recent years has focussed on the concept of 'populism'. Typically this involves a charismatic leader who seeks power on the basis of offering an end to politics as we know it. This leader is presented as of a new type, either because s/he is not a professional politician, or is one who somehow claims exclusively to know and understand the 'people' and promises to champion them against the political 'establishment', the 'elite' who have been in power for so long and achieved so little. There is an overlap with the much older category of 'strong man' leader, the protecting father who is not a populist in today's sense but in whom the 'people' have a confidence that transcends their broken trust in political institutions and democratic process.

Not all forms of contemporary populism are of the 'Right': 'Left' populisms can and do occur, as the era of Chavez and Maduro in Venezuela can be seen to illustrate, and perhaps also the 2016 electoral campaigns of Corbyn and Sanders in the UK and US respectively, though neither of these posed a sharp 'us the people vs. the elite' dichotomy. Syriza in Greece and Podemos in Spain are seen by some as examples of 'Left' populism, while the Five Star Movement (M5S) in Italy defies placing on that axis (which as we have noted is of limited usefulness in describing politics today). Leftist populism can be seen as at least partially adhering to the principles of safety and dignity, though in different ways to Rightist versions: material security rather than border security is often the guarantee of safety, via state provision for health and welfare, while dignity may also be materially defined in terms of better pay, secure employment and housing, rather than being seen culturally.

One feature which all varieties of 'populism', including the M5S, have in common, and which therefore is often taken in academic discussions of the term to be its defining characteristic, is a deep disaffection with the political 'establishment'. The populist leader's appeal is that of the outsider, someone untainted by the complacency or corruption of the elite, someone who can be in touch with the 'people', and so really offers something different. Psychologically, this is the wish for purity, a narcissistic impulse of reaching for the perfect world, in response to a collapse of trust in politics in the real world. As such, the enthusiasm for the new order, the 'Golden Dawn' promised by the extremist party of that name in Greece, is condemned to eventual collapse, as the promise of purity cannot be delivered.

The extent to which contemporary populism is a new development in leader-follower relations is debatable. Has there not for a long time been an us vs. them at the heart of human society, ready to be stirred up by leaders who believe in themselves as forces of renewal, and now more easily stirred via the direct and fevered channels of social media? Or are we seeing a new kind of leadership, facilitated by modern communications but with a new emotional dynamic?

At the psychological level, there is nothing new about today's populisms. Their basic dynamic appears to be one in which the parental figures (the incumbent political class, the 'elite') are felt to have comprehensively failed, even to have betrayed those for whom they are responsible. A deep, amorphous anger fills the political air and people feel various combinations of abandoned, deceived and exploited. As we saw in Chapter 1, feelings of distrust and rage against parental figures of early life are universal. So how can we understand the rise of cynicism and anger in popular attitudes towards politics, to the point where elections are won by parties or leaders whose key promise is to overthrow the establishment, to replace the actual, bad parents with an ideal, good one?

For many, economic recession is the key explanation, bringing as it does attacks on the well-being and dignity of the unemployed and the low waged, and a sense of insecurity to many others. Others see globalisation and rapid cultural change as the main problem, disrupting the stable communities which offered a sense of safety and self-respect. So combine austerity regimes with the surge in migration, and you may have the two crises which bring to a head long-standing popular disaffection at the underlying trends of growing inequality and increasing globalisation. There may seem to be little need for expert psychology to contribute to understanding where the swell of anger comes from.

But there is still important psychological work to do. Nations similarly affected by the two crises have responded in different ways, which psychosocial analysis may help to explain. And the specific content and focus of public feeling in individual countries is important to understand. Just how do people experience their difficulties, what troubles them most, who do they blame, what do they want most? The core argument of this book would suggest that the central issues are ones of safety and dignity: somehow people feel that their societies now are unsafe for them, and do not endow them with dignity. Without reliable understanding of the emotional profiles of regressive populist movements, it is difficult for political leaders opposing them to develop the best strategies for doing so.

Also, feelings of safety and dignity are gained and lost in many areas of life, not only in the political sphere. What changes might there have been at deeper levels of society, in family life and everyday culture, and in the various societal provisions that bear on early development, which may have been impacting on our early experience and making us more insecure in our core emotional selves? At least since the 1970s, there have been suggestions that, for various reasons, the presence in many societies of narcissistic traits has been increasing. If that is so, then even without economic crisis and cultural fragmentation there would be an increasing need amongst the public for leaders who would collude with or invite narcissistic defences, and promise painlessly and simply to deliver the safety and dignity which people feel they lack.

AND SO TO TRUMP AND KIM JONG-UN

Speaking of which, at the time of writing the most obvious and con-sequential example of a populist leader is Donald Trump, elected as president of the US in 2016. Trump, perhaps like Duterte, also elected in 2016, and some others in the wave of populist arrivals, brings a new dimension to the idea of personalised politics. The idea of 'per-sonalisation' as we encountered it earlier usually refers to the way in which citizens 'consume' their politics, with the personalities or personas of leaders being of as much or more interest to voters than the policies they are attached to and the parties and ideologies they represent. It is something that happens in the media sphere, and it reflects an important change in how citizens relate to their political leaders, as well as in the increased attention which many politicians pay to their appearance and social behaviour. But Trump seems to have brought his personality through and beyond style into the content of politics, so that strategy and sometimes objectives are defined by who he is. So there is a mutation of leadership best described not as per-sonalisation but as a 'personisation' of statecraft, similar in some ways to a kind of autocracy. To some extent, in Trump's case this involves a fragmentation of strategy and objectives, due to his emotional lability and superficiality and also, a recent report by Bob Woodward sug-gests,[10] to ad hoc restraints which some of those around him are able to impose.

Thus when Donald Trump met Kim Jong-Un in June 2018, it was not a summit in the usual sense of the term, that is, a meeting at which the participants represent large and complex bodies of strate-gic interests and expertise. This was a meeting that somehow sprang from the self-centred calculations of two highly narcissistic individu-als, aided it seems by more conventional diplomatic efforts on the part of South Korea to transform the unhappy situation on the Korean Peninsula. The calculations of the two men converged in that both saw a dramatic mould-breaking meeting being to their individual advan-tage. It would not actually have to change anything, but would enable each to offer their own people a better world, any subsequent failure of which to arrive could later be blamed on the other, or explained in some other way (perhaps riskier for Trump as the US has free media).

The meeting in Singapore was an encounter between the two major types of narcissism of the twentieth century, continuing into the present. Trump embodies the narcissistic tendency inherent in market-based societies, while Kim is the apotheosis of the collectivised form of narcissism generated by totalitarian societies. But the psychological root of each man is the same. We must remind ourselves that narcissism is not a simple excess of self-regard, but a defence against fear, against what would otherwise be an overwhelming internal sense of vulnerability and weakness. It is a mode of experience in which the intrinsic dependency of the self on others is so terrifying that it has to be denied. We all engage in this manoeuvre to some extent, but when narcissism becomes the founding principle of a personality, the fear against which it defends is firmly sealed off in the unconscious.

Trump's contemptuous intolerance of the complexities and uncertainties of politics was clear in the abrupt and aggressive manner of his departure from the G7 summit en route to the Singapore meeting, which was more of his own, simpler design, based on the performance of success rather than its achievement. Narcissism in leaders does not necessarily bring disaster; on the contrary, some measure of it may be necessary for the self-belief required to succeed in the arduous work of progressive politics. But for that to happen the leader's narcissistic self must be identified with some ideal of the common good – a vision of real reconciliation, say, in a leader whose task is to resolve a conflict. In the cases of Trump and Kim, their narcissistic selves appear to be expressed through visions of their own importance as paragons of what they believe their societies to be about – Trump, the feral property developer; Kim, the dynastic godhead. In this case, whatever the consequences of the 'summit', it demonstrated that in this psychological age, the importance of a psychological understanding of politics has never been so great.

NOTES

1 www.aljazeera.com/news/2017/02/duterte-kill-rid-drugs-170202073247477.
html, accessed 27.7.18.

2 www.reuters.com/article/us-philippines-drugs/philippines-duterte-says-hes-
been-demonized-over-drugs-war-idUSKBN1CU1QY, accessed 27.7.18.

3 www.hrw.org/tag/philippines-war-drugs, accessed 27.7.18.

4 See www.ipsos.com/ipsos-mori/en-uk/politicians-remain-least-trusted-
profession-britain, accessed 11.9.18.

5 See https://cms.edelman.com/sites/default/files/2018-01/2018%20Edelman%
20Trust%20Barometer%20Global%20Report.pdf, accessed 11.9.18.

6 This was in his essay 'Politics as a Vocation', reprinted in *From Max Weber. Essays
in Sociology.*

7 For many of us there is some degree of difference between our outward
persona and inner character, and this difference is likely to be greater for
public figures whose public image is deliberately crafted. Still, the outside is
usually heavily influenced by the inside, so basically we are looking at the
relationship between leader character and public emotion. I choose to use
the term 'character' here instead of 'personality'. In some contexts the two
are synonymous, but 'personality', since it is often assessed by behavioural
checklists and self-report, may be less able to capture the idea of a deep inner
self. Also 'character' has connotations of the person as a *moral* agent, and so is
appropriate for psychological analysis in political contexts, especially in the
study of leaders.

8 This phrase, an important one in the psychosocial literature, was first
deployed by the cultural theorist Raymond Williams – see his 1977 book
Marxism and Literature.

9 www.americanrhetoric.com/speeches/jensstoltenbergbombingmemorial.
htm, accessed 27.7.18.

10 *Fear: Trump in the White House* (2018), the veteran journalist's intensively
researched book on the Trump administration, was an instant best-seller.

REFERENCES

Adlam, J., Kluttig, T. & Lee, B., eds. (2018) *Violent States and Creative States.* 2 vols.
London: Jessica Kingsley.

Anderson, B. (1983) *Imagined Communities. Reflections on the Origin and Spread of Nationalism.* London: Verso.

Bar Tal, D. (2013) *Intractable Conflicts. Socio-Psychological Foundations and Dynamics.* Cambridge: Cambridge University Press.

Bowlby, J. (1988) *A Secure Base.* Abingdon: Routledge, revised edn., 2005.

Cooper, A. (2018) *Conjunctions. Social Work, Psychoanalysis, and Society.* Abingdon: Routledge.

Elias, N. (1939) *The Civilising Process.* Oxford: Blackwell, revised edn., 1994

Erikson, E. (1950) *Childhood and Society.* Harmondsworth: Penguin, revised edn., 1965.

Frank, J. (2004) *Bush on the Couch. Inside the Mind of the US President.* London: Politico's.

Frank, J. (2012) *Obama on the Couch: Inside the Mind of the President.* New York: Free Press.

Freud, S. (1921) Group psychology and the analysis of the ego. In *Penguin Freud Library, Vol. 12: Civilization, Society and Religion.* Harmondsworth: Penguin, 1991.

Fromm, E. (1949) *Man for Himself.* London: Ark, revised edn., 1986.

Gellner, E. (1983) *Nations and Nationalism.* Ithaca, NY: Cornell University Press.

Gerodimos, R. (2015) The ideology of far left populism in Greece: Blame, victimhood, and revenge in the discourse of Greek anarchists. *Political Studies* 63, 608–625.

Gray, J. (2003) *Al Qaeda and What it Means to be Modern.* London: Faber & Faber.

Greenfeld, L. (2016) *Advanced Introduction to Nationalism.* Cheltenham: Edward Elgar.

Hayek, F. (1944) *The Road to Serfdom.* London: Ark Paperbacks, revised edn., 1986.

Hobsbawm, E. & Ranger, T., eds. (1983) *The Invention of Tradition.* Cambridge: Cambridge University Press, revised edn., 1992.

Hoggett, P. (2011) Climate change and the apocalyptic imagination. *Psychoanalysis, Culture and Society* 16(3), 261–275.

Hoggett, P. & Thompson, S. (2012) *Politics and the Emotions.* London: Continuum.

Honneth, A. (1995) *The Struggle for Recognition,* Cambridge: Polity.

Lauenstein, O., Murer, J., Boos, M. & Reicher, S. (2015) 'Oh motherland I pledge to thee . . . ': A study into nationalism, gender and the representation of an imagined family within national anthems. *Nations and Nationalism* 21(2), 309–329.

Lindner, E. (2006) *Making Enemies: Humiliation and International Conflict.* Westport, CT: Praeger Publishers.

Macpherson, C.B. (1962) *The Political Theory of Possessive Individualism. Hobbes to Locke.* Oxford: Oxford University Press.

Margalit, A. (1996) *The Decent Society.* Cambridge, MA: Harvard University Press.

Mintchev, N. & Hinshelwood, R.D. (2017) *The Feeling of Certainty. Psychosocial Perspectives on Identity and Difference.* Cham, Switzerland: Palgrave.

Richards, B. (2017) *What Holds Us Together.* London: Karnac.

Sandler, J. (1987) *From Safety to Superego. Selected Papers of Joseph Sandler.* New York: Guilford Press.

Sennett, R. (2003) *Respect: The Formation of Character in an Age of Inequality*. Harmondsworth: Penguin, revised edn., 2004.

Smith, A. (2009) *Ethno-Symbolism and Nationalism: A Cultural Approach*. Abingdon: Routledge.

Szasz, T. (1961) *The Myth of Mental Illness*. New York: Harper, revised edn., 2010.

Theweleit, K. (1987) *Male Fantasies*. Cambridge: Polity.

Volkan, V. (2001) Transgenerational transmission and chosen traumas: An aspect of large-group identity. *Group Analysis* 34, 79–97.

Volkan, V. (2004) *Blind Trust. Large Groups and their Leaders in Times of Crisis and Terror*. Charlottesville, VA: Pitchstone Publishing.

Volkan, V., Itzkowitz, N. & Dod, A. (1997) *Richard Nixon. A Psychobiography*. New York: Columbia University Press.

Weber, M. (1919) *From Max Weber. Essays in Sociology*. Abingdon: Routledge, revised edn., 2009.

Weintrobe, S., ed. (2013) *Engaging with Climate Change: Psychoanalytic and Interdisciplinary Perspectives*. London: Routledge.

Wieland, C. (2015) *The Fascist State of Mind and the Manufacturing of Masculinity*. Hove: Routledge.

Wilkinson, R. & Pickett, K. (2009) *The Spirit Level*. London: Penguin.

Williams, R. (1977) *Marxism and Literature*. Oxford: Oxford University Press.

Winnicott, D. (1986) *Home Is Where We Start From. Essays by a Psychoanalyst*. Harmondsworth: Penguin.

Woodward, B. (2018) *Fear: Trump in the White House*. New York: Simon & Schuster.

Wouters, C. (2007) *Informalization: Manners and Emotions since 1890*. London: Sage.

Yates, C. (2015) *The Play of Political Culture, Emotion and Identity*. Basingstoke: Palgrave Macmillan.

2

TRUST AND POLITICS

The Emperor's not very new clothes

Ken J. Rotenberg

"The Emperor's New Clothes", a story by Hans Christian Andersen written in 1837, is about a vain Emperor who cared only about wearing and displaying clothes. In the story, two weavers produce for the Emperor what they say is the finest, best suit of clothes made from a fabric that is invisible to anyone who is unfit for his position or hopelessly stupid. The clothes are non-existent, but the Emperor wears them for fear of being thought unfit for his position or stupid. The Emperor's ministers pretend to see the new clothes for the same reason. The Emperor wears his new clothes in a procession through the town before his subjects, who go along with the pretence because they also did not want to appear unfit or stupid. During the procession, a naïve young child in the crowd blurts out that the Emperor is wearing nothing at all – which is then taken up by others in the crowd. Although the Emperor thinks the assertion is true, he continues the procession. The story has been made into a play and a movie, to the delight of many generations.

In its simplicity, the Emperor's New Clothes story depicts a leader who is deceived. The deception is perpetuated by himself, his ministers, and the people in the town for the sake of their self-esteem and public respect. The consensual deception is challenged by a young child, who is naïve to societal pressures. The story may be regarded as a metaphor for political leadership and political power in contemporary times. Political leaders collaborate with their ministers on deceptive policies that by social communications achieve a consensual acceptance by their citizens. The veracity of those communications and actions may be challenged by opposing political parties and by vigilant media – the metaphorical child. Is the Emperor's (now not so) New Clothes an accurate description of politics and government in contemporary times? It represents a *very* cynical view of no-truth politics – a political cynicism presumably shown in Australia and the US (see Leigh, 2002).

THE FALL OF DEMOCRACY?

It is often stated that a degree of political cynicism is required for political health, but a wide array of authors believe that a fundamental trust in politicians and government is required for democracy to work (see Warren, 1999, 2004). The lack of trust in government by citizens in democracies undermines their participation in the political process and adherence to government policies (see Garen & Clark, 2015). Trust in government has been viewed as social capital, which promotes people's political involvement among other forms of civic activities (see Chapter 1). The purpose of this chapter is to review psychological research, as well as other sources, regarding the factors that affect citizens' trust in politicians and government and the consequences of that trust.

Trust in politicians/government is multi-levelled. This issue can be described, in part, by the two target dimensions of the BDT Framework (see Chapter 1). This includes specificity that ranges from specific to general, and familiarity that ranges from somewhat familiar to very familiar. For example, some political scholars have concluded that citizens' trust in Congress is at an all-time low but that citizens' trust in their own congressman or congresswoman is quite strong (Fisher, van Heerde, & Tucker, 2010). Trust in leaders (e.g., a President or Prime Minister) is conventionally different from trust in individual members of the same political party and the leader's political party (see Rotenberg, 2016). Other researchers have found that people's trust in the nature of government (i.e., as a democracy) is distinct from people's trust in an existing government (e.g., Schiffman, Thelen, & Sherman, 2010). The target of trust is an important consideration.

Other researchers have proposed that there are different forms or types of trust. For example, Fisher, van Heerde, and Tucker (2010) proposed that there are three different types of trust: strategic trust, moral trust, and deliberative trust. These researchers tested their hypothesis using the data gathered from YouGov's weekly online British Omnibus survey (n = 1,753; July 2007) and the British Election Study Continual Monitoring Panel (n = 1,018; March 2009). The survey included 13 questions designed to assess each type of trust judgment, including the following: on balance, politicians deliver on their promises (strategic trust); politicians share the same goals and values as me (moral trust); and parties represent supporters, not funders (deliberative trust). The participants reported how much trust they had in parties and politicians on an 11-point scale. In support of their formulations, the researchers found that items assessing each of the different types of trust (as identified above) statistically predicted the individuals' rating of how much they trusted the government.

DOES TRUST IN GOVERNMENT AFFECT CITIZENS' BEHAVIOUR IN DEMOCRATIC COUNTRIES?

In order to address that question, Martin (2010) used data gathered from the 2007 Australian Election Study. The citizens were administered scales assessing their trust in government. The majority of the public expressed an untrusting attitude towards government, with 58% of respondents saying members of the government usually or sometimes look after themselves. By contrast, only 43% of the public agreed that government can usually or sometimes be trusted to do the right thing. Finally, only 15% of respondents expressed the most trusting attitude (i.e., that the government can usually be trusted to do the right thing). The findings were interpreted as the Australian public demonstrating political cynicism. It was found, though, that the measure of trust in politicians was positively associated with positive attitudes towards democracy, positively associated with voting when it is not compulsory, and negatively associated with voicing frustration through challenging forms of activities (e.g., engaging in protests). The findings support the contention that trust in the government contributes to democracy.

IT WAS THE BEST OF TIMES, IT WAS THE WORST OF TIMES! (MOSTLY THE LATTER)

There is evidence indicating that political trust has been declining since the mid-1960s in many democratic countries (Blind, 2007). Cheng, Bynner, Wiggins, and Schoon (2012) have proposed that that decline is a global phenomenon. Evidence for changes in political trust and the factors affecting it have been found in a study by Hetherington and Rudolph (2008). These researchers carried out a time-series analysis, from 1976–2006, on the factors that affected political trust in the US. Trust in the government was assessed by individuals' reports that "the government in Washington will do what is right". Overall, the researchers reported that trust in government declined over time. It was found, though, that political trust increased when the public viewed international issues as vital (e.g., terrorism, national security, war, and the Middle East). Furthermore, it was found that political trust decreased when the public thought that there were problems with the economy (i.e., a period of depression). The effects of economic concern were found to result in asymmetry, insofar as relatively few people regard the economy as good, even in good times. According to the authors, the positive effects of a good economy on political trust were relatively weak and thus they failed to offset the effects of bad economies, which resulted in the decline in citizens' trust in government. The findings may indicate that the US public is on the path to viewing politicians as emperors in new clothes.

DO POLITICAL SCANDALS MATTER?

It was around 50 years ago that Watergate burst upon us. The bitter political path spanned the period from the bugging of the Democratic National Committee headquarters at the Watergate hotel on May 28, 1971 to the resignation of President Richard Nixon on August 9, 1974. Hetherington and Rudolph (2008) found that government scandals (e.g., the Clinton impeachment proceedings) predicted declines in trust in government across time. The effects were not as substantial, though, as the effects of economic and international issues on trust in government. There is evidence that government scandals have negative effects on trust in government in countries other than the US. For example, qualitative research carried out by Isotalus and Almonkari (2014) indicates that political scandals had negative effects on citizens' trust in Finland.

WHAT CAUSES THE PUBLIC TO VIEW A POLITICIAN AS TRUSTWORTHY?

The trustworthiness of political candidates emerged, for example, during the 2016 US presidential race. Perceptions of the trustworthiness of politicians have been the focus of surveys and those have been the source of discussion in the media (e.g., Kolbert, 2016). It has been noted that many politicians lacked trustworthiness during the campaign regarding whether the UK should remain in or leave the European Union – called Brexit (Rotenberg, 2016).

The primary role of politicians is to persuade voters to endorse their views on everything and ultimately to vote for them (see Combs & Keller, 2010). The goal of their communication just happens to coincide with the conditions under which children and adults lie (see Chapter 2). Indeed, politicians engage in an exaggerated form of faking positivity in order to please others and attain approval. One way of undermining those effects is for the politician to present their communication as contrary to their self-interest – even compatible with the views of their opponents. This principle is supported by the study by Combs and Keller (2010). Their study was guided by the premise that a politician who engages in communications contrary to his or her self-interest violates expectations – in a positive fashion – which promotes perceptions of his or her trustworthiness.

In the first of three studies by those researchers, university undergraduates read an advertisement by a candidate (a fictional politician by the name of John Dixon) which was highly critical of his opponent (a fictional politician named David Hunter). The advertisement suggested that Hunter was a liar and that his policies would damage the state's economy. The undergraduates read one of three responses by David Hunter (all of which rejected the allegations at the onset): one went on to attack the moral values of his opponent (*counterattack*); one praised his own economic policies (*praised self*); and the third praised his opponent's policies as agreeing with his own and promised to take those forward to government if elected (*praised opponent*). It was found that the undergraduates judged the candidate as more trustworthy (i.e., showing trustworthiness, integrity, and honesty) and were more likely to vote for him when he had praised his opponent than when he counterattacked him. Furthermore, it was found that perceived trustworthiness was responsible, in part, for the pattern of voting. The three studies carried out by Combs and Keller (2010) provided support for the conclusion that people trust politicians and vote for them when they view the politician as acting against their own self-interest and positively violating expectations. From my perspective, this coincides with the principle that such acts decrease the likelihood that the politician is viewed as faking and thus deceiving others.

THE BDT FRAMEWORK

Guided by the BDT Framework, my colleagues and I (Rotenberg & Bierbrauer, in preparation) have examined trust beliefs in politicians. We have developed the Trust in Politicians (TP) Scale composed of scenarios that depict politicians potentially displaying three types of behaviour: reliability (e.g., keeping campaign promises), emotional trustworthiness (e.g., maintaining the confidentiality of information conveyed to government officials), and honesty (e.g., telling the truth about government spending). In our study, undergraduates were administered the TP scale and it was found, as expected, that the scale was composed of the three types of trust beliefs: reliability, emotional, and honesty. Also, we found that the undergraduates' honesty trust beliefs in politicians were associated with their willingness to vote for the Labour Party.

SUMMARY

The chapter began with the consideration of the Emperor's New Clothes story and its implications for the lack of trust in politicians today. The chapter reviews the research supporting the conclusion that some trust in government is essential for democracies and that trust is affected by international issues, economic issues, and political scandals. The chapter examined the attributes that potentially contribute to perceptions of politicians as trustworthy, such as acting against self-interest. Finally, the chapter culminates in the description of a BDT investigation of trust in politicians.

REFERENCES

Blind, P. K. (2007). Building trust in government in the twenty-first century: Review of literature and emerging issues. 7th *Global Forum on Reinventing Government*, 26–29 June, Vienna Austria.

Cheng, H., Bynner, J., Wiggins, R., & Schoon, I. (2012). The measurement and evaluation of social attitudes in two British Cohort studies. *Social Research Council*, 107, 351–371.

Combs, D. J. Y., & Keller, P. S. (2010). Politicians and trustworthiness: Acting contrary to self-interest enhances trustworthiness. *Basic and Applied Social Psychology*, 32, 328–339. doi:10.1080/01973533.2010.519246

Fisher, J., van Heerde, J., & Tucker, A. (2010). Does one trust judgment fit all? Linking theory and empirics. *The British Journal of Politics and International Relations*, 12, 161–188. doi:10.1111/j.1467–856X.2009.00401.x

Garen, J., & Clark, J. R. (2015). Trust and the growth of government. *CATO Journal*, 35(3), 549–580.

Hetherington, M. J., & Rudolph, T. J. (2008). Priming, performance, and the dynamics of political trust. *Journal of Politics, 70*, 498–512.

Isotalus, P., & Almonkari, M. (2014). Political scandal tests trust in politicians. *Nordicom Review*, 35(2), 3–16. doi:10.2478/nor-2014–0011

Kolbert, E. (2016, November 3). How can Americans trust Donald Trump? *The New Yorker*. Retrieved from www.newyorker.com/news/daily-comment/how-can-americans-trust-donald-trump

Leigh, A. (2002). Explaining distrust: Popular attitudes towards politicians in Australia and the United States. In D. Burchell & A. Leigh (Eds.), *The Prince's new clothes: Why do Australians dislike their politicians?* Sydney: UNSW Press.

Martin, A. (2010). Does political trust matter? Examining some of the implications of low levels of political trust in Australia. *Australian Journal of Political Science*, 45, 705–712. doi:10.1080/10361146.2010.517184

Rotenberg, K. J. (2016, June 13). The EU referendum: It is a matter of trust. *Conversations*.

Schiffman, L., Thelen, S. T., & Sherman, E. (2010). Interpersonal and political trust: Modeling levels of citizens' trust. *European Journal of Marketing*, 44(3/4), 369–381.doi:10.1108/03090561011020471

Warren, M. E. (Ed.). (1999). *Democracy and trust*. New York and Cambridge: Cambridge University Press.

Warren, M. E. (2004). What does corruption mean in a democracy? *American Journal of Political Science*, 48(2), 328–343.

Chapter 3

Community as social ties

Carolyn Kagan, Mark Burton,
Paul Duckett, Rebecca Lawthom
and Asiya Siddiquee

Summary

In the previous chapter we examined theories of community and explored its various dimensions, including sentiment (the way community exists symbolically), space (the way community is defined by a physical or temporal space) and social structure (the way community is defined by social features of a group – such as its membership rules). In this chapter, we explore in more detail the social structural dimension to community by examining the nature of the social ties between people that define the concept of community and then consider how the concept is employed to prescribe rather than describe the behaviours of its members.

Social ties

Social ties are the social connections that bond people. These might be both malign and benign. The nature of the social ties that we are bound by (the relationships we have with our family, friends, peers, community and so on) has a dramatic impact upon our psychological and our physical health (Kawachi & Berkman, 2001; Wilkinson & Pickett, 2009). Underpinning theories of social ties is importance of others' perception of us for our sense of self.

> Other people's perception of us is evaluative and judgmental: they like or dislike, they accept or reject, they trust or don't trust, they look up to or down on us. So essential is this intimate monitoring of others' reactions to us for our security, safety, socialization, and learning that instead of experiencing it as their reactions to us, we often experience it as if it were our experience of ourselves. When we do something that is shameful in others' eyes, we can hate ourselves for it, and when we do something that others admire, value, and appreciate, we can get a glowing sense of self-realization.
>
> (Wilkinson, 2005, p. 91)

More generally, the studies of social networks point to the importance social ties play in our sense of well-being.

> ... being embedded in a network of supportive relationships is associated in general with health and psychological well-being.
>
> (Dalton et al., 2001, p. 234)

The social ties between people are greatly influenced by social systems and, as such, the social structural dimension to community both teases out the nature of those ties and suggests ways in which those ties are formed. Below, we examine three types of social tie: those based on affection (such as in social groups), functional interdependence (such as shared needs) and coercion (such as in work places where an employee might be punished for failing to attend work). The nature of social ties might be seen as extraordinarily complex. However, it is easier to discern the ways that bonds of affection, functional interdependence and coercion inform the assumptions of researchers and policy makers and how these theories that relate to community carry assumptions about the social ties that constitute community. After a brief introduction to these three types of social ties, we consider how each might become expressed in social policy – as prescriptions of how people should live.

Reflect!

Do you like to spend time alone – how might the amount of time you spend alone be related to life stage? Babies, school age children, young adults, adults, older adults participate differently in family life and institutional life.

Social ties of affection

Studies of affection refer to the ways people are bonded together through a concern for one another's welfare, built out of a liking for each other. Here we find friendship groups but also philanthropic groups. Often, when bonds are believed to be largely based on affection, we find studies that search for the existence of informal, sustained voluntary associations between people and social policies that see community as built on voluntarism (such as active citizenship, volunteering schemes, the role of the charitable sector and so on). Here people are bonded together because they want to help others. So, to trace the degree to which a group forms a community when carrying these assumptions, we would measure the degree to which the group engages in voluntarism and philanthropy. These social ties are most likely to be affected by homophily – the love of sameness. Thus, such ties can become concentrated in groups that share characteristics based on gender, ethnicity, class, disability status and so on. People form ties of liking because they feel they are alike. The social identity upon which likeness is based can be manipulated – such as the manipulation of national identity to increase or decrease social ties of affection within and between groups. In the UK, the 'Leave' campaign behind 'Brexit' in the UK was quite successful at manipulating social ties of affection at a supranational level – creating antagonism between UK citizens and citizens in the European Union. In the USA, the Trump administration's pledge to 'Build the Wall' on its border with Mexico invoked and inflamed existing racial tensions in the populace. In Australia, social ties of affection between indigenous and non-indigenous people have been effectively disrupted to such an extent that Australia has, for 200 years, avoided establishing a treaty with indigenous people to negotiate sovereignty and has sustained a perverse cultural ritual of celebrating the invasion of Aboriginal and Torres Strait Islanders' land each year on 'Australia Day'.

Social platforms like Facebook and Twitter have been criticised for manipulating people's social ties of affection by asking users to like or dislike other users' content and then building communities on the basis of this that sharpen differences between group members and non-members; enable victimisation and social exclusion through 'unfriending' a member; create content feed algorithms that reduce the contact between group members and non-group members; and create toxic spaces where groups can engage in confrontation and antagonism with non-group members. All of this is done not to forge communities but to monetise social ties through selling to advertisers information on the social ties that the platform has created. These social platforms remind us how creating communities through ties of affection can create sharp boundaries between those that are alike and those that are not and how for those outside, the severance from a group's ties of affection can lead to indifference at best and hatred at worst (e.g. online 'trolling'). Political discourses around immigration in the USA, UK and Australia, as well as elsewhere, can also be seen as direct manipulations of social ties of affection, essentially severing those ties by exaggerating differences between immigrants and non-immigrants. In Australia, these discourses have sustained the practice of the indefinite detention of asylum seekers in off-shore processing centres.

Social ties of interdependence

Where the belief is that social ties are based on interdependence among members, research often searches for patterns of exchange between group members such as through LETS (Local Exchange Trading Scheme) and self help organisations. It is here that we see theories of social capital. Thus, when networks between people are strong and there are strong norms of reciprocity (people helping each other out) it is said there is strong social capital amongst people. This is generally thought to be a good thing and to lead to positive well-being and good health, with lots of people being involved with others in different ways and on a range of activities (Gilchrist, 2004). In the UK an example of community forming through the social ties of interdependence was the tragedy of the Grenfell Tower in London in 2017. Grenfell Tower was a 23-storey residential tower block where a fire in the early hours of the morning of July 14, 2017 spread rapidly through the whole tower block, killing 72 people. The fire was initially blamed on the use of dangerous cladding and insulation on the building, poorly maintained fire safety equipment in the building and an inadequate fire evacuation plan for the building. During the tragedy people living in the tower block and in the surrounding community assisted in the rescue of tower block residents and in the aftermath, the surviving residents and people in the surrounding community worked together to support each other materially and to hold to account those who were responsible for the tragedy politically.

These ties can develop between people not because they like one another, but because they feel they need one another.

It is easy to see that such strong links between people could easily turn inwards and the distinction between those inside and those outside the community becomes important. Indeed, strong inward looking communities might positively exclude new people, leading to conflict, or make excessive claims on 'insiders'; restrict access to opportunities and individual freedoms; and promote a 'downward levelling of norms' (Evans, 1997). The most obvious manifestation of this can be seen in the 'gated community'. Gated communities have become more prevalent across Australia, Europe, the United States of America and major cities in China (see Figure 1.3 in Chapter 1 for a gated community in Manchester). Hutton (2002) reported that at the turn of the century 3 million people in the USA were living in gated communities. Branic and Kubrin (2018) stipulate that more recent estimations of the number of people living in gated communities is difficult to obtain; but there is little doubt that the figure has considerably increased from earlier estimations. Some of these have high levels of interdependence between residents and independence from the state such that residents organise their own community tax to pay for rubbish collection and policing and do not pay state taxes for such services. Thus, residents of these gated communities become highly dependent upon one another in terms of relying on each other to provide the funding to keep their neighbourhood clean and secure. They also become bound together by their own membership rules which can include specific bylaws. The latter can, for example, specify a minimum age for children who are permitted to enter the community, and security provisions.

Social ties of coercion

When the assumption is that social ties will be coercive, the focus of research is often on the imposition of structures on a group that seek to maintain social order or of social ties that operate as a form of resistance against patterns of exclusion and domination. Typically, the focus is on a community as a place of confinement from which people cannot escape rather than a place where people are bonded by affection or co-dependence: the processes that bind people together are negative. Pahl (1970) outlines a form of community to which people have strong allegiances, due to shared social and economic disadvantage. These communities are often close knit but are difficult to leave due to the circumstances people find themselves in. Pahl notes that such communities can be stifling for some but comforting to others, anticipating the UK Government's framing of neighbourhoods as communities experiencing different levels of social deprivation, as described through the Indices of Deprivation (UK Government, 2015). Whilst these descriptions offer objective assessments of some dimensions of community life, they do not necessarily correspond to perceived deprivation by those living in particular neighbourhoods. In Australia, government assessments of indigenous social deprivation identified the neglect and abuse of indigenous children in indigenous communities. That assessment justified the imposition of 'the intervention' in 73 indigenous communities in Australia's Northern Territory that made, inter alia, changes to welfare provision, law enforcement and land tenure. This was enacted through enforced alcohol and pornography bans, compulsory health checks and increased social and economic surveillance, and gave the government the right to seize indigenous land. In 2010, a United Nations investigation concluded that many of those measures constituted racial discrimination and violations of human rights against indigenous people.

In reality, the different kinds of social ties co-exist and might evolve into each other. For example, a community bound together by ties of coercion might transform into ties of affection and mutual interdependence if the cause for the negative effects of their being bound together as a community becomes focused on those outside. This can be realised in scapegoating of other marginalised groups in one form and in another more progressive form can be the development of political awareness of the social structures that causes the problems people are experiencing, as in processes of 'conscientisation' (see Chapter 3). So, the ties between people can be multi-layered but also transitional.

Theory prescriptions for community

It is said that philosophers, politicians and the 'public' provide prescriptions of community while social scientists provide descriptions and definitions of community which are prescriptions in disguise. Thus, theories of community and theoretical frameworks used to study communities are often normative and ideological – they say something about how the theorists or researchers think community should be.

Since the early 1900s, social scientists have increasingly moved from making theoretical venturings about what communities might be to empirical observation of what communities are. Some of these studies have sought to understand the complexity of community by having researchers immerse themselves in a community for substantial periods of time. There have been a number of such intensive studies (for example Lynd & Lynd, 1929; Jahoda, Lazarsfeld & Zeisel, 2002; Whyte, 1943; Harrison 2008). Such studies point to the complexity of community and how different dimensions of community become meaningful for people at different times and in different contexts. What is perhaps clearer to define is how the different dimensions of community affect the empirical and theoretical work of social scientists and social policy makers, that is how social scientists perceive community rather than necessarily how people experience community. This gives us an insight into the preconceptions of those who study community, including community psychologists, as well as the socio-economic context in which those preconceptions develop.

For example, Tönnies' theory of community (see Chapter 4) was located in conservative thought at the time of the industrial revolution in the West. This was a time of dramatic social upheavals during which the regulation of society by nature (employed at the time when the economy was organised around the farming community and the traditions of the craftsperson) was shifting to a regulation of society by bureaucratic social administration and the mechanisation of working practices (production lines and factories). Conservative thought was hostile to the growing process of urbanisation and the fear that the destruction of rural communities and their replacement by urban communities could loosen social control and lead to a threat to the social order by the masses. Thus, the theory that Tönnies gave voice to was grounded in a normative prescription that was against forms of social regulation that were at that time new.

Thus, the distinction between Gemeinschaft and Gesellschaft draws our attention to the role that social structures play in defining our sense of community. People's sense of shared identity, loyalty, allegiance and so on changes as their patterns of work and mobility change. In making those distinctions, Tönnies was berating the loss of one type of sense of community (Gemeinschaft) that was happening under the rapid process of economic and social change through industrialisation.

Up until the 1970s, much of what was written about communities based in Europe and North America continued to focus, in one way or another, on the transformation that has happened to urban and to rural life through the social and economic changes that occurred during the industrial revolution. Prior to this, danger was perceived to largely exist outside of the city walls. The city protected you from harsh conditions of rural life (where you were at risk of being raided by bandits, attacked by wild animals and battered by storms). Since the 1900s, the perception of danger has shifted to inside the city walls (Bauman, 2007a). The spatial dimension of community was central to such work. As we describe in Chapter 4, since the 1970s we have seen an increasing focus on the importance of the symbolic nature of community following the latest major economic and social transformation (the shift in the West from a capitalist producer society to a capitalist consumer society).

Both the focus on the spatial dimension of community and that on the symbolic nature of community could be viewed as based upon changes in social structure (in terms of global socio-economic transformations). These social structures have had a dramatic impact upon the social ties between people in communities and it is here that we can perhaps see at its most pronounced how theorists can prescribe rather than describe what those social relations might be. Thus, we contrast two approaches to theorising and researching community based first on social ties of affection and co-operation and second on social ties of coercion.

Ties of affection and co-operation: community as social capital

Social support has usually been understood and measured as a process occurring between two individuals. This has kept much of the research on social support at the individual level (Felton & Shinn, 1992). The various types of support are described in Table 5.1. Clearly, social support also occurs in groups (Maton, 1989), especially in microsystems (focusing on friendships). Those groups provide support to their members even when the individual members change. The sense of belonging within such organisations or microsystems may be as important as social support from individuals (Felton & Shinn, 1992). Recognition of this has led to increasing interest in the concept of social capital.

In 1995, Putnam reflected upon the decline of organised bowling leagues in the USA and how these were being replaced with people going to bowling alleys to bowl with friends and family instead. This

Table 5.1 Types of social support

Type of support	Example
Material	Child care, money lending, running errands, help with transport, DIY jobs
Social integration	Companionship
Emotional	Informal counselling, 'a shoulder to cry on'
Esteem	Making someone feel good about themselves by complementing them and displaying other forms of respect towards them

became a metaphor to describe what many commentators saw as US citizens' withdrawal from actively engaging in civil life (in sports clubs, voluntary organisations, neighbourhood associations and so on). Putnam's work is part of a body of social commentary that has focused on the consequences of modern individualism that characterises the dominant cultural mode of living in the US the UK, Australia and elsewhere (see Chapters 2 and 3) and the loss of social support at community and societal levels.

Reflect!

If you were asked to tell someone who had come to live in your country from abroad about how to take part in community groups, interest groups or local politics, what would you tell them? How did you learn about this?

Putnam's work created a considerable level of interest from academics and social policy makers who have used the concept to promote various policies (such as active citizenship in the UK).

> By 'social capital' I mean features of social life – networks, norms, and trust – that enable participants to act together more effectively to pursue shared objectives ... To the extent that the norms, networks, and trust link substantial sectors of the community and span underlying social cleavages – to the extent that the social capital is of a bridging sort – then the enhanced cooperation is likely to serve broader interests and to be widely welcomed.
>
> (Putnam, 1995, pp. 664–665)

For Putnam, increasing levels of trust between people arises from the strengthening of norms of co-operation such as the belief in the importance of reciprocity (the belief that if you do good acts for others, others will do good acts for you) and the growth of networks of civic engagement. Putnam identified two forms of social capital. Bonding capital is that which occurs between people who are 'like' one another (that is, it happens within the one community rather between two different communities). Bridging capital occurs between people and groups where co-membership of one particular community plays no necessary part (that is, it happens between different communities). For Putnam, bridging social capital was the key to promoting civil life (increased civil engagement in a democratic political system).

Putnam's thesis is that increases in social capital and increased levels of trust among people will all lead to higher levels of civic engagement (see Figure 5.1) and that this will result in a society character- ised by high levels of democratic polity (a political system that seeks to promote high levels of citizen representation and participation in executive decision making processes).

The epidemiologist Richard Wilkinson incorporates the notion of social capital to explain his find- ings that societies that are less egalitarian are less healthy.

> ... egalitarian societies ... have ... social cohesion. They have a strong community life. Instead of social life stopping outside the front door, public space remains a social space ... People are more likely to be involved in social and voluntary activities outside the home...
>
> Social capital ... lubricates the working of the whole society and economy. There are fewer signs of anti-social aggressiveness, and society appears more caring. In short, the social fabric is in better condition.
>
> (Wilkinson, 1996, p. 4)

Wilkinson's work would add to the conceptual model proposed by Putnam, as illustrated by Figure 5.2.

So, researchers such as Wilkinson point to the corrosive effects on social cohesion of income inequali- ties. However, the popular focus upon social capital has tended to neglect this aspect, and discussion about social capital by social policy makers and social scientists alike often fails to acknowledge how social capital might be largely dependent upon levels of social equality and that declines and rises in social capital are likely to be inversely related to the declines and rises in social inequalities (Wilkinson,

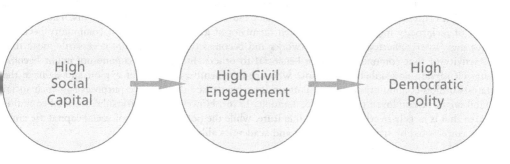

Figure 5.1 Income equality and social capital.

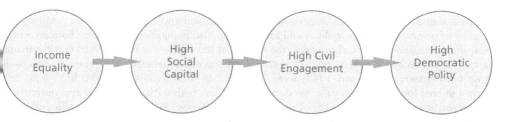

Figure 5.2 Income equality, social capital and democracy.

2005). Another element that is largely absent from Putnam's work, highlighted by drawing upon Wilkinson's work, is the importance of 'respect' and a consideration that respect might precede trust. Thus, before you can establish trust between people, there needs to be mutual respect and that the feeling that you or your group is disrespected by others is reason for a deterioration of social cohesion (Szreter, 2002; Wilkinson, Kawachi & Kennedy, 1998). That feeling of respect might be read by the ways your community is valued in comparison with another group or in comparison with how your group appeared valued in the past to how it is now. This might be measured by the degree to which your community is represented in the political system (is your voice heard in Parliament or are your people recognised in your country's constitution?), in cultural institutions (are your stories told through the popular arts and the mass media?) and the degree to which your community has access to economic and material resources (are you paid a decent wage, do you have access to good education, health, housing and social services?).

The criticism here is that the theory of social capital is somewhat blinkered to the broader socio-economic and political context and insufficiently engages with the problem posed by political and ideological systems that create social inequalities. For example, Putnam's thesis that increases in social capital result in increased civil engagement and a more democratic political system somewhat ignores the structural and ideological systems in which such processes occur. Moreover, civic engagement can be widespread in non-democratic political systems and such engagement is not bound to result in an increase in democratic political processes (Boggs, 2001). Also, highly democratic systems can lead to social inequalities and discrimination (such as the Swiss deciding in 2009 through a democratic referendum to ban the building of minarets, various European countries since 2004 banning the burqa, and in the UK a referendum on membership of the European Union leading to a result that has produced political turmoil and strong political divisions across the UK – known as Brexit). Indeed, increases in social capital and civil engagement can result in a deterioration of democratic polity if that engagement is through street gangs, religious cults and reactionary political movements. The fact that norms of reciprocity might develop between members of a community, and a community becomes increasingly interconnected by social networks and becomes trusting, does not necessarily mean that the activity of that community will be beneficial to others. Indeed, that community might become quite self serving and unhelpful to those who are not members – it might exploit and damage the interests of non-community members. Putnam later recognised the negative purposes to which social capital might be employed (see Portes & Landolt, 1996). However, the 'dark side' of social capital is an area that is largely overlooked in the literature, while the positive aspects of social capital are commonly emphasised by social policy makers and academics alike.

Think!

Draw up a table of positive and negative aspects of social capital. On balance, do you think social capital should be encouraged? Why is this?

This lack of understanding of the importance of socio-political and economic context – namely the influence of power, economics, politics and ideology – is also highlighted in the way Putnam writes about the deterioration in social capital in the USA since the 1960s. Putnam believed that the major reason for the decline was the effect of generational succession whereby the pre-war generation (those born between 1910 and 1940) were succeeded by later generations who have been less engaged in civil life, placed less value on duty and held less faith in the ability and appropriateness of government to intervene in the life of the individual. However, Putnam fails to consider why this has happened and to consider the socio-political events and processes that might have contributed to this change in values and loss of faith in political institutions and a growing culture of competitive individualism.

The notion of social capital has also been criticised in a number of other ways. For example, it is somewhat gender blind. Much of the initial research into social capital focused on support systems used largely by men during the 1970s (such as sports clubs) and women's systems of support were largely ignored and/or considered irrelevant to the political world and to citizenship (James cited in Lowndes, 2000).

Also, most social support research has been middle class focused and biased against non-dominant groups (Mickelson & Kubzansky, 2003). The privatised and individualised lifestyle of middle class USA may seem less familiar to those who are not middle class and not living in the USA (Szreter, 2002) where the 'we' is used by and to signify a liberal/cosmopolitan elite. The 'Me Too' movement is an interesting case in point. The movement began in 2006 and was focused on black women's experience of sexual abuse, particularly in socio-economically deprived communities. In 2017 the movement effectively became re-appropriated by middle class American women – notably by Hollywood actors. The reframing of 'Me Too' has led critics to berate dilution of the movement as its focus has shifted away from issues of race and class. Class also impacts upon the way social capital is distributed, valued and used. Writers like Bourdieu (1986) have pointed out how the poor generally have more access to social capital because they have little access to any other form of capital. Also, by accessing social capital the poor might in fact find that it might lock them into poverty (such as on housing estates where social capital is provided by street gangs and so on, which might disconnect them from other social networks that might offer them a way out of their poverty). This is the problem of bonding social capital (which links us together with those in our designated community) in comparison with bridging social capital (which links us to people outside of our specified community). Both the rich and the poor tend to have more bonding social capital than bridging social capital which results in people becoming locked into poverty or wealth and power being locked up with small pockets of elite groups. Indeed, bridging capital may be difficult to create where deeply embedded and somewhat change resistant social inequalities and historical antagonisms create distrust and disrespect between groups.

We now consider what might happen if the social ties are strong between people but that these are largely characterised as ties of coercion rather than affection and co-operation.

Reflect!

Consider your local community – can you discern bridging and bonding ties? How do they come about? Which is stronger, bonding or bridging capital? Why is this?

Ties of coercion: community as ghetto

A contrasting vision of a community tied together by bonds of affection and co-operation is that of people being connected by ties of coercion and exploitation and such a picture of a community is provided by descriptions of communities as ghettos.

> Ghettos and prisons are two varieties of the strategy of 'tying the undesirables to the ground', of confinement and immobilization. In a world in which mobility and the facility to be on the move have become principal factors of social stratification, this is (both physically and symbolically) a weapon of ultimate exclusion and degradation.
>
> (Bauman, 2001, p. 120)

A ghetto is a community into which people are placed involuntarily and from which people are prevented from leaving. Ghettos contrast with gated communities (described earlier) where residents cut themselves off from the outside voluntarily and residents are free to leave, but non-residents are not free to enter. Gated communities are constructed to keep those inside secure and free from threat and their residents are usually resource rich, while ghettos are constructed to keep those outside secure and free from threat and the residents are usually resource poor.

Among the most prominent historical examples of ghettos are the Jewish ghettos (for example, Budapest, Kovno, Łódź, Vilna and Warsaw), in Nazi occupied Europe during the 1930s and 1940s. These ghettos were internment areas built on the previously existing ghettos where Jewish people had been required to live in Eastern Europe.

Conditions in these Jewish ghettos under Nazi control were wretched. Large numbers of people were crammed into small areas where food was scarce and amenities were minimal. For example, the Warsaw ghetto was just over four hundred hectares in area and housed 400,000 Jewish people. Ironically the most prominent contemporary examples of a ghetto are parts of the Occupied Territories of Palestine – the Israeli political administration subjecting the Palestinians to the treatment Jewish people were subjected to by the Nazis.

Among modern day ghettos are the 'black ghettos', particularly prevalent in the USA, and immigrant ghettos that are becoming widespread across Europe. In Australia, ghettos were created for indigenous people when they were moved onto small parcels of land (reserves, missions and stations). This was the Australian government's political response to the dispossessions of indigenous people from their native lands.

Ghettos are often those communities that are experiencing multiple levels of economic deprivation. It is not the absence of resource per se that makes such communities ghettos, but the effect such material deprivation has on their residents' ability to leave. The situation faced by some people living on council (or public housing) estates in the UK reflects this. These estates have long been characterised as places of heightened crime and delinquency and those that live there are commonly caricatured as criminals and delinquents (they are often called 'sink estates'). Such representations have continually been reinforced through mass media portrayals (in documentaries, dramas, literature, music and cinema). These communities gain negative reputations which are then transferred onto those who live there. It is difficult to find a city or a town in the UK that does not have an area within it stigmatised in this way.

Example: Community leadership

We worked, and a group of students, worked with some residents who lived on the edge of a prosperous market town in the North West of England. There were few facilities in this area: no schools, doctors' surgeries, community meeting places, or libraries. There was a small parade of shops with most units empty and one rough public house. The estate was called Broadheath (a pseudonym). All the houses and flats were simply called Broadheath no. 1 or 203, or 1,130. There were no names to the roads. Residents were of the firm belief that as soon as they gave their address as Broadheath, when applying for jobs and so on, they got no further, due to the negative reputation attached to Broadheath. They could not give their address without naming Broadheath, whereas everywhere else in the town could just give their house number and road and did not need to name the district.

Blanden, Gregg & Machin (2005) reported on the decreasing levels of intergenerational social mobility in the UK, showing that a child born in the 1970s was less likely to move out of the poverty of its parents than a child born in the 1950s. The report further concluded that social mobility in the UK and USA were both lower than in Germany, which had the middle rate of social mobility in the countries surveyed by the report, and were substantially lower than in Canada and the Nordic countries, which had the highest level of social mobility. To be poor in the UK is to inherit the poverty of parents and to bequeath poverty to children. Sprigings and Allen (2005, p. 389) argue that one of the paradoxical effects of the UK Government's policies on community building

> restricts the residential mobility of poorer households and exacerbates (rather than combats) their social exclusion because a key indicator of social inclusion is their ability to take advantage of the social, cultural and economic opportunities that so often exist elsewhere.

As we briefly described in Chapter 4, people can also find that while they themselves do not move, their communities (both social settings and social identities) move (or shape-shift) around them, transformed by socio-economic and political forces into something unrecognised and unwanted. You might find that you are not placed into a ghetto, but that the place in which you live or the social identity you are given becomes transformed in such a way that you become ghettoised. For example, many communities that developed around the coal mining and manufacturing industries were economically and socially devastated following the policy of disinvestment in manufacturing in the UK. Another example is how the social identity of Muslims has shifted since the terrorist attacks on the USA in 2001 such that racism and Islamophobia can make daily life difficult for many Muslim people in the West. Here a ghetto does not need to be a physical space – it can be a symbolic space, a representation or stereotype (see section on ghetto walls below).

The restrictions on the freedom to leave can make ghettos resemble a form of prison or mental institution. Indeed, the process of 'ghettoisation' runs in parallel with a penal system with an ongoing mutual exchange occurring between residents in each as part of a systemic criminalisation and pathologisation of the poor (Duckett & Schinkel, 2008). Bauman (2001) argues that the ghetto serves as the dumping ground for those for whom society has no economic or political use.

The ghetto walls

Ghettos can exist without the need for physical barriers to keep people inside. Barriers can be attitudinal or social. For example, there may be no physical barrier that stops black residents from crossing the street and walking into a nearby white neighbourhood. But if they do, they may be watched and then reported by white residents, and then trailed, stopped and searched by the police.

Social attitudes can ghettoise. Whilst physical barriers to social inclusion for disabled people, for example, have greatly reduced in the UK, their exclusion is maintained through attitudinal barriers. Similarly, a diagnosis of 'mental illness' can transform social identity to the extent that employment is restricted and people are perceived as a potential threat to others. They become ghettoised by a medical label. People can find themselves locked into a social identity (based on ethnicity, disability, gender, sexuality, social class and so on).

Reflect!

Which social identities do you have which:

- You have chosen?
- Have been chosen for you?
- You can change?
- You cannot change?

In this way, a community might be a bad place to be because of the people who you are placed there with (whether that is a place or a social identity). To be placed in a ghetto often means you are being placed in with those whom society has either labelled as 'bad' or 'mad'. This is the way that problem places are seen as inhabited by problem people (Johnston & Mooney, 2007). So, people find themselves placed in these physical settings or social identities against their will and once there are unable to leave.

> The truth is that council housing is a living tomb. You dare not give up the house because you might never get another, but staying is to be trapped in a ghetto of both place and mind.
> (Hutton, 2007, www.guardian.co.uk/commentisfree/2007/feb/18/comment.homeaffairs)

The 'favelas', 'barrios', 'bustees', 'townships' and 'slums' which characterise majority world cities (Neuwirth, 2006) all illustrate similar processes of ghettoisation.

Think!

Can you think of people who lack the social mobility to move out of their stigmatised identity? What might be the reasons for this? What consequences does this have for their lives?

In a ghetto, social relations will often be characterised more by antagonism than by affection and co-operation. Ghetto residents can turn in on themselves and distance themselves from others to whom they attribute blame for the stigma their place (or identity) attracts. Newly arrived immigrants, disabled people, people diagnosed with a mental illness, unemployed people and so on may all be targeted for discrimination in disadvantaged communities. Bauman (2001) captures this process:

> To regain a measure of dignity and reaffirm the legitimacy of their own status in the eyes of society, residents … overstress their moral worth as individuals (or as family members) and join in the dominant discourse of denunciation of those who undeservingly 'profit' from social programmes, faux pauvres and 'welfare cheats'. It is as if they could gain value only by devaluing their neighbourhood and their neighbours. They also engage in a variety of strategies of social distinction and withdrawal which converge to undermine neighbourhood cohesion.
> (Bauman, 2001, p. 121)

Here, the social relations between people are not characterised by affection or co-operation but by antagonism. Indeed, the whole analysis rests on the assumption that the social ties between people in such settings are hostile, not harmonious. These different ways of thinking about social ties can also be found in how social boundaries around communities are seen.

Social boundaries: benign or benevolent?

The construction of social and cultural borders can be a reminder of the benign side to community – social safety – or of its less than benign side – social division. The identification of the very things that people have in common with each other (whatever that might be) also has the effect of marking out those with whom people have less in common. Thus, the construction of community around 'sameness' (shared interests, shared space, shared identity and so on) denotes a place where you are around people who are similar to you and apart from people who are dissimilar to you (the Other). Often the homogeneity of both those inside and those outside of a community becomes amplified, as does the perceived deviance of the outsiders and righteousness of the insiders. In this way, community can involve the construction of barriers (not only physical, but also social and cultural) that are closely monitored to maintain the protection of those on the inside and the persecution of those outside. Uncritically constructing community as a place of safety and security can lead to a justification for this process of 'Othering' and boundary making.

> ...the unrelenting processes of social differentiation which reflect and amplify social hierarchy are fundamentally important in any analysis of social integration and community. It is these processes which create social exclusion, which stigmatise the most deprived and establish social distances throughout society.
>
> (Wilkinson, 1996, p. 171)

If we assume that the social ties between people in communities are based on affection and co-operation we might see those boundaries as more benevolent than benign. Community psychologists often do just that – focusing on the positive effects of community and the barriers that are created around them. For example, McMillan and Chavis point to the positives of constructing boundaries as a means to offset the harmful effects such social divisions might create:

> Social psychology research has demonstrated that people have boundaries protecting their personal space. People need these barriers to protect against threat ... While much sympathetic interest in and research on the deviant have been generated, group members' legitimate needs for boundaries to protect their intimate social connections have often been overlooked ... the harm which comes from the pain of rejection and isolation created by boundaries will continue until we clarify the positive benefits that boundaries provide to communities.
>
> (McMillan & Chavis, 1986, p. 4)

Here, the Other becomes the deviant whom 'we' (the cosmopolitan elite) need to be protected against with boundaries. However, McMillan and Chavis interpret social barriers as providing emotional safety.

These differences in perspective and lived reality (whether we view or experience communities as sites of social capital and places which can enable and empower, or as ghettos which marginalise and stigmatise) are inextricably linked to social power at a structural level. One of the criticisms of Putnam's theory of social capital is that communities are largely seen as doing it for themselves and the role of the state in creating the conditions for this to happen or not to happen is largely overlooked (Szreter, 2002).

Community and social policy

Not only is it possible to trace the ideological and theoretical underpinnings of the various ways community is defined, it is also important to consider how the concept of community has been employed to achieve particular political ends. Indeed, 'community' has largely been defined over the last two hundred years for political and administrative purposes and once placed in its historical context we find that it is a concept that "...*has been contested, fought over and appropriated for different uses and interests to justify different politics, policies and practices*" (Mayo, 1994, p. 48). This perspective states that the concept of community conveys not a description of but a prescription for social organisation. Below we list a number of examples of how community has been prescribed in this way.

● Under colonial direct rule in East Africa in the late nineteenth and early twentieth centuries, the concept of 'community' was used to classify and regulate South Asian immigrant skilled manual workers. The construct 'tribe' was used to administer the African workforce but this was inappropriate for the South Asian workers so a new concept had to be created and used to classify and regulate the Asian population (Bauman, 1996).

- In the UK during the mid twentieth century the concept of community was used in urban planning as a tool for social engineering. Community was invoked to smooth social resistance against a social programme that sought 're-development' of working class areas and mass movement of working class neighbourhoods to new housing estates following 'slum clearances'. These urban planning initiatives deployed the symbolic association of community with safety, security and extended family to promote their social planning agenda and placate working class concerns that their lives were being re-ordered at the behest of and for the benefit of the political classes.
- In Europe during the 1950s 'community' was used in the Paris Treaty of 1951 and the Rome Treaty of 1957 to proffer an organisational structure that would supersede the concept of the 'nation state' – the European Community. The use of the concept of community functioned to focus attention on mutual aid and protection and deflect attention from the attempts to create a superpower to compete economically, politically and militarily in global order.
- In the UK, the disappearance of 'community' from the political lexicon during the neo-conservative emphasis on individualism was epitomised by Thatcher's 'no such thing as society' speech (see Chapter 1). When the Labour Party came to power in the UK in 1997, the concept of community became re-introduced into social policy discussion and was used, specifically in programmes of 'urban regeneration/renewal', to signify 'bottom up' programmes of social and economic reform and the political process of decentralisation and devolution. More generally, it was used to promote the development of 'third-way politics' – a transfer of responsibility away from the social institution and from the individual and onto the collective of individuals – the community. Thus, 'community' became the site of a political project that sought to leave society unbound from both the tyranny of being governed by the dictates of social institutions and the self-interest of the individual and thus 'community' would mediate between the individual and the social institution and become the site where the individual would become re-shackled by moral responsibility to the political economy of the nation state.

Thus, it is important to understand the socio-economic and cultural context in which attempts are made to anchor the meaning of the concept of community and the ideological purposes for which it is invoked. Such an understanding points to the historical and political malleability of the concept (for example, in the policies of 'community care', 'urban regeneration' and 'New Deal for communities' in the UK, and 'community renewal' in Australia, Canada and the USA). Common to all of these modern initiatives that invoke community is the notion of 'participation', a key process in critical community psychology.

Nature of participation

As with the concept of 'community', participation is a complex and problematic concept (Cooke & Kothari, 2001; Cornwall, 2008). Cooke (2001) distinguished between participation as a means and as an end. Participation as means, he argues, builds a sense of commitment and enhances effectiveness of service delivery. This kind of participation would be as part of externally defined, top down agendas. Participation as an end, on the other hand, is said to increase empowerment, or control over development activities from which people had hitherto been excluded. This kind of participation is driven bottom up and will often originate with marginalised people themselves. Beetham, Blick, Margetts and Weir (2008) suggest that participation can be characterised along four different dimensions: individual versus collective action or initiative; unstructured versus structured through existing organisations and channels; time-bound or one-off versus ongoing through time; and reactive versus proactive.

Although they argue that widening and deepening participation leads to greater social justice, they point out that any form of participation in the UK is as unequal as the distribution of power and resources throughout society. Participation does not necessarily have a levelling effect.

Reflect!

Think about your own participation in any activities or groups which aim to contribute to social change. What do you do and with whom?

In much of community psychology action there are elements of both types of participation. Kagan (2006a, 2006b) suggests that it is bottom up participation and collective action or those participation practices that include bottom up processes that are likely to have the greatest impact on both well-being and potential for changing the material circumstances of life. This type of participation does several things (Campbell & Jovchelovitch, 2000; Campbell & Murray, 2004).

First, the group's critical awareness and development of critical thinking is enhanced. Second, members of the group re-negotiate their collective social identity and varied, associated perspectives and views of the world. They do this by people developing shared understanding, information and ways of talking about themselves and others. Lastly, people's confidence and ability to take control of their lives is reinforced. People are *empowered* to make changes to their lives. With this type of participation it is necessary to have access to power, and resources, and this is the role of the external agents, community psychologists or other professionals.

Montero (2004a) discusses participation from the perspective of those who are participating. She conceptualises participation as a process closely connected to the concept of 'commitment'. Rather than a linear ladder with its metaphor of higher and lower forms of participation, Montero conceptualises a dynamic system of concentric circles with the nucleus of maximum participation and commitment at the centre. The circles radiate through different levels of participation-commitment to the outer layer of positive friendly curiosity with no commitment (see Figure 5.3).

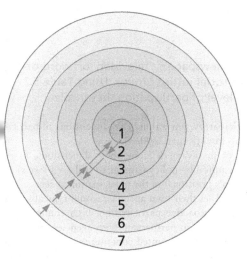

1. Nucleus of maximum participation and commitment
2. Frequent participation and high commitment
3. Specific participation, medium commitment
4. Sporadic participation, low commitment
5. New and tentative participation, low commitment
   (e.g. financial support material)
6. Tangential participation, unclear
   (e.g. approval, agreement)
7. Positive, friendly curiosity. No commitment.

↗ People moving in and out with greater or lesser levels of commitment

Figure 5.3 Levels of participation and commitment in the community.
Source: Montero, 2004a. Reproduced with permission of the author.

Table 5.2 Stances of participation

Level of participation	Activity
1. Information	Tell people what is planned
2. Consultation	Offer a number of options and listen to the feedback
3. Deciding together	Encourage others to provide some additional ideas and options, and join in deciding what is the best way forward
4. Acting together	Not only do different interests decide together what is best, they also form a partnership to carry it out
5. Supporting independent community initiatives	Others are helped to do what they want (perhaps within a framework of grants advice and support provided by the resource holder)

Source: adapted from Wilcox, 1994, p. 4. Licensed under CC BY-ND-NC 1.0.

Note: Levels 3–5 involve substantial participation.

Thus, for Montero, participation is a dynamic system wherein individuals or groups can move in and out. Part of the task of trying to gain participation is to enable movement from the outer to the inner levels, and a further task is to support those at the inner levels so that they are able to retain their levels of commitment.

Wilcox (1994) builds on Arnstein's (1969) 'ladder of participation' to suggest a more static five levels, or stances towards participation, which offer increasing degrees of control to those involved. Table 5.2 summarises the five levels. It is the levels of 'deciding' and 'acting together' and 'supporting community initiatives' that are most likely to lead to transformative change.

Act!

Using a variety of methods (e.g. the web, newspapers, television or word-of-mouth) identify a number of social action or social justice groups. Using Table 5.2 decide what their key features are and what level of participation they involve.

We have combined these approaches and think of participatory work along two dimensions of participation (proactive and passive) and commitment (high to low) (Kagan, 2006a).

We can then map different activities and degrees of involvement along these dimensions, as in Figure 5.4. We can position the types of participation required by policy (similar to Wilcox's levels) as well as participation roles in practice (similar to Montero's positions) in the participation space.

Community activists, who identify their own needs and set their own agendas, would typically find that their own strategies for achieving change are in the proactive participation, high commitment quadrant. Community members and representatives who work in partnership with agencies on policy agendas can also be situated in this quadrant, whereas those self-appointed community representatives who get co-opted into activities with agendas set by professionals could be situated in the proactive participation, low commitment quadrant. Professionals who are committed to working on community issues but who work weekdays only and go home at night can also be placed in this quadrant. This mapping of participation and commitment can be useful for exploring movement over time, and for

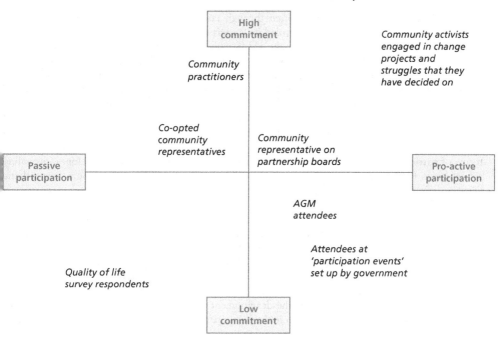

Figure 5.4 Mapping participation in terms of pro-activity and commitment.

identifying those most at need of support for their activities, lest they risk stress, disaffection or burnout – those in the top right, high commitment, proactive participation quadrant.

One of the difficulties inherent in the term 'participation' is that the term is contested and used in different ways by different people. Brodie, Cowling and Nissen (2009) distinguish between public, social and individual participation. Public participation is *"the engagement of individuals with the various structures and institutions of democracy"*. Sometimes this is referred to as political or civic participation or participatory governance. Examples of public participation include voting; becoming an elected politician or joining a political party; becoming involved in the governance of a school, hospital or other public institution. Social participation refers to collective activities that people might get involved in, such as residents' groups, clubs and societies, solidarity groups, local protest campaigns and so on. Individual participation refers to the choices and actions that individuals make and which are reflections of their values and concerns. They include, for example, buying fair trade goods, volunteering time to a local good cause, donating money to charities, writing letters in response to a campaign and so on. Clearly the modes of participation overlap. Community psychology might be concerned with them all, though perhaps is more focused on social and public participation.

Ife (1995) identifies a number of conditions under which people are most likely to participate and these can help to assess the likelihood of genuine participation being achieved.

1 People will participate if they feel the issue or activity is important. Clearly, this is more likely if people themselves have been involved in identifying the issue and had a say in any action to be taken, from the outset. It will be more difficult to encourage participation in relation to an issue that others have defined as important, and more difficult still if people have been given an

opportunity to express their views – often through consultation processes, rather than genuine participative processes – only to be overruled by 'experts'.

2   People must feel that their action will make a difference. If there seems to be little opportunity of success it will be difficult to encourage people to participate. This is linked to the ways in which people have been involved in deciding on action to be taken, but also to the degree to which they can see that they or people close to them will benefit. In this case, there may be a role to be played in helping translate a general community benefit into tangible benefits for individuals or groups.

3   Different forms of participation must be acknowledged. Formal participation, in committees and formally constituted groups, is only one kind of participation. It is important that people's different skills, talents, interests, available time and energy are taken into account and more informal forms of participation recognised. This might include posting leaflets, stuffing envelopes, providing refreshments for events or meetings, art work, childminding, helping with transport, sympathetic listening, contributing to discussions, keeping notes of events and so on.

4   People must be enabled to participate and be supported in their participation. This means that help with care (of children, elders etc.), transport, availability of translation and interpretation as necessary, the timing and location of events, the involvement of gatekeepers and community leaders, or advocates as necessary will all need to be taken into account to enable participation.

5   Structures and processes must not be alienating. Participation that relies on writing, confidence in speaking in a group, involvement in formal meetings, the articulation of complex experiences and ideas, and so on may be alienating to those not used to such activities. On the other hand, participation that is linked to an activity or the development of more naturally occurring relationships might be more enabling. It is possible to make participation fun and stimulating so that the activities themselves can be positive experiences.

Example: Gardening as a tool for participation

A community group was concerned with the appearance of the local environment. There was little interest from local people in doing anything about it. A small group of activists began clearing and planting up some of the flower beds around the residences. Gradually more residents got involved as they saw the results of the work and how the environment around people's homes improved. Children with reputations for troublesome behaviour locally also showed interest and were given tasks to do. Other residents began to offer refreshments to the 'gardeners', including the children with whom they had recently been in some conflict. When the group entered and won awards in a local competition, still more people got involved and the project extended beyond gardening to other physical improvements of the locality. After two years the most active people had not participated at the start and the original activists were able to withdraw.

As participation is a relational and dynamic process, it is particularly important that we engage in constant processes of reflection to ensure we are inclusive, enabling and supportive, and can recognise signs of exhaustion and fatigue, due to the emotional toll that participating in community action can take (Kagan 2006a, 2006b). Boundary critique (see Chapter 7) can help us reflect upon whether there are some people whose participation is essential, without whom the problem will be defined in a restrictive way and the action implemented will be inappropriate.

Working participatively does not mean that we ask people what they want and how in an uncritical way, and then go and make this happen. Instead, it is a process wherein expert (community psychological) knowledge is combined with lay knowledge through processes of collaborative working (Kagan, Duggan, Richards & Siddiquee, 2011). Through this process,

> ...two forms of knowledge merge: the 'ordinary' or common knowledge, transmitted through traditions and everyday life contributed by community members; and the scientific knowledge of the community psychologists, derived from their learning and experience.

Montero (1998) argues that this process of sharing different forms of expertise is guided by the principles of reality (how circumstances are perceived and experienced) and possibilities (assessment of what kinds of changes are needed and goals to be sought). Both are necessary.

> 'Reality' without 'possibilities' leads to helplessness and passivity. 'Possibilities' without 'reality' lead to confusion and loss of perspective, therefore inducing failure and helplessness.
>
> (Montero, 1998, p. 66)

Thus, participation is more a process of facilitating discussion, exploring differences and reaching agreement amongst people affected by an issue, where people hold different world views, attitudes and beliefs about the issue, themselves in relation to it, and possibilities for change.

However, there are dangers in focusing on participation in this way which are connected to our critique of community. The danger is if community psychologists carry with them the idea that community is largely a positive, safe place where people are bonded together by a sense of affection and functional interdependence, they may either be shocked or be unable to understand those communities (and there are many of them) that do not function in this way.

As critical community psychologists we need to take care we do not inadvertently use processes of participation to promote the illusion of choice and voice for those whose social reality is that they have neither, whilst remembering that participation can still serve as route to empowerment (Zambrano, 2007).

In this chapter we looked critically at the nature of social ties and how the different ways of thinking about connections between people are used to prescribe community in a variety of ways. We examined the ways in which communities are boundaried, in particular in relation to ghettoisation, and the links between community and social policy. Lastly we looked positively and critically at the notion of participation and its role in critical community psychology.

The importance of maintaining a critical perspective on both the concept of community and the concept of participation is part of the process of challenging oppression and marginalisation and we need to maintain this perspective as we move into Part 2 of the book, Act!

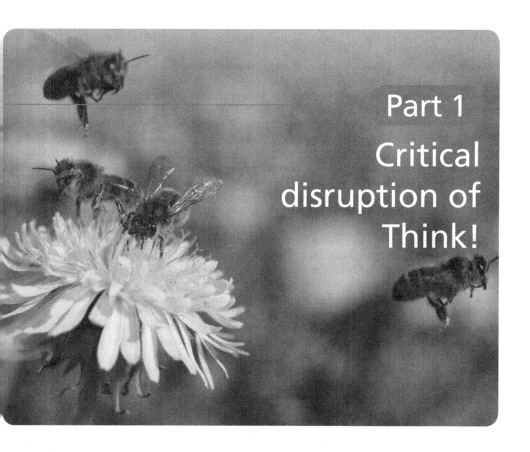

Part 1
Critical disruption of Think!

In this first critical disruption chapter we seek to problematise some of the material in Part 1 so as to illustrate how theory (thinking) can lead us into problems if our thoughts are not accompanied by action and reflection. That is not to say that the materials in Part 1 are based solely on theory (much of what we have written is grounded in action and reflection), but that action and reflection are not so much discussed here as in Parts 2 and 3.

In Part 1 we have discussed the importance of systems thinking for critical community psychology and how psychology should be considered a 'systems discipline' and have at its focus the social systems (family, peer group, community, economy, state and so on) that shape and are shaped by human behaviour. The question this begs is: 'to what extent have we acknowledged the social systems that have shaped the content of our book?' Such a question allows us to critically disrupt the explicit and implicit historical accounts we provide in Part 1 (both the construction of the history of community psychology and historical accounts of the theories and applications of 'community') and the critique of individualism embedded throughout Part 1. We hope to show how our thoughts might result in unintended action and how our arguments take on a different appearance once situated into their cultural and political context. We first consider how our thoughts on individualism might be disrupted by reflecting on where such thoughts come from. We then consider how our history of community psychology might be used (that is, put into action) in ways we do not intend.

Critically disrupting the challenge to individualism

Our critique of mainstream psychology is that it is individualistic at its heart because it purports to study individuals decontextualised from their historical, social, political, economic and cultural surroundings. In this, we share our perspective with other critical thinkers (who are cited throughout our book). Our challenge to individualism is not just about method or about theory, but is also an ideologically based challenge to the dominant cultural norms carried by the most economically and politically powerful social institutions (such as corporations and government bodies). However, such challenges against the ideology of individualism largely come from academics located in the university systems of the core capitalist countries, who are relatively well funded and have privileged access to publish their work in the dominant journals in the field.

This is a problem because one of the main concerns about the dominance of individualism in psychology (and more broadly in the social sciences) highlighted by such critical thinkers is that individualism promotes the belief that you can separate the observer from the observed (that is, the belief that psychologists can objectively rather than subjectively study individuals and that such observations can be held as 'facts' that exist independent of the social conditions under which the 'facts' were gathered). This results in the work of psychologists being stripped of its cultural and political heritage and obscures the way that the gender, class, race, disability status and so on of those who practise psychology impacts upon their work. But, in rejecting this doctrine of neutral observers, critical thinkers become subject to their own critique – we need to consider how their criticism of individualism is shaped by the individualistic culture in which they operate. Thus, we cannot hold up our own criticism of psychology without subjecting ourselves to our own critique. The critique we need to consider is whether our thoughts on individualism are themselves individualistic (given we are located in an individualistic culture) and to more broadly consider the impact of individualism on our own work.

It has been argued that a discussion of individualism can only be entertained under an individualistic framework – that the dichotomy between individualism and collectivism (which we allude to often in our book) is an individualistic construct (Sampson, 2000). A collectivist perspective would view both the individual and the collective as part of an indivisible whole and would thus view individualism and collectivism as not separate processes, but part of one process with neither the individual nor the collective having the possibility of dominating over or having conflict with the other. Thus, under a collectivist framework the notion of individualism as an alternative to collectivism is based on a false dichotomy – in essence, it cannot exist. We deal with this issue in Chapter 3 (see the treatment of Bhaskar's approach which argues for a transformational approach to the individual–society question), but it is for the reader to judge how successful this is.

The second problem is that the case against individualism is likely to have become somewhat exaggerated. We believe it to be true that the doctrine of individualism has been adopted wholesale by the dominant political and economic social institutions in the West. For example:

● Government: the marginalisation of socialism and promotion of active citizenship (whereby responsibilities for promoting well-being are shifted from the state and onto the individual); personal freedom is given precedence and public spaces and public services are increasingly privatised.
● Economic institutions: the adoption of a model of human behaviour that views consumers as autonomous actors who are motivated by self-interest.
● Mass media: the cult of the celebrity where individual life stories dominate and personality supplants politics.
● Science: the dominance of positivism which has promoted the view of the scientist as independent, objective observer detached from culture and politics and from the observed, mimicking the way self is conceptually separated from society.

Yet none of this means that individualism is the only cultural *value* in the West. As Billig (2008) points out, the modern era was never fully individualistic and this remains so. Outside of dominant political and economic systems and of the epistemological paradigms deployed by scientists, collectivism thrives – people are still willing to pay taxes that fund health services and education and to engage in mass participation (such as through mass boycotts, petitions and protests). The collective continually confounds the individualistic culture that capitalism was supposed to have spawned.

So, despite the relative dominance of individualism as normative model and theory of society, we are able to find ways to disengage from the imposed cultural norms. Indeed, our focus on the dominance of individualism might say more about how we, the authors of this book, are particularly dominated by powerful institutions. This might be because we work closely with (or at least in similar social circles to) people in positions of power who can influence us, we have money and reputations that can be lost if we upset those in power, and we read lots so we are at risk of soaking up the propaganda produced by the system.

> Propaganda very often works better for the educated than it does for the uneducated. This is true on many issues. There are a lot of reasons for this, one being that the educated receive more of the propaganda because they read more. Another thing is that they are the agents of propaganda. After all, ... they're supposed to be the agents of the propaganda system so they believe it. It's very hard to say something unless you believe it. Other reasons are that, by and large, they are just part of the privileged elite so they share their interests and perceptions, whereas the general population is more marginalized. It, by and large, doesn't participate in the democratic system, which is overwhelmingly an elite game.
>
> (Chomsky, 1992, p. 119)

So, it might be the case that those who are working in those social institutions (such as ourselves as academics working in the scientific community) might find disengagement from an individualistic culture harder as recipients of the most intense individualistic propaganda – we matter more to the people in power as we write, we teach and are in positions of influence.

Critically disrupting our history of community psychology

The way we have laid out our account of individualism might function rhetorically, using hyperbole to strengthen our argument or at least to make our arguments clearer. So too our construction of a history of community psychology and a history of the contested nature of community needs to be reflected upon. Our histories, and those we have inherited from others, might say as much about what we would like the history to be rather than describe what the history is (if the latter is ever possible).

It has been said that history is written by the victor (an aphorism sometimes attributed to Churchill who did write such history). We might extend that to saying that history is written by the powerful – those who have the cultural, economic, political and social resources to ensure their version of history sticks. Historical accounts are always subject to disagreements; for example, feminists have renamed history as herstory when analysing the past with a gendered lens. This is because history is as much about the discarding of information as it is about archiving information – separating out the trivial events (such as what you ate for breakfast) from the important events (such as decisions made by Parliament). But decisions over what is and is not important are based on the presumptions and preferences of particular interest groups and on their particular tastes, values, politics, belief systems and so on. So, history can become a series of distortions bent towards the interest of particular social groups and by the features of the archiving processes). At worst, historical events might be based on fabrications of or denial of events for the purpose of propaganda.

Many of the struggles of the powerless against the powerful, which we describe in this book, are not only for an adequate share of resources, but also to ensure recorded history does justice to their stories. Kundera summed this up in the following quote that has become a clarion call for the poor and dispossessed around the world:

> The struggle of man against power is the struggle of man against forgetting.
>
> (Kundera, 1978, p. 3)

The version of history that wins is likely to be the one that portrays those who have the greatest power in the most benign light. So, the history of the Second World War portrays the Germans and Japanese as war criminals (the Holocaust, the torture and summary execution of prisoners and so on), while the British, US and Soviet armies have their actions extolled as virtuous. Thus, the bombing of Dresden has not been recorded in history as a war crime, nor was dropping the atomic bomb on Hiroshima and then on Nagasaki three days later, nor the collateral damage – for example the Bengal famine. Churchill himself, rather than being cast as a racist, drunken war criminal has been cast as a hero (even though there is as much evidence to support the former as a more accurate characterisation). Churchill's involvement in war crimes is largely written out of the history books and only exists in radical texts that sit at the edge of mainstream consciousness.

This critical reading of history recalls Foucault's work that connects power and knowledge (see Chapter 11), that is, it is always possible to take apart an intellectual system and trace its component parts to the interests of certain social groups (Parker, 1999). The feminist community psychology approach emphasises the following characteristics:

> A willingness to make explicit the implicit assumptions embedded in our most sacred and taken for granted concepts; an acceptance that all knowledge is socially produced and therefore can never be value free; interests, however implicit, are always being served; an awareness that there is an inescapable relationship between knowledge and power.
>
> (Cosgrove & McHugh, 2000, p. 817)

So, what is important is not what is said, but *who* says *what* about *whom*. Applying this reflection we can consider how our history of community psychology might be enacted in a way that serves particular interest groups. In turning to the histories of community psychology that have been written, the one history that is most dominant is that of the Swampscott conference (see Chapter 2). This became the globally dominant account of where community psychology came from; it has become dominant as Swampscott is regularly cited as the birthplace for community psychology and manifestations of community psychology outside of the USA are largely described as developing after Swampscott (see Fryer, 2008). Whose interests does this serve? Well, to be cited as a founder of community psychology can accrue for you and those associated with you (your colleagues, your institution, your publisher, your students and so on) considerable social prestige within the field of community psychology. Indeed, in the USA there are regular events and projects that celebrate the achievements of the great, founding fathers (they were all men) of community psychology who were present at Swampscott (a history not a herstory). Given the dominance of the USA in the world, due to the power and reach of its publishing industry and the relatively resource rich status of its academic institutions, it might be difficult to unseat the way Swampscott has been written into the history of community psychology.

Finally, is there a problem in the histories we have constructed or reconstructed because we might have constructed our history of community in a way distorted by the encroachment of an individualistic perspective? For one, as academics we are locked into a convention of academic practice where ideas are believed to belong to individuals who need to be cited and referenced. Indeed, not to do so is viewed as at best either academic sloppiness or at worst plagiarism. That is why throughout this book you will see this practice observed (our text would not be published otherwise). For an interesting cultural and political critique of plagiarism see Martin (1994). This can lead to history being structured around individual biographies (individual academics or small groups of academics) and about singular events (an individualised history). As Eskin (1999 cited in Sampson, 2000) put it, we write our own autobiographies as though they are about a person who is in full command of his or her own person, thereby deleting the cast of hundreds (perhaps thousands) who make our own life stories what they are. This is notable in how we recognise scholarship with individual degrees predicated on the concept of the autonomous worker. Recent doctoral candidates of Maori origin in Aotearoa/New Zealand have articulated the need to author their work in a culturally appropriate way, invoking a historical family tree indicating where one comes from and multiple authors. Universities are struggling with this notion as individual ownership of intellectual property is a fundamental plank of scholarship.

Think!

Only five names appear in the authorship of our book. Can you think of any feasible way in which we could have given recognition to the wider network of those who have contributed to its genesis and production?

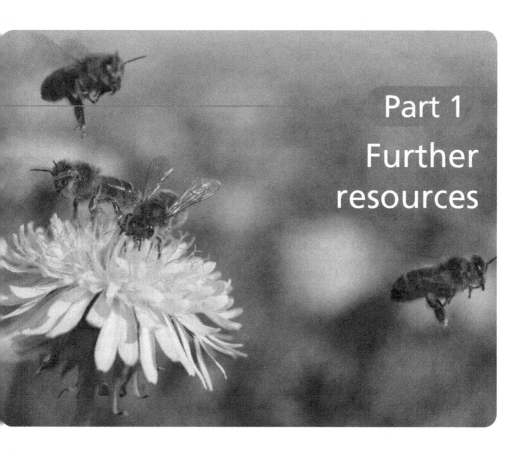

Here is a collection of some resources with a short description to assist in your reading of Part 1 (Chapters 1, 2, 3, 4 and 5).

Films

- Works by documentary maker Adam Curtis: http://watchdocumentaries.com/tag/adam-curtis/
- *Peterloo* (2018). Directed by Mike Leigh: a film about everyday people caught up in the 1819 Peterloo Massacre, Manchester. Good for some of the speeches on why political representation matters and for thinking about the similarities with contemporary pro-democracy protests. www.peterloofilm.co.uk/
- *Embrace of the Serpent* (2016). Directed by Ciro Guerra. This is a highly acclaimed film that tells the story of the invasion of a sacred site in the Amazon jungle from an indigenous perspective. Prepare to be mesmerised.
- *Raining Stones* (1993). Directed by Ken Loach. This is a film set on the outskirts of Manchester (in an area where we have worked with residents) during the 1990s. It tells the story of a family's experience of poverty. Dealing with life on the margins, it shows how unemployment and money impact upon the whole family.

Watch these two films together:

- *Crude* (2009). Directed by Joe Berlinger, this is a documentary on the class action suit against Chevron/Texaco by indigenous people in the Amazon region of Ecuador. The film is available at a number of sources on the internet – try searching for 'Crude', and 'film' or 'movie'.
- *Erin Brockovich* (2000). Directed by Steven Soderbergh, this film is based on the real-life story of a woman's legal battle against a California power company accused of polluting a city's water supply.
- *The Boy in the Striped Pyjamas* (2008). Directed by Mark Herman. This film focuses on issues around the treatment of Jewish people in Nazi Germany by telling the story of a friendship between a Jewish boy in a concentration camp and a German boy who is the son of the camp's commandant.
- *The Children of Gaza* (UK Channel 4 documentary) by documentary filmmaker Jezza Neumann. This documentary looks at the lives of children in Gaza who live under the occupation of the Israeli government.
- *The BlacKkKlansman* (2018). Directed by Spike Lee, this is both funny and a thought-provoking and provocative examination of racism in the USA. It is based on a true story of a black police officer in the 1970s who infiltrated the Ku Klux Klan. The film concludes with footage from the 2017 'Unite the Right' rally in Charlottesville which powerfully connects the racism of the past to the racism of the present.
- *Wall Street* (1987). Directed by Oliver Stone. A young and impatient stockbroker is willing to do anything to get to the top, including trading on illegal inside information taken through a ruthless and greedy corporate raider who takes the youth under his wing. The 'Greed is Good' speech in the movie came to symbolise the excesses of neoliberal economic politics.
- *The Big Short* (2015). Directed by Adam McKay. The story of the events behind the Global Financial Crisis. It tells the story of four financial outsiders who saw the corruption of the financial dealings of banks in the USA and how they saw it as an opportunity to make some money out of the impending global collapse. The story is both funny and shocking.
- *Jellyfish* (2018). Directed by James Gardener. With a life under duress as a teenager responsible for siblings and a mother with mental health difficulties, stand up comedy is the road to survival.

Theatre

- *Les Miserables*. If you can, go and see the musical theatre production of *Les Miserables* (or get hold of a DVD – or even read the book!). What does this tell us about power and powerlessness the ways in which marginalisation and misery can be turned into commodities for commercial organisations to gain profits?

Books

- Davies, N. (1998). *Dark Heart: The Shocking Truth about Modern Britain*. London: Vintage. Nick Davies' *Dark Heart* is a wonderful book that shows how appalling life for the poor in the UK is.
- Fanon, F. (1967). *Black Skins, White Masks*. New York: Grove. Classic text on the damage of coloniality.
- Hanley, L. (2017). *Estates: An Intimate History*. London: Granta Books. This is an account of what it is like growing up and living on a social housing estate near Birmingham, UK. Read it and you can really feel what it must have been like. How might you design an area of social housing?
- Klein, N. (2015). *This Changes Everything*. London: Penguin Books/Simon Schuster. Klein argues that the climate catastrophe facing us cannot be dealt with by the neoliberal, high consumption patterns of living in the rich world. Essential reading about climate change.

There is a documentary directed by Avi Lewis of the issues raised in the book at https://this changeseverything.org/the-documentary/

- Mckenzie, L. (2015). *Getting By: Estates, Class and Culture in Austerity Britain*. Bristol: Policy Press. A good ethnographic account of how women and men live poverty differently in austerity Britain.
- Wainwright, H. (2009). *Reclaim the State: Experiments in Popular Democracy*. London: Seagull Books. This book gives example of popular participation that has contributed to transformational change in different ways in different parts of the world. Well worth a look!

Other relevant resources

- *Wars With and Without Bullets*: a *Special Issue* of *The Journal of Critical Psychology, Counselling and Psychotherapy* (March 2019). *The Journal of Critical Psychology, Counselling and Psychotherapy* 19(1), 1–85. All the contributions are written from an anti-capitalist standpoint and contributions include those from community, disability and human rights activists.
- See what you can find out about the philanthropic work of Bill and Melinda Gates' use of profits from the Microsoft industry. What does this tell you about participation, people's voice and autonomy? The Bill and Melinda Gates Foundation is at www.gatesfoundation.org
- How do you think the approaches promoted by the World Bank contribute to transformational change (or not)? Look at the website of the World Bank Academy which houses online courses at https://olc.worldbank.org/wbg-academy. You might also like to look at some of their documents, such as the *World Bank Participation Sourcebook*, http://documents.worldbank.org/curated/ en/289471468741587739/The-World-Bank-participation-sourcebook. As you look at these resources ask yourself "*what is the wider agenda here?*"
- If you want to check information about a think tank or similar organisation try Source Watch at www.sourcewatch.org/. Look at their critical reviews of the Bill and Melinda Gates Foundation and the World Bank Institute. What does this add? You might also find the Corporate Watch site interesting: https://corporatewatch.org/
- Look at the Climate Psychology Alliance (CPA). Central to the vision behind CPA is that they are seeking to place human science alongside natural science in the cause of ecologically informed living, through understanding and facing difficult truths. Members set out to understand the unconscious feelings and attitudes preventing human action on climate change. Try exploring the site and discuss the extent to which the approach taken by the Climate Psychology Alliance is, or is not, community psychological. What makes it so? www.climatepsychologyalliance.org
- See what you can find out about the Zapatista revolution by looking at some of the websites listed below. Ask yourself "*why is the Zapatista revolution of relevance to critical community psychology?*" See http://la.utexas.edu/users/hcleaver/Chiapas95/zapsincyberwebsites.html

Relevant networks/online groups

- http://communitypsychologyuk.ning.com/
- www.bps.org.uk/member-microsites/community-psychology-section
- www.compsy.org.uk/
- www.jiscmail.ac.uk/cgi-bin/webadmin?A0=COMMUNITYPSYCHUK
- http://libpsy.org
- www.ecpa-online.com
- http://list.waikato.ac.nz/mailman/listinfo/compsychwaikato
- www.scra27.org
- https://psysr.net/

References

All links checked and working on 22 March 2019.

Agger, I., & Buus Jensen, S. (1996). *Trauma and healing under state terrorism*. London England: Zed.

Ahmed Iqbal Ullah Race Relations Resource Centre. (2013). *Wangari Maathai & th green belt movement*. Available at https://prezi.com/ilx0yojudfjb/wangari-maathai-the green-belt-movement/.

Akhurst, J., Kagan, C., Lawthom, R., & Richards, M. (2016). Community psychology practic competencies: Some perspectives from the UK. *Global Journal of Community Psycholog Practice, 7*(4), 1–15, online.

Aldrich, C. (2005). *Learning by doing: A comprehensive guide to simulations, computer games and pedagogy in e-learning and other educational experiences*. Chichester, England: Wiley

Alinsky, S. (1971). *Rules for radicals: A pragmatic primer for realistic radicals*. New York, NY Vintage.

American Evaluation Association (AEA). (2018). *Guiding principles for evaluators (updated)* Fairhaven, MA: American Evaluation Association. Available at www.eval.org/p/cm/ld fid=51.

American Evaluation Association (AEA). (2011). *Statement on cultural competence in eval uation*. Fairhaven, MA: American Evaluation Association. Available at www.eval.org ccstatement.

Angelique, H., & Culley, M. (2007). History and theory of community psychology: An inter national perspective of community psychology in the United States. In S. Reich, M. Rieme I. Prilleltensky & M. Montero (Eds.), *International community psychology: History an theories*. New York, NY: Springer.

Archibald, T. (2019). What's the problem represented to be? Problem definition critique as tool for evaluative thinking. *American Journal of Evaluation*. doi:109821401882404.

Arcidiacono, C., Tuozzi, T., & Procentese, F. (2016). Community profiling in participator action research. In L.A. Jason & D.S. Glenwick (Eds.), *Handbook of methodologica approaches to community-based research: Qualitative, quantitative and mixed methods* New York, NY: Oxford University Press.

Argyle, M., Furnham, A., & Graham, J.A. (1981). *Social situations*. Cambridge, England Cambridge University Press.

Argyris, C., & Schön, D. (1996). *Organizational learning II: Theory, method and practice* Reading, MA: Addison Wesley.

Argyris, C., & Schön, D. (1978). *Organizational learning: A theory of action perspective* Reading, MA: Addison-Wesley.

Armistead, N. (ed.) (1974). *Reconstructing social psychology*. Harmondsworth, England Penguin.

Arnstein, S.R. (1969). A ladder of participation. *Journal of the American Planning Association 35*(4), 216–224.

Audit Commission (1998). *A fruitful partnership. Effective partnership working*. Managemen Paper. London, England: Audit Commission.

Austin, A. (2018). *Social exclusion: Black people have everything to lose under Trump*. Avail able at www.demos.org/publication/social-exclusion-black-people-have-everything-lose under-trump.

Australian Bureau of Statistics (2018). Press release issued on 29th November 2018 cat. nc 3302.0.55.003: Life tables for Aboriginal and Torres Strait Islander Australians, 2015–2017

Canberra, Australia: Australian Bureau of Statistics. Available at www.abs.gov.au/ausstats/abs@.nsf/Lookup/by%20Subject/3302.0.55.003~2015-2017~Media%20Release~Life%20expectancy%20lowest%20in%20remote%20and%20very%20remote%20areas%20(Media%20Release)~15.

Baachi, C. (2012). Introducing the 'what's the problem represented to be?' approach. In A. Bletsas & C. Beasley (Eds.), *Engaging with Carol Bacchi: Strategic interventions & exchanges* (pp. 21–24). Adelaide, Australia: University of Adelaide Press.

Bagni, F., Bojic, I., Duarte, T., Preis Dutra, J., Gaule, S., van Heerden, A., . . . Psaltoglou, A. (2017). Design principles for co-creating inclusive and digitally mediated public spaces. In C. Smaniotto Costa & K. Ionnidis (Eds.), *The making of the public space: Essays on emerging urban phenomena. Culture & territory.* (pp. 25–40). Lisbon, Portugal: Edições Universitárias Lusófona.

Balloch, S., & Taylor, M. (2001). *Partnership working: Policy and practice.* Bristol, England: Policy Press.

Banister, P., Burman, E., Parker, I., Taylor, M., & Tindall, C. (1997). *Qualitative methods in psychology: A research guide.* Buckingham, England: Open University Press.

Barker, R.G. (1968). *Ecological psychology: Concepts and methods for studying the environment of human behavior.* Stanford, CA: Stanford University Press.

Barreto, A.P. (2011). *Terapia comunitária passo a passo.* Fortaleza, Brazil: Grática LCR.

Bauman, Z. (2007a). *Liquid times: Living in an age of uncertainty.* Cambridge, England: Polity Press.

Bauman, Z. (2007b). *Consuming life.* Cambridge, England: Polity Press.

Bauman, Z. (2005). *Liquid life.* London, England: Wiley.

Bauman, Z. (2001). *Community. Seeking safety in an insecure world.* Cambridge, England: Polity Press.

Bauman, Z. (2000). *Liquid modernity.* Cambridge, England: Polity Press.

Bauman, Z. (1996). *Alone again – Ethics after certainty.* London, England: Demos.

Bauman, Z. (1989). *Modernity and the Holocaust.* New York, NY: Cornell University Press.

Beebeejaun, Y., Durose, C., Rees, J., Richardson, J., & Richardson, L. (2014). 'Beyond text': Exploring ethos and method in co-producing research with communities. *Community Development Journal, 49*(1), 37–53.

Beetham, D., Blick, A., Margetts, H., & Weir, S. (2008). *Power and participation in modern Britain: A literature review for Democratic Audit.* Wembley, England: Creative Print Group.

Bell, B. (2014). *The global disability rights movement: Winning power, participation and access.* Available at www.huffingtonpost.com/beverly-bell/the-global-disability-rig_b_5651235.html?guccounter=1.

Bell, D.M. (2016). A raison d'être for making a reggae opera as a pedagogical tool for psychic emancipation in (post)colonial Jamaica. *International Journal of Inclusive Education, 20*(3), 278–291.

Bellamy Foster, J. (2009). *The ecological revolution: Making peace with the planet.* New York, NY: Monthly Review Press.

Bender, M.P. (1976). *Community psychology.* London, England: Methuen.

Benner, P., Hooper-Kyriakidis, P., & Stannard, D. (1999). *Clinical wisdom and interventions in critical care.* Philadelphia, PA: W.B. Saunders.

Bennett, K., Beynon, H., & Hudson, R. (2000). *Coalfields regeneration: Dealing with the consequences of industrial decline.* Bristol, England: Policy Press and the Joseph Rowntree Foundation.

Benneworth, P. (2013). University engagement with socially excluded communities: Toward the idea of the 'engaged university.' In P. Benneworth (Ed.), *University engagement with socially excluded communities* (pp. 3–32). New York, NY: Springer.

Bhambra, G.K., & Holmwood, J. (2018). Colonialism, postcolonialism and the liberal welfare state. *New Political Economy, 23*(5), 574–587.

Bhana, A., Petersen, I., & Rochat, T. (2008). Community psychology in South Africa. In S. Reich, M. Riemer, I. Prilleltensky & M. Montero (Eds.), *International community psychology: History and theories.* New York, NY: Springer.

Bhaskar, R. (1998). *The possibility of naturalism: A philosophical critique of the contemporary human sciences* (3rd ed.). London, England: Routledge.

Bhaskar, R. (1979). On the possibility of social scientific knowledge and the limits of naturalism. In J. Mepham & D.H. Ruben (Eds.), *Issues in Marxist philosophy: Epistemology, science, ideology* (Vol. 3) (pp. 107–139). Brighton, England: Harvester.

Bhatia, S., & Sethi, N. (2007). History and theory of community psychology in India: A international perspective. In S.M. Reich, M. Riemer, I. Prilleltensky & M. Montero (Eds.), *International community psychology* (pp. 180–199). Boston, MA: Springer. https://doi.org/10.1007/978-0-387-49500-2_9.

Billig, M. (2008). *The hidden roots of critical psychology.* London, England: Sage.

Bishop, A. (2002). *Becoming an ally: Breaking the cycle of oppression in people* (2nd ed.). Nova Scotia, Canada: Fernwood Publishing.

Bishop, B.J., Dzidic, P.L., & Breen, L.J. (2013). Multiple-level analysis as a tool for policy: A example of the use of contextualism and causal layered analysis. *Global Journal of Community Psychology Practice, 4*(2), 1–13.

Blake, R., & Mouton, J. (1961). *The managerial grid.* Houston, TX: Houston Gulf.

Blanchard, A. (2006). Virtual behavior settings: An application of behavior setting theories to virtual communities. *Journal of Computer-Mediated Communication, 9*(2), online.

Blanden, J., Gregg, P., & Machin, S. (2005). *Intergenerational mobility in Europe and North America.* London, England: Centre for Economic Performance, London School of Economics and Political Science.

Blickstead, J.R., Lester, E., & Shapcott, M. (2008). *Collaboration in the third sector: From co-opetition to impact driven cooperation.* Toronto, Canada: Wellesley Institute. Available at www.wellesleyinstitute.com/wp-content/uploads/2011/11/collaborationinthethirdsector.pdf.

Boal, A. (1995). *The rainbow of desire: The Boal method of theatre and therapy* (Adrian Jackson, Trans.). London, England: Routledge.

Boggs, C. (2001). Social capital and political fantasy: Robert Putnam's 'Bowling alone'. *Theory and Society, 30*(2), 281–297.

Bond, M.A., & Mulvey, A. (2000). A history of women and feminist perspectives in community psychology. *American Journal of Community Psychology, 28*(5), 599–630. doi:10.1023/A:1005141619462.

Boudon, R. (1986). *Theories of social change: A critical analysis.* London, England: Polity Press.

Bourdieu, P. (1986). The forms of social capital. In J. Richardson (Ed.) *Handbook of theory and research for the sociology of education* (pp. 241–258). New York, NY: Greenwood.

Boyd, A., Geerling, T., Gregory, W.J., Kagan, C., Midgley, G., Murray, P., & Walsh, M.P. (2007). Systemic evaluation: A participatory, multi method approach. *Journal of the Operational Research Society, 58*(10), 1306–1320.

Boyd, A., Geerling, T., Gregory, W.J., Kagan, C., Midgley, G., Murray, P., & Walsh, M.P. (2003). Participative learning for evaluation: A systems approach to the development of evaluatio capability in community health projects. In A. Erasmus & P. du Toit (Eds.), *Proceedings of Action Learning, Action Research and Process Management/Participatory Action Research (ALARPM/PAR) Conference, Pretoria*. Available at https://e-space.mmu.ac.uk/25916/.

Boyd, A., Geerling, T., Gregory, W., Midgley, G. Murray, P., Walsh, M., & Kagan, C. (2001). *Capacity building for evaluation: Report to the Manchester, Salford and Trafford Health Action Zone*. Hull, England: University of Hull.

Boyd, N.M., & Bright, D.S. (2007). Appreciative inquiry as a mode of action research for community psychology. *Journal of Community Psychology, 35*(8), 1019–1036. doi:10.1002/jcop.20208.

Boyle, D., & Harris, M. (2009). *The challenge of co-production. How equal partnerships between professionals and the public are crucial to improving public services*. London, England: NESTA. Available at https://media.nesta.org.uk/documents/the_challenge_of_co-production.pdf.

Bradshaw, J.R. (2015/1972). The taxonomy of social need. In R. Cookson, R. Sainsbury & C. Glendinning (Eds.), *Jonathan Bradshaw on social policy: Selected writings 1972–2011* (pp. 1–12). York, England: University of York/White Rose Research Online. Available at http://eprints.whiterose.ac.uk/112541/.

Brandenburger, A., Nalebuff, B. (1996). *Co-opetition: A revolution mindset that combines competition and cooperation*. New York, NY: Currency Doubleday.

Brandes, D., & Norris, J. (1998). *The gamesters' handbook 3*. London, England: Nelson Thornes.

Brandon, D., Brandon, A., & Brandon, T. (1995). *Advocacy: Power to people with disabilities*. Birmingham, England: Venture Press.

Branic, N. & Kubrin, C. (2018). Gated communities and crime in the United States. In G. Bruinsma & S. Johnson (Eds.), *The Oxford handbook of environmental criminology* (pp. 405–427). Oxford, England: Oxford University Press.

Bridger, A.J., Emmanouil, S., & Lawthom, R. (2017). Trace.space: a psychogeographical community project with members of an arts and health organisation. *Qualitative Research in Psychology, 14*(1), 42–61.

British Psychological Society. (2018). *Code of Ethics and Conduct*. Leicester, England: British Psychological Society. Available at www.bps.org.uk/news-and-policy/bps-code-ethics-and-conduct.

Brodie, E., Cowling, E., & Nissen, N. (2009). *Understanding participation: A literature review*. London, England: NCVO. Available at www.bl.uk/collection-items/understanding-participation-a-literature-review.

Bronfenbrenner, U. (1994). Ecological models of human development. In *International encyclopedia of education* (Vol. 3, 2nd ed.). Oxford, England: Elsevier. Reprinted in M. Gauvain & M. Cole (Eds.), *Readings on the development of children* (2nd ed., 1996, pp. 37–43). New York, NY: Freeman. Available at http://edfa2402resources.yolasite.com/resources/Ecological%20Models%20of%20Human%20Development.pdf.

Bronfenbrenner, U. (1979). *The ecology of human development*. Cambridge, MA: Harvard University Press.

Brown, J., & Isaacs, D. (1994). The core processes of organizations as communities. In P.M. Senge, A. Kleiner, C. Roberts, R.B. Ross & B.J. Smith (Eds.), *The fifth discipline fieldbook: Strategies and tools for building a learning organization*. London, England: Nicholas Brealey Publishing.

Brown, R. (2015). The marketisation of higher education: Issues and ironies. *New Vistas, 1*(1), online.

Brown, R., & Carasso, H. (2013). *Everything for sale? The marketisation of UK higher education*. Abingdon, England: Routledge.

Bruno, I., Didier, E., & Vitale, T. (2014). Statactivism: Forms of action between disclosure and affirmation. *PArtecipazione e COnflitto – PArticipation and COnflict, 7*(2), 198–220.

Büchs, M., & Koch, M. (2017). *Postgrowth and wellbeing.* Cham, Switzerland: Springer International Publishing.

Burchardt, T., Le Grand, J., & Piachaud, D. (1999). Social exclusion in Britain 1991–1995. *Social Policy and Administration, 33*(3), 227–244.

Burns, D. (2007). *Systemic action research: A strategy for whole system change.* Bristol, England: Policy Press.

Burrell, G., & Morgan, G. (1979). *Sociological paradigms and organisational analysis.* London, England: Heinemann.

Burton, M. (2016a). *New evidence on decoupling carbon emissions from GDP growth: What does it mean?* Available at https://steadystatemanchester.net/2016/04/15/new-evidence-on-decoupling-carbon-emissions-from-gdp-growth-what-does-it-mean.

Burton, M. (2016b). *Intervening at the regional level: Building momentum for another possible regional economy: opportunities and traps.* Paper presented at the 5th International Degrowth Conference, Budapest. Available at www.academia.edu/28426063/Intervening_at_the_regional_level_Building_momentum_for_another_possible_regional_economy_opportunities_and_traps.

Burton, M. (2015). Building consensus for another possible economy at municipal level. In J. Condie & A.M. Cooper (Eds.) *Dialogues of sustainable urbanisation: Social science research and transitions to urban contexts* (Chapter 63, pp. 282–285). Penrith, Australia: University of Western Sydney. Available at www.academia.edu/attachments/38876891/download_file?st=MTQ0Nzc2Mz Q4Nyw3OC4xNDkuMjEwLjE1LDEwMzk5OTM%3D &s=swp-toolbar.

Burton, M. (2014a). *Less levity Professor Stern! Economic growth, climate change and the decoupling question.* Available at https://steadystatemanchester.net/2014/09/21/less-levity-professor-stern-economic-growth-climate-change-and-the-decoupling/question/.

Burton, M. (2014b). Social reproduction. In T. Teo (Ed.), *Encyclopedia of critical psychology* (pp. 1802–1804). New York, NY: Springer. Available at https://link.springer.com/referenceworkentry/10.1007/978-1-4614-5583-7_266.

Burton, M. (2013a). A renewal of ethics. *The Psychologist, 26*(11), 802–807. Available at https://thepsychologist.bps.org.uk/volume-26/edition-11/renewal-ethics.

Burton, M. (2013b). The analectic turn: Critical psychology and the new political context. *Les Cahiers de Psychologie Politique, 23*, online. Available at http://lodel.irevues.inist.fr/cahierspsychologie politique/index.php?id=2465.

Burton, M. (2013c). Liberation psychology: A constructive critical praxis. *Estudos de Psicologia (Campinas), 30*(2), 249–259.

Burton, M. (2013d). In and against social policy. *Global Journal of Community Psychology Practice, 4*(2). Available at www.gjcpp.org/pdfs/burton-v4i2-20130522.pdf.

Burton, M. (2009a). *A green deal for the Manchester-Mersey bioregion: An alternative regional strategy.* Manchester, England. Available at http://greendealmanchester.wordpress.com/about/.

Burton, M. (2009b). *Concepts for bioregional development.* Available at http://greendealmanchester.wordpress.com/concepts-for-bioregional-development/.

Burton, M. (2009c). *Sustainability: Utopian and scientific.* Available at https://greendealmanchester.wordpress.com/sustainability-utopian-and-scientific/.

Burton, M. (2004a). Viva nacho! Liberating psychology in Latin America. *The Psychologist, 17*(10), 584–587.

Burton, M. (2004b). Liberation social psychology: Learning from the Latin American experience. *Clinical Psychology (Clinical Psychology Forum), 38*(June 2004), 32–37.

Burton, M. (2000). Service development and social change: The role of social movements. In C. Kagan (Ed.), *Collective action and social change*. Manchester, England: IOD Research Group. Available at www.compsy.org.uk/conf11.doc.

Burton, M. (1999). *Service development and social change: The role of social movements*. Paper presented to UK National Community Psychology Conference, Manchester, January. Available at www.compsy.org.uk/Community%20Psychology%20Conference,%20Manchester,%201999.pdf.

Burton, M. (1994). Towards an alternative basis for policy and practice in community care – with special reference to people with learning disabilities. *Care in Place: International Journal of Networks and Community, 1*(2), 158–174.

Burton, M., & Kagan, C. (2009). Towards a really social psychology: Liberation psychology beyond Latin America. In M. Montero & C. Sonn (Eds.), *The psychology of liberation. Theory and application* (pp. 51–73). New York, NY: Springer.

Burton, M., & Kagan, C. (2008). *Societal case formulation*. Available at www.compsy.org.uk/Societal%20case%20formulation%20expanded%20version%202008.pdf.

Burton, M., & Kagan, C.M. (2007). Psychologists and torture: More than a question of interrogation. *The Psychologist, 20*(8), 484–487.

Burton, M., and Kagan, C. (2006). Decoding Valuing People. *Disability and Society, 21*(4), 219–313.

Burton, M., & Kagan, C. (2005). Liberation social psychology: Learning from Latin America. *Journal of Community and Applied Social Psychology, 15*(1), 63–78.

Burton, M., & Kagan, C. (2003). Community psychology: Why this gap in Britain? *History and Philosophy of Psychology, 4*(2), 10–23.

Burton, M., & Kagan, C. (2000). *Edge effects, resource utilisation and community psychology*. Paper presented at European Community Psychology Conference, Bergen, Norway. Available at www.compsy.org.uk/edge.htm.

Burton, M., & Kagan, C. (1998). Complementarism versus incommensurability in psychological research methodology. In M. Cheung-Chung (Ed.), *Current trends in history and philosophy of psychology*. Leicester, England: British Psychological Society.

Burton, M., & Kagan, C. (1996). Rethinking empowerment: Shared action against powerlessness. In I. Parker and R. Spears (Eds.), *Psychology and society: Radical theory and practice*. London, England: Pluto Press.

Burton, M., & Kagan, C. (1995). *Social skills and people with learning disabilities: A social capability approach*. London, England: Chapman and Hall.

Burton, M., & Kagan, C. (1982). Looking at environments (i). The physical and social environments of the mental health services. *Nursing Mirror*, August.

Burton, M., & Kellaway, M. (Eds.). (1998). *Developing and managing high quality services for people with learning disabilities*. Aldershot, England: Ashgate.

Burton, M., Irvine, B., & Emanuel, J. (2014). *The viable economy* (1st ed.). Manchester, England: Steady State Manchester. Available at https://steadystatemanchester.files.wordpress.com/2014/11/the-viable-economy-master-document-v4-final.pdf.

Burton, M., Kagan, C.M., & Duckett, P. (2012). *Making the psychological political: Challenges for community psychology*. Presented at the 2nd International Conference of Community Psychology 2008, Lisbon. *Global Journal of Community Psychology Practice. 3*(4), online.

Burton, M., Boyle, S., Harris, C., & Kagan, C. (2007). Community psychology in Britain. In S. Reich, M. Riemer, I. Prilleltensky & M. Montero (Eds.), *International community psychology: History and theories*. New York, NY: Springer.

Call for Real Action Collective (2009). *Call for real action: First report*. Available at http:/ calltorea-laction.wordpress.com/first-report/.

Camarotti, M.H., Siva, M.H., Medeiros, R.A., Lins, R.A., Barros, P.M., Camorotti, J., & Rodgruigues, A. (2004). Terapia comunitaria: Relato de la experiencia en Brasilio-Distrit¢ Federal [Community therapy: Report of an experience in Brasilia-Distrito Federal]. In A Sanchez Vidal, A. Zambrano Constanzo & M. Palacín Lois (Eds.), *Psicología comunitari¢ Europa: Communidad, poder, ética y volores* [European community psychology: Commu nity, power, ethics and values] (pp. 362–376). Barcelona, Spain: Publicacions de la Univer sitat de Barcelona.

Campbell, C.D. (2000). Social structure, space, and sentiment: Searching for common groun¢ in sociological conceptions of community. In Chekki, D.A. (Ed.), *Community structure an¢ dynamics at the dawn of the new millennium*. Connecticut: JAI Press Inc.

Campbell, C., & Jovchelovitch, S. (2000). Health, community and development. *Journal o Community and Applied Social Psychology, 10*, 255–270.

Campbell, C., & Murray, M. (2004). Community health psychology: Promoting analysis an¢ action for social change. *Journal of Health Psychology, 9*(2), 187–195.

Canagarajah, A.S. (1996). 'Nondiscursive' requirements in academic publishing, materia¢ resources of periphery scholars, and the politics of knowledge production. *Written Com munication, 13*, 435–472.

Carlquist, E., Nafstad, H.E., & Blakar, R.M. (2007). Community psychology in a Scandina vian welfare society: The case of Norway. In S.M. Reich, M. Riemer, I. Prilleltensky & M Montero (Eds.), *International community psychology* (pp. 282–298). Boston, MA: Springe: https://doi.org/10.1007/978-0-387-49500-2_14.

Carmen, R. (2000). A future for the excluded? Learning from Brazil. *Development, 43*, 47–5(

Carmen, R., & Sobrado, M. (2000). *A future for the excluded: Job creation and income gen eration by the poor. Clodomir Santos de Morais and the organization workshop*. Londor England: Zed Books.

Carson, R. (1962). *Silent Spring*. New York, NY: Houghton Mifflin.

Case, A.D. (2017). Reflexivity in counterspaces fieldwork. *American Journal of Communit Psychology, 60*(3–4), 398–405.

Chatterjee, H.J., & Camic, P.M. (2015). The health and well-being potential of museums an art galleries. *Arts & Health, 7*(3), 183–186. doi:10.1080/17533015.2015.1065594.

Checkland, P., & Scholes, J. (1990). *Soft systems methodology in action*. Chichester, Englanc John Wiley.

Cheong, P.H. (2006). Communication context, social cohesion and social capital buildin among Hispanic immigrant families. *Community, Work and Family, 9*(3), 367–387.

Chilisa, B. (2012). *Indigenous research methodologies*. Thousand Oaks, CA: SAGE Publication:

Chilisa, B., Major, T.E., & Khudu-Petersen, K. (2017). Community engagement with a postcc lonial, African-based relational paradigm. *Qualitative Research, 17*(3), 326–339.

Chomsky, N. (1992). *Chronicles of dissent: Interviews with Noam Chomsky by David Bars amlan*. Boston, MA: South End Press.

Chouchani, N., & Abed, M. (2018). Online social network analysis: Detection of commun: ties of interest. *Journal of Intelligent Information Systems* (Aug 2018a), online. Available a https://link.springer.com/article/10.1007/s10844-018-0522-7.

Clennon, O. (2018). *Black scholarly activism between the academy and grassroots*. New Yorl NY: Palgrave Macmillan.

Clennon, O.D., Kagan, C., Lawthom, R., & Swindells, R. (2016). Participation in commu nity arts: Lessons from the inner-city. *International Journal of Inclusive Education, 20*(3 331–346.

Clifford, J., & Marcus, G. (1986). *Writing culture: The poetics and politics of ethnography.* Berkeley: University of California Press.

Cohen, A. (1986). *Symbolising community boundaries. Identity and diversity in British cultures.* Manchester, England: Manchester University Press.

Cohen, A.P. (1985). *The symbolic construction of community.* London, England: Routledge and Kegan Paul.

Coleman, R. (2000). Self-help and social change. In C. Kagan (Ed.), *Collective action and social change.* Retrieved from www.compsy.org.uk.

Collective of Authors. (2007). *The Birmingham Manifesto.* Available at www.compsy.org.uk/ The%20Birmingham%20Manifesto.pdf.

Collins, K., & Ison, R. (2009). Jumping off Arnstein's ladder: Social learning as a new policy paradigm for climate change adaptation. *Environmental Policy and Governance, 19*(6), 358–373.

Committee on the Rights of Persons with Disabilities. (2017). Observations by the United Kingdom of Great Britain and Northern Ireland on the report of the Committee on its inquiry carried out under article 6 of the Optional Protocol. United Nations, Convention on the Rights of Persons with Disability. Available at https://tbinternet.ohchr.org/_layouts/ treatybodyexternal/TBSearch.aspx?Lang=e n&TreatyID=4&DocTypeCategoryID=7.

Cook, J.R. (2015). Using evaluation to effect social change: Looking through a community psychology lens. *American Journal of Evaluation, 36*(1), 107–117.

Cooke, B. (2001). The social psychological limits of participation? In B. Cooke & U. Kothari (Eds.), *Participation: The new tyranny?* London, England: Zed Books.

Cooke, B., & Kothari, U. (2001). *Participation: The new tyranny?* London, England: Zed Books.

Cooperrider, D.L., & Whitney, D.K. (2005). *Appreciative inquiry: A positive revolution in change.* San Francisco, CA: Berrett Koehler.

Corbett, C.J. (2011). Review of pracademics and community change: A true story of nonprofit development and social entrepreneurship during welfare reform by O. Cleveland and R. Wineburg [Lyceum Books; www.lyceumbooks.com]. *Global Journal of Community Psychology Practice, 1*(3), online.

Corbett, T., & Noyes, J.L. (2008). *Human services systems integration: Conceptual framework.* Institute for Research on Poverty Discussion Paper 133–98. Available at www.irp. wisc.edu/publications/dps/pdfs/dp133308.pdf.

Cornwall, A. (2008). Unpacking participation: Models, meanings and practices. *Community Development Journal, 43*(3), 269–283.

Cosgrove, L., & McHugh, M.C. (2000). Speaking for ourselves: Feminist methods and community psychology. *American Journal of Community Psychology, 28*, 816–838.

Craig, G., Gaus, A., Wilkinson, M., Skøivánková, K., & McQuade, A. (2007). *Contemporary slavery in the UK.* York, England: Joseph Rowntree Foundation.

Crespo, I., Pallí, C., Lalueza, J. (2002). Moving communities: A process of negotiation with a Gypsy minority for empowerment. *Community, Work and Family, 5*(1), 49–66.

Creswell, J.W. (2002). *Educational research: Planning, conducting, and evaluating quantitative and qualitative research.* Upper Saddle River, NJ: Merrill-Pearson Education.

Crosby, A. (2009). Anatomy of a workshop: Women's struggles for transformative participation in Latin America. *Feminism and Psychology, 19*(3), 343–353.

Crow, G., Allan, G., & Summers, M. (2001). Changing perspectives on the insider/outsider distinction in community sociology. *Community, Work and Family, 4*(1), 29–48.

Crowther, J., Martin, I., & Shaw, M. (1999). *Popular education and social movements in Scotland today.* Leicester, England: NIACE.

Dabelstein, N. (2003). Evaluation capacity development: Lessons learned. *Evaluation, 9*(3) 365–369.

Daher, M., & Haz, A.M. (2011). Changing meanings through art: A systematization of a psy chosocial intervention with Chilean women in urban poverty situation. *American Journa of Community Psychology, 47*(3–4), 322–334.

D'Alisa, G., Demaria, F., & Kallis, G. (Eds.). (2014). *Degrowth: A vocabulary for a new era* Abingdon, England: Routledge.

Dalton, J., & Wolfe, S. (2012). Education connection and the community practitioner: Com petencies for community psychology practice – draft, August 15th 2012. *The Communit Psychologist, 45*(4), 7–14.

Dalton, J., Elias, M., & Wandersman, A. (2001). *Community psychology: Linking individual and communities*. Belmont, CA: Wadsworth.

Daly, H.E., & Farley, J. (2011). *Ecological economics: Principles and applications*. Washing ton, DC: Island Press.

Danziger, K. (1994). Does the history of psychology have a future? *Theory and Psychology 4*, 467–484.

Danziger, K. (1990). *Constructing the subject: Historical origins of psychological research* Cambridge, England: Cambridge University Press.

Darling, F.F. (1970). *Wilderness and plenty*. London, England: Oxford UP.

Davey, B. (2015). *An introduction to ecological economics. University of Nottingham/FEASTA* Available at www.feasta.org/2015/09/14/an-introduction-to-ecological-economics/.

Davies, N. (1998). *Dark heart: The shocking truth about hidden Britain*. London, England Vintage Press.

Deal, M. (2003). Disabled people's attitudes toward other impairment groups: A hierarchy o impairments. *Disability and Society, 18*(7), 897–910.

Dearing, R. (1997). *National Committee of Inquiry into Higher Education*. Norwich, England HMSO.

Debord, G. (1983). *Society of the spectacle* (K. Knabb, Trans.). London, England: Rebe Press.

Değirmencioğlu, S.M. (2007). Moving but not yet talking: Community psychology in Turkey. I S.M. Reich, M. Riemer, I. Prilleltensky & M. Montero (Eds.), *International community psy chology* (pp. 356–362). Boston, MA: Springer. https://doi.org/10.1007/978-0-387-49500 2_19.

Department of Health (2001). *Valuing People: A strategy for learning disability services in th 21st century* (Cm 5086). London, England: Department of Health.

Desai, P., & Riddlestone, S. (2002). *Bioregional solutions: For living on one planet*. Schum acher Briefings 8. Dartington, England: Green Books.

Devine, P., Pearmain, A., & Purdy, D. (Eds.). (2009). *Feelbad Britain: How to make it better* London, England: Lawrence and Wishart.

Dewey, J. (1946). *The problems of men*. New York, NY: Philosophical Library.

Dewey, J. (1916/1966). *Democracy and education. An introduction to the philosophy of edu cation*. New York, NY: Free Press. (First published in 1916 in New York by Macmillan).

Douglas, K., & Carless, D. (2013). An invitation to performative research. *Methodologica Innovations Online, 8*(1), 53–64.

Doyal, L., & Gough, I. (1991). *A theory of human need*. Basingstoke, England: Macmillan.

Duckett, Paul (2012). Seroxat: A story about UK pharmacological corporations, UK polit cians, academics and other corrupt bastards. In C. Walker, K. Johnson & L. Cunningha (Eds.), *Community psychology and the socio-economics of mental distress: Internationa perspectives* (pp. 16–31). Basingstoke, England: Palgrave Macmillan.

Duckett, P.S. (2009). Critical reflections on key community psychology concepts: Off-setting our capitalist emissions? *Forum Gemeindepsychologie, 14*(2). Available online from: www.gemeindepsychologie.de/fg-2-2009_06.html.

Duckett, P.S. (2005). Globalised violence, community psychology and the bombing and occupation of Afghanistan and Iraq. *Journal of Community and Applied Social Psychology, 15*(5), 414–423.

Duckett, P. (2002). Community psychology, millennium volunteers and UK higher education: A disruptive triptych? *Journal of Community and Applied Social Psychology, 12*(2), 94–107.

Duckett, P.S. (1998). What are you doing here? 'Non disabled' people and the disability movement, a response to Fran Bransfield. *Disability and Society, 13*(4), 625–628.

Duckett, P.S., & Schinkel, M. (2008). Community psychology and injustice in the criminal justice system. *Journal of Community and Applied Social Psychology, 18*, 518–526.

Duckett, P., Sixsmith, C., & Kagan, C. (2008). Researching pupil well-being in UK secondary schools: Community psychology and the politics of research. *Childhood, 15*(1), 91–108.

Duff, W.M., Flinn, A., Suurtamm, K.E., & Wallace, D.A. (2013). Social justice impact of archives: A preliminary investigation. *Archival Science, 13*(4), 317–348.

Duncan, G., Zlotowitz, S., & Stubbs, J. (2017). *Meeting us where we're at. Learning from INTEGRATE's work with excluded young people.* London, England: Centre for Mental Health. Available at www.centreformentalhealth.org.uk/sites/default/files/centreformentalhealth_meeting_us_where_were_at_briefing_.pdf.

Duncan, N., Bowman, B., Naidoo, A., Pillay, J., & Roos, V. (2007). *Community psychology: Analysis, context and action.* Capetown, South Africa: UCT Press.

Durkheim, É. (1894/1982). *The rules of sociological method and selected texts on sociology and its method.* London, England: Macmillan (Original publication 1894).

Durose, C., & Richardson, L. (2015). *Designing public policy for co-production: Theory, practice and change.* Bristol, England: Policy Press.

Dussel, E. (2013). *Ethics of liberation in the age of globalization and exclusion* (A.A. Vallega, Ed.). Durham, NC: Duke University Press.

Dussel, E. (2008). *Twenty theses on politics.* Durham, NC: Duke University Press.

Dussel, E. (2000). Europe, modernity and eurocentrism. *Nepantla: View from the South, 1*(3), 465–478.

Dussel, E. (1995). *The invention of the Americas: Eclipse of 'the other' and the myth of modernity.* New York, NY: Continuum.

Dzidic, P., Breen, L.J., & Bishop, B.J. (2013). Are our competencies revealing our weaknesses? A critique of community psychology practice competencies. *Global Journal of Community Psychology Practice, 4*(4), 1–10, online.

Edge, I., Kagan, C., & Stewart, A. (2004). Living poverty: Surviving on the edge. *Clinical Psychology, 38*(June), 28–31.

Ellis, J. (2009). *Monitoring and evaluation in the third sector: Meeting accountability and learning needs.* Paper presented to NCVO/VSSN Conference: Researching the Voluntary Sector, 2009. www.ces-vol.org.uk retrieved 29 September 2009.

Engeström, Y. (1999). Activity theory and individual and social transformation. In Y. Engeström, R. Miettinen & R-L. Punamäki (Eds.), *Perspectives on activity theory* (pp. 19–38). Cambridge University Press.

Engeström, Y., & Miettinen, R. (1999). Introduction. In Y. Engeström, R. Miettinen & R-L. Punamäki (Eds.), *Perspectives on Activity Theory* (pp. 1–16). Cambridge University Press.

Escobar, A. (2007). Worlds and knowledges otherwise: The Latin American modernity/coloniality research program. *Cultural Studies, 21*(2), 179–210.

Estrada, A.M., Ibarra, C., & Sarmiento, E. (2007). Regulation and control of subjectivity and private life in the context of armed conflict in Colombia. *Community, Work and Family* 10(3), 257–281.

European Environment Agency. (2013). *Late lessons from early warnings: Science, precaution innovation* (Publication 1/2013). Copenhagen, Denmark: European Environment Agency. Available at www.eea.europa.eu/publications/late-lessons-2.

Evans, K. (1997). "It's alright round here if you're local": Community in the inner city. In I Hoggett (Ed.), *Contested communities: Experiences, struggles, policies* (pp. 33–50). Bristol England: Policy Press.

Evans, S.D., Malhotra, K., & Headley, A.M. (2013). Promoting learning and critical reflexivit through an organizational case study project. *Journal of Prevention & Intervention in th Community, 41*(2), 105–112.

Evans, S.D., Duckett, P., Lawthom, R., & Kivell, N. (2017). Positioning the critical in com munity psychology. In M.A. Bond, I. Serrano-García, C.B. Keys & M. Shinn (Eds.), *AP/ handbook of community psychology: Theoretical foundations, core concepts, and emergin, challenges* (pp. 107–127). Washington, DC: American Psychological Association.

Falkembach, E.M.F., & Torres, A.C. (2015). Systematization of experiences: A practice o participatory research from Latin America. In H. Bradbury (Ed.), *The SAGE handbook o action research* (3rd ed., pp. 76–82). London, England: SAGE Publications Ltd.

Fals Borda, O. (1988). *Knowledge and people's power: Lessons with peasants in Nicaragua Mexico and Colombia*. New York, NY: New Horizons Press.

Fals Borda, O., & Rahman, M.A. (1991). *Action and knowledge: Breaking the monopol of power with participatory action-research*. London, England: Intermediate Technolog Publications.

Fang, M.L., Sixsmith, J., Lawthom, R., Mountian, I., & Shahrin, A. (2015). Experiencin 'pathologized presence and normalized absence'; understanding health related experience and access to health care among Iraqi and Somali asylum seekers, refugees and person without legal status. *BMC Public Health, 15*(1), online. Available at http://bmcpublichealth biomedcentral.com/articles/10.1186/s12889-015-2279-z.

Fanon, F. (1967). *Black skins, white masks*. New York, NY: Grove.

Farias, L., & Perdomo, G. (2004). Moral dilemmas of community leaders and sense of com munity. *Journal of Prevention and Intervention in the Community, 27*(1), 25–37.

Feeney, M. (2019). Tea in the Pot, 'third place' or social prescription? Exploring the positiv impact on mental health of a voluntary women's group in Glasgow. In L. McGrath & I Reavey (Eds.), *The handbook of mental health and space: Community and clinical applica tions*. Oxford, England: Routledge.

Felton, B.J., & Shinn, M. (1992). Social integration and social support: Moving 'social*sup port' beyond the individual level. *Journal of Community Psychology, 20*(2), 103–115 doi:10.1002/1520-6629(199204)20:2<103::AID-JCOP2290200202>3.0.CO;2-4.

Ferreira Moura, J., Morais Ximenes, V., Camurça Cidade, E., & Barbosa Mepomuceno, B. (i press, 2019). *Psychosocial implication of poverty: Diversities and resistances*. New York NY: Springer.

Fetterman, D., Rodríguez-Campos, L., Wandersman, A., & O'Sullivan, R.G. (2014). Collabor ative, participatory, and empowerment evaluation: Building a strong conceptual foundatio for stakeholder involvement approaches to evaluation (A response to Cousins, Whitmor and Shulha, 2013). *American Journal of Evaluation, 35*(1), 144–148.

Fetterman, D.M., & Wandersman, A. (Eds.). (2005). *Empowerment evaluation principles i practice*. New York, NY: Guildford Press.

Filipe, A., Renedo, A., & Marston, C. (2017). The co-production of what? Knowledge, values, and social relations in health care. *PLOS Biology, 15*(5), e2001403. doi:10.1371/journal. pbio.2001403.

Fisher, A.T., Sonn, C., & Bishop, B.J. (Eds.). (2002). *Psychological sense of community. Research, applications, and implications.* New York, NY: Springer.

Fisher, J., Lawthom, R., & Kagan, C. (2016). Delivering on the Big Society? Tensions in hosting community organisers. *Local Economy: The Journal of the Local Economy Policy Unit, 31*(4), 502–517.

Fisher, J., Lawthom, R., & Kagan, C. (2014). Revolting tales of migrant workers and community organisers: A UK community psychological perspective. *Australian Community Psychologist, 26*(1), 37–50.

Fisher, J., Lawthom, R., Hartley, S., Koivunen, E., & Yeowell, G. (2018). *Evaluation of Men in Sheds for Age UK Cheshire final report.* Manchester, England: Manchester Metropolitan University.

Flores, J.M. (2009). Praxis and liberation in the context of Latin American theory. In M. Montero & C. Sonn (Eds.), *Psychology of liberation: Theory and applications.* New York, NY: Springer.

Fook, J., & Askeland, G.A. (2006). The 'critical' in critical reflection. In S. White, J. Fook & F. Gardner (Eds.), *Critical reflection in health and social care.* Maidenhead, England: Open University Press/McGraw Hill Education.

Foot, J., & Hopkins, T. (2010). *A glass half-full: How an asset approach can improve community health and well-being* (p. 32). London, England: IDeA (Improvement and Development Agency). Available at www.assetbasedconsulting.net/uploads/publications/A%20glass%20 half%20full.pdf.

Ford, J. (1995). Middle England: In debt and insecure? *Poverty, 92,* 11–14.

Foster-Fishman, P.G., & Behrens, T.R. (2007). Systems change reborn: Rethinking our theories, methods, and efforts in human services reform and community-based change. *American Journal of Community Psychology, 39*(3/4), 191–196.

Foster-Fishman, P.G., Nowell, B., & Yang, H. (2007). Putting the system back into systems change: A framework for understanding and changing organizational and community systems. *American Journal of Community Psychology, 39*(3/4), 197–216.

Foster-Fishman, P., Berkowitz, B., Lounsbury, D.W., Jacobson, S., & Allen, N.A. (2001). Building collaborative capacity in community coalitions: A review and integrative framework. *American Journal Community Psychology, 29*(2). 241–261.

Foucault, M. (1980). Two lectures. In C. Gordon (Ed.), *Power/knowledge: Selected interviews.* New York, NY: Pantheon.

Foucault, M. (1976). *The history of sexuality, Volume 1: An introduction* (R. Hurley, Trans.). London, England: Penguin.

Foweraker, J. (1995). *Theorizing social movements.* London, England: Pluto.

Francescato, D. (2000). Community psychology intervention strategies as tools to enhance participation in projects promoting sustainable development and quality of life. *Gemeindepsychologie, 6*(2), 49–58.

Francescato, D., & Aber, M.S. (2015). Learning from organizational theory to build organizational empowerment. *Journal of Community Psychology, 43*(6), 717–738. doi:10.1002/ jcop.21753.

Francescato, D., & Zani, B. (2013). Community psychology practice competencies in undergraduate and graduate programs in Italy. *Global Journal of Community Psychology Practice, 4*(4), 1–12, online.

Francescato, D., Arcidiacono, C., Albanesi, C., & Mannarini, T. (2007). Community psychology in Italy: Past developments and future perspectives. In S.M. Reich, M. Riemer, I Prilleltensky & M. Montero (Eds.), *International community psychology* (pp. 263–281) Boston, MA: Springer. https://doi.org/10.1007/978-0-387-49500-2_13.

Francescato, D., Gelli, B., Mannarini, T., & Taurino, A. (2004). Community development Action research through profiles analysis in a small town in Southern Italy. In A. Sanche: Vidal, A. Zambrano Constanzo & M. Palacin Lois (Eds.), *Psicologia comunitaria Europa Communidad, poder, ética y valores* (pp. 247–261). Barcelona, Spain: Publicacions Univer sitat de Barcelona.

Freire, P. (1994). *Pedagogy of hope*. New York, NY: Routledge.

Freire, P. (1972a). *Pedagogy of the oppressed*. Harmondsworth, England: Penguin.

Freire, P. (1972b). *Cultural action for freedom*. Harmondsworth, England: Penguin.

Freire, P., & Faundez, A. (1989). *Learning to question: A pedagogy of liberation*. Geneva Switzerland: World Council of Churches.

Freitas, M.F. de Q. (1994). Prácticas en comunidad y psicología comunitaria [Practices in com munity and community psychology]. In M. Montero (Ed.), *Psicología Social Comunitaria Teoría, método y experiencia*. Guadalajara, Mexico: Universidad de Guadalajara.

Freitas, M.F.Q. (2009). (In) Coerências entre prácticas psicossocias em comunidade e projeto de transormação social: Aproximaçãos entre as psicologias socais da libertação e comuni taria. *Psico, 36*(1), 47–54.

Freitas, M.F.Q. (2000). Voices from the South: The construction of Brazilian community socia psychology. *Journal of Community and Applied Social Psychology, 10*(4), 315–326.

French, J.R.P., & Raven, B.H. (1959). The bases of social power. In D. Cartwright (Ed.), *Stua ies in social power*. Ann Arbour, MI: University Michigan Press.

French, R.S. (2019). *Policy and politics: Evidence-based policy – Older than advertised an weaker than we could wish*. Available at https://discoversociety.org/2019/01/02/policy-and politics-evidence-based-policy-older-than-advertised-and-weaker-than-we-could-wish/.

Fricker, M. (2007). *Epistemic injustice: Power and the ethics of knowing*. Oxford, Englanc Oxford University Press.

Fryer, D. (2008). Some questions about 'the history of community psychology'. *Journal c Community Psychology, 36*(5), 572–586.

Fukuoka, M. (1985a). *The one-straw revolution: An introduction to natural farming*. Nev York, NY: Bantam Books.

Fukuoka, M. (1985b). *The natural way of farming: The theory and practice of green ph losophy*. Tokyo, Japan: Japan Publications, 1985. Available at www.rivendellvillage.org Natural-Way-Of-Farming-Masanobu-Fukuoka-Green-Philosophy.pdf.

Fynn, A. (2013). Using appreciative inquiry (AI) to evaluate an education support ngo i Soweto. *Psychology in Society, 44*, online.

Gaotlhobogwe, M., Major, T.E., Koloi-Keaikitse, S., & Chilisa, B. (2018). Conceptualizin evaluation in African contexts: Conceptualizing evaluation in African contexts. *New Dire tions for Evaluation, 2018*(159), 47–62.

Gates, A. (1998). *Letter from Alice Gates*. Available at www2.oberlin.edu/external/EOC SEPA/Gates-letter.html.

Geertz, C. (1973). *Thick description: Towards an interpretative theory of culture*. New Yor! NY: Basic Books.

Gergen, M., & Gergen, K.J. (2011). Performative social science and psychology. *Forum Qual tative Sozialforschung/Forum: Qualitative Social Research, 12*(1), online. Available at www qualitative-research.net/index.php/fqs/article/view/1595.

Gilchrist, A. (2004). *The well connected community: A networking approach to community development*. Bristol, England: Policy Press.

Global Footprint Network. (n.d.). *Ecological footprint: Global Footprint Network*. Available at www.footprintnetwork.org/our-work/ecological-footprint/.

Glyn, A. (2006). *Capitalism unleashed*. Oxford, England: Oxford University Press.

González Rey, F. (2017). The topic of subjectivity in psychology: Contradictions, paths and new alternatives. *Journal for the Theory of Social Behaviour, 47*(4), 502–521.

González Rey, F. (2015). Human motivation in question: Discussing emotions, motives, and subjectivity from a cultural-historical standpoint: Human motivation in question. *Journal for the Theory of Social Behaviour, 45*(4), 419–439.

Goodings, L., & Tucker, I. (2019). Social media and mental health: A topological approach. In L. McGrath & P. Reavey (Eds.), *The handbook of mental health and space: Community and clinical applications*. Oxford, England: Routledge.

Goodley, D., & Lawthom, R. (2011). Disability, community and empire: Indigenous psychologies and social psychoanalytic possibilities *International Journal of Inclusive Education, 15*(1), 101–115.

Goodley, D.A., & Lawthom, R. (2005). Epistemological journeys in participatory action research: Alliances between community psychology and disability studies. *Disability and Society, 20*(2), 135–151.

Gough, I. (2017). *Heat, greed and human need: Climate change, capitalism and sustainable wellbeing*. Cheltenham, England: Edward Elgar Publishing.

Gramsci, A. (1971). *Selections from the prison notebooks* (Q.H. a. G.N. Smith, Trans.). London, England: Lawrence and Wishart.

Gramsci, A. (1968). Soviets in Italy (Writing from 1919 and 1920). *New Left Review* (1st series), *51*, 28–58.

Gray-Rosendale, L.A., & Harootunian, G. (2003). *Framing feminisms: Investigating histories, theories, and moments of fracture*. New York: State University of New York Press.

Gregory, A. (2000). Problematizing participation. A critical review of approaches to participation in evaluation theory. *Evaluation, 6*(2), 179–199.

Gregory, A. (1997). Evaluation practice and the tricky issue of coercive contexts. *Systems Practice, 10*(5), 589–609.

Gridley, H., & Breen, L. (2008). So far and yet so near? Community psychology in Australia. In S. Reich, M. Riemer, I. Prilleltensky & M. Montero (Eds.), *International community psychology: History and theories*. New York, NY: Springer.

Grieger, I., & Ponterotto, J.G. (1998). Challenging intolerance. In C.C. Lee & G.R. Walz (Eds.), *Social action: A mandate for counsellors* (pp. 17–50). Alexandra, VA: American Counselling Association and ERIC Counselling and Student Services Clearinghouse.

Griseri, P. (1988). *Managing values: Ethical change in organisations*. Basingstoke, England: Macmillan.

Grosfoguel, R. (2008). Transmodernity, border thinking, and global coloniality: Decolonizing political economy and postcolonial studies. *Revista Crítica de Ciências Sociais, 80*. Available from *Eurozine*. at www.eurozine.com/transmodernity-border-thinking-and-global-coloniality/?pdf.

Grover, R. (1995). *Communities that care: Intentional communities of attachment as a third path in community care*. Brighton, England: Pavilion Publishing.

Guba, E.G., & Lincoln, Y.S. (2001). *Guidelines and checklist for constructivist (A.K.A. fourth generation) evaluation*. Evaluation Checklists Project. www.wmich.edu/evalctr/checklists/constructivisteval.pdf retrieved 2 January 2009.

Guba, E.G., & Lincoln, Y.S. (1989). *Fourth generation evaluation*, Newbury Park, CA, Sag Publications.

Gutiérrez, G. (1988). *A theology of liberation*. Maryknoll, NY: Orbis Books (Revised from firs English translation in 1973 published by Orbis from the original Teologia de la liberación Perspectivas: CEP, Lima).

Gutiérrez, G. (1973). *A theology of liberation* (M. O'Connell, Trans.). New York, NY: Orbis

Habermas, J. (1984). *The theory of communicative action: Reason and rationalisation in soci ety*. Boston, MA: Beacon Press.

Hagan, T., & Smail, D. (1997). Power-mapping: Background and basic methodology. *Journa of Community and Applied Social Psychology, 7*, 257–267.

Hallsworth, M., & Sanders, M. (2016). Nudge: Recent developments in behavioural scienc and public policy. In F. Spotswood (Ed.), *Beyond behaviour change: Key issues, interdisci plinary approaches and future directions*. Bristol, England: Policy Press.

Halpern, D. (2019, January 24). Chances are you've been nudged by the government with out realising. *The Times*. Available at www.thetimes.co.uk/article/chances-are-you-ve-been nudged-by-the-government-without-realising-vznvb2gq0?utm_source=newsletter&utm campaign=newsletter_119&utm_medium=email&utm_content=119_5010928&CMP= NLEmail_118918_5010928_119.

Hamber, B., Masilela, T.C., & Terre Blanche, M. (2001). Towards a Marxist community psy chology: Radical tools for community psychological analysis and practice. In M. Seeda (Ed.), N. Duncan & S. Lazarus (Cons. Eds.), *Community psychology: Theory, method an practice* (pp. 51–66). Cape Town, South Africa: Oxford University Press.

Hanks, K., & Belliston, L. (2006). *Rapid Viz: A new method for the rapid visualization o ideas*. Menlo Park, CA: Crisp Publications.

Hanley, L. (2017). *Estates: An intimate history*. London, England: Granta Books.

Harré, N. (2011). *Psychology for a better world. Strategies to inspire sustainability*. Auck land, New Zealand: Auckland University Press. Available at http://elibrary.bsu.az books_400/N_350.pdf.

Harré, N., Madden, H., Brooks, R., & Goodman, J. (2017). Sharing values as a foundation fo collective hope. *Journal of Social and Political Psychology, 5*(2), 342–366.

Harré, R. (1993). *Social being* (2nd ed.). Oxford, England: Blackwell.

Harrison, A.K. (2008). Racial authenticity in rap music and hip hop. *Sociology Compass, 2*(6 1783–1800.

Harvey, D. (2007). *A brief history of neoliberalism*. Oxford, England: Oxford Universit Press.

Harvey, D. (2005a). *Spaces of neoliberalization*. Heidelberg, Germany: University of Heide berg Press.

Harvey, D. (2005b). The sociological and geographical imaginations. *International Journal o Politics, Culture and Society, 18*(3/4), 211–255.

Hassan, A., Fatimilehin, I., & Kagan, C. (2019). 'Geedka shirka' (under the tree): Cultura migratory and community spaces for preventive interventions with Somali men and the families. In L. McGrath & P. Reavey (Eds.), *The handbook of mental health and space Community and clinical applications*. Oxford, England: Routledge.

Hawe, P., Shiell, A., & Riley, T. (2009). Theorising interventions as events in systems. *America Journal of Community Psychology, 43*(3–4), 267–276.

Haworth, J.T., & Roberts, K. (2007). Leisure: The next 25 years. For *Science review for th DTI Foresight project on Mental Capital and Mental Wellbeing*. London, England: DTI.

Hawtin, M., Hughes, G., & Percy-Smith, J. (1994). *Community profiling: Auditing socia needs*. Buckingham, England: Open University Press.

Hernández, E. (2004). Metadecision: Training community leaders for effective decision making. *Journal of Prevention and Intervention in the Community, 27*(1), 53–70.

Hillery, G.A. (1955). Definitions of community: Areas of agreement. *Rural Sociology 20*, 111.

Himmelman, A. (2001). On coalitions and the transformation of power relations: Collaborative betterment and collaborative empowerment. *American Journal of Community Psychology, 29*(2), 277–284.

Hodgson, F.C., & Turner, J. (2003). Participation not consumption: The need for new participatory practices to address transport and social exclusion. *Transport Policy, 10*(4), 265–272.

Holland, S. (1992). From social abuse to social action. In J. Ussher & P. Nicholson (Eds.), *Gender issues in clinical psychology* (pp. 68–77). London, England: Routledge.

Holland, S. (1991). From private symptom to public action. *Feminism and Psychology, 1*(1), 58–62.

Hollander, N.C. (1997). *Love in a time of hate: Liberation psychology in Latin America.* New Brunswick, NJ: Rutgers University Press.

Holmgren, D. (2008). *Future scenarios: Mapping the cultural implications of peak oil and climate change.* www.futurescenarios.org/, retrieved 3 October 2009.

Holmgren, D. (2007). *Essence of permaculture.* Hepburn, Australia: Holmgren Design Services. Available at https://holmgren.com.au/essence-of-permaculture-free/.

Hook, D., Kiguwa, P., & Mkhize, N. (2004). *Introduction to critical psychology.* Lansdowne, South Africa: UCT Press.

Howlett, M., Kekez, A., & Poocharoen, O.-O. (2017). Understanding co-production as a policy tool: Integrating new public governance and comparative policy theory. *Journal of Comparative Policy Analysis: Research and Practice, 19*(5), 487–501.

Hu, C., Zhao, L., & Huang, J. (2015). Achieving self-congruency? Examining why individuals reconstruct their virtual identity in communities of interest established within social network platforms. *Computers in Human Behavior, 50*, 465–475.

Humphrey, J.C. (2000). Cracks in the feminist mirror: research and reflections on lesbians and gay men working together. *Feminist Review, 66*, 95–130.

Hutton, W. (2007, February 18). 'Open the gates and free people from Britain's ghettos', *The Observer*; also available online at http://observer.guardian.co.uk/comment/story/0,2015638,00.html (Accessed 5 June 2009).

Hutton, W. (2002). *The world we are in.* London, England: Little Brown.

Hutton, W. (1995). *The state we're in.* London, England: Little Brown.

Hytner, B., D'Cocodia, L., Kagan, C., Spencer, L., & Yates, W. (1981). *Report of the Moss Side Enquiry to the Leader of the Greater Manchester Council.* Manchester, England: Greater Manchester Council.

Ife, J. (1995). *Community development. Creating community alternatives: Vision, analysis and practice.* Melbourne, Australia: Longman.

Illich, I., Zola, I., McKnight, J., Caplan, J., & Shaiken, S. (1977). *Disabling professions.* London, England: Marion Boyars.

Imagine. (2016). *Marsh Farm organisation workshop: Evaluation report.* Bristol, England: Imagine/Office for Civil Society. Available at www.corganisers.org.uk/what-is-community-organising/stories/marsh-farm-organisation-workshop/.

Intergovernmental Panel on Climate Change (IPCC). (2018). *Global warming of 1.5°C: Summary for policymakers.* Geneva, Switzerland: United Nations Intergovernmental Panel on Climate Change. Available at www.ipcc.ch/report/sr15/.

Jackson, K.T., Burgess, S., Toms, F., & Cuthbertson, E.L. (2018). Community engagement: Using feedback loops to empower residents and influence systemic change in culturally diverse communities. *Global Journal of Community Psychology Practice, 9*(2), 1–21.

Jackson, L., Peters, M.A., Benade, L., Devine, N., Arndt, S., Forster, D., . . . Ozoliņš, J. (John)
(2018). Is peer review in academic publishing still working? *Open Review of Educationa*
Research, 5(1), 95–112.

Jackson, M. (2003). *Systems thinking: Creative holism for managers.* Chichester, England
John Wiley.

Jackson, T. (2017). *Prosperity without growth: Foundations for the economy of tomorrou*
(2nd ed.). London, England: Routledge. Preface available online at www.book2look.com
embed/eFJiPjyMKG&euid=68185891&ruid=68174127&referurl=www.routledge.com&
lickedby=H5W&biblettype=html5.

Jahoda, M., Lazarsfeld, P., & Zeisel, H. (2002). *The sociology of an unemployed community*
Chicago, IL: Aldine.

Jambeck, J.R., Geyer, R., Wilcox, C., Siegler, T.R., Perryman, M., Andrady, A., . . . Law, K.L
(2015). Plastic waste inputs from land into the ocean. *Science, 347*(6223), 768–771.

Jameson, F. (2009). Ideological analysis: A handbook. In F. Jameson (Ed.). *Valences of th*
dialectic (pp. 215–363). London, England: Verso.

Janis, I. (1982). *Groupthink* (2nd ed.). Boston, MA: Houghton-Mifflin.

Jara, O. (2012). Systematization of experiences, research and evaluation: Three differen
approaches. *International Journal for Global Development Education Research (Revista*
Internacional sobre Investigación En Educación Global y para el Desarrollo), 1(February)
71–84.

Jara, O. (n.d.). *Orientaciones teórico-practicas para la sistematizatión de experiencias* [*i*
theory-practice guide to the systematisation of experiences]. San José, Costa Rica: Cen
tro de Estudios y Publicaciones Alforja. Available at http://centroderecursos.alboan.org
ebooks/0000/0788/6_JAR_ORI.pdf.

Johnson, B. (1992). *Polarity management: Identifying and managing unsolvable problems*
Amherst, MA: HRD Press. www.polaritymanagement.com.

Johnson, D. (2000). Laying the foundation: Capacity building for participatory monitoring an
evaluation. In M. Estrella, J. Blauert, D. Campilan, J. Gaventa, J. Gonsalves, I. Gujit, D. Johnson &
R. Ricafort (Eds.), *Learning from change: Issues and experiences in participatory monitorin*
and evaluation (pp. 217–228). London, England: Intermediate Technology Publications.

Johnson, D.W., & Johnson, F.P. (1996). *Joining together: Group theory and group skills* (6t
ed.). Boston, MA: Allyn and Bacon.

Johnston, C., & Mooney, G. (2007). 'Problem' people, 'problem' places? New Labour an
council estates. In R. Atkinson & G. Helms (Eds.), *Securing an urban renaissance.* Bristo
England: Policy Press.

Joseph Rowntree Foundation (JRF). (2018). *Budget 2018: Tackling the rising tide of in-wor*
poverty. York, England: Joseph Rowntree Foundation. Available at www.jrf.org.uk/repor
budget-2018-tackling-rising-tide-work-poverty.

Jovchelovitch, S. (2007). *Knowledge in context: Representations, community and culture*
London, England: Routledge.

Junqué, M., & Baird, K.S. (Eds.). (2018). *Ciudades sin miedo: guía del movimiento munic*
palista global (Primera edición). Barcelona, Spain: Icaria Editorial (English edition is *Fea*
less cities: Guide to the global municipalist movement. (2019). London, England: Nev
Internationalist).

Jurgenson, N. (2009). Facebook, the transumer and liquid capitalism. *Sociology Lens.* www
sociologylens.net/article-types/opinion/facebook-the-transumer-and-liquid-capitalism/310£

Kagan, C. (2013). *Co-production of research: For good or ill?* Presented at the Postgradu
ate Policy Research Conference, Edge Hill University. Available at https://e-space.mmu
ac.uk/609524/1/Co%20production%20reserach%20ormskirk%20b%2013.pdf.

Kagan, C. (2008). Broadening the boundaries of psychology through community psychology. *Psychology Teaching Review, 14*, 28–31.

Kagan, C. (2007). Working at the 'edge': Making use of psychological resources through collaboration. *The Psychologist, 20*(4), 224–227.

Kagan, C. (2006a). *Making a difference: Participation, well-being and levers for change* (intelligence report). Liverpool, England: RENEW.

Kagan, C. (2006b, January 11). Health hazards. *New Start.* Available at www.compsy.org.uk/stress.html.

Kagan, C. (2002). *Have we been here before? A community psychological perspective on regeneration and empowerment.* Paper presented to Harvester Housing Seminar, Manchester, England.

Kagan, C. (1997a). *Agencies and advocacies: Experience in the North West.* Whalley, England: North West Training and Development Team.

Kagan, C. (1997b). *Regional development for inclusion: Community development and learning disabled people in the North West of England.* Manchester, England: IOD Research Group.

Kagan, C. (1990). *Network development: An experiment in case management?* Whalley, England: North Western Regional Health Authority (N.W.D.T.).

Kagan, C. (1986). *Towards leisure integration and advocacy (BLISS).* Manchester, England: Manchester Polytechnic.

Kagan, C., & Burton, M.H. (2018). Putting the 'social' into sustainability science. In W. Leal Filho (Ed.), *Handbook of sustainability science and research* (pp. 285–298). Cham, Switzerland: Springer International Publishing.

Kagan, C., & Burton, M. (2014). Culture, identity and alternatives to the consumer culture. *Educar Em Revista (Brazil), 53*(Dossier: Educação, Cotidiano e Participação: desafios e contribuições para a formação). Available at http://ojs.c3sl.ufpr.br/ojs/index.php/educar/article/view/36583.

Kagan, C., & Burton, M. (2010). Marginalisation. In Nelson & Prilleltensky (Eds.), *Community psychology: In pursuit of liberation and well-being* (2nd ed.). Basingstoke, England: Palgrave Macmillan.

Kagan, C., & Burton, M. (2000). Prefigurative action research: An alternative basis for critical psychology. *Annual Review of Critical Psychology, 2*, 73–87.

Kagan, C., & Diamond, J. (2019). *Rethinking university-community engagement: Reflections on higher education policy and practice in England.* London, England: Palgrave Macmillan.

Kagan, C., & Duggan, K. (2011). Creating community cohesion: The power of using innovative methods to facilitate engagement and genuine partnership. *Social Policy and Society, 10*(03), 393–404.

Kagan, C., & Duggan, K. (2010). *Birley Fields development: Impact on the local community. Working paper 1: Context setting.* Manchester, England: Research Institute for Health and Social Change. Available at https://e-space.mmu.ac.uk/117657/1/978-1-900139-43-4.pdf.

Kagan, C., & Duggan, K. (2009). *Breaking down barriers: Universities and communities working together. Urban regeneration: Making a Difference – Community Cohesion Thematic Evaluation Report.* Manchester, England: RIHSC. Available at https://e-space.mmu.ac.uk/83457/1/978-1-900139-29-8.pdf.

Kagan, C., & Friends of Hough End Hall. (2015). *Community alliances against big business.* Presented at the 2nd UK Community Psychology Festival, Manchester, England.

Kagan, C., & Kilroy, A. (2007). Community psychology and well-being. In J. Haworth & G. Hart (Eds.), *Wellbeing: Individual, community and social perspectives.* London, England: Palgrave Macmillan.

Kagan, C., & Lawthom, R. (2014). *From competencies to liberation.* Presented at the Symposium on Liberation Psychology, International Congress Community Psychology, Fortaleza, Brazil. Available at www.researchgate.net/publication/308967854_From_Competencies_to_Liberation_community_ psychology_learning.

Kagan, C., & Lewis, S. (1995). Families, empowerment and social change: Empowerment and counter-hegemonic action. In S. Lewis, C. Kagan & M. Burton (Eds.), *Families, work and empowerment: Coalitions for social change.* Manchester, England: IOD Research Group. https://e-space.mmu.ac.uk/41686/.

Kagan, C., & Lewis, S. (1990). 'Where's your sense of humour?' Swimming against the tide in higher education. In E. Burman (Ed.), *Feminists and psychological practice.* London, England: Sage. Out of print but online at https://ericaburmancom.files.wordpress.com/2013/01/fppmerged.pdf.

Kagan, C., & Scott-Roberts, S. (2002). *Family based intervention for children with cerebral palsy and their inclusion in the community: Occupational and community psychological perspectives.* Manchester, England: COP Research Group. Available at https://e-space.mmu.ac.uk/41781/.

Kagan, C., & Siddiquee, A. (2005). *Review of the East Manchester Neighbourhood Nuisance Team.* RIHSC occasional papers 03/05. Manchester, England: RIHSC. Available at https://e-space.mmu.ac.uk/24693/.

Kagan, C., & Siddiquee, A. (2004). *Final report of evaluation of the Standing Conference for Community Development web-site.* RIHSC occasional papers. Manchester, England: RIHSC/SCCD. https://e-space.mmu.ac.uk/24636/.

Kagan, C., & Stewart, A. (2007). *The In Bloom competition: Gardening work as a community involvement strategy.* Presented at the 2nd International Community, Work and Family conference, Lisbon.

Kagan, C., Burton, M., & Siddiquee, A. (2017). Action research. In C. Willig & W. Stainton-Rogers (Eds.), *The Sage handbook of qualitative research in psychology* (2nd ed., pp. 55–73). Thousand Oaks, CA: SAGE Inc.

Kagan, C., Caton, S., & Barnett, M. (Eds.). (2005). *Regenerating professionals? Report of Sustainable Communities Summit 2005 fringe event.* RIHSC occasional papers on community engagement. Manchester, England: RIHSC. https://e-space.mmu.ac.uk/41863/.

Kagan, C., Caton, S., & Amin, A. (2001). *The need for witness support.* Manchester, England: IOD Research Group. https://e-space.mmu.ac.uk/41755/.

Kagan, C., Lewis, S., & Heaton, P. (1998). *Caring to work: Accounts of working parents of disabled children.* London, England: Family Policy Studies Centre/Joseph Rowntree Foundation.

Kagan, C., Tindall, C., & Robinson, J. (2009). Community psychology: Linking the individual with the community. In R. Woolfe, S. Strawbridge & B. Douglas (Eds.), *Handbook of counselling psychology* (3rd ed.). London, England: Sage.

Kagan, C., Caton, S., Amin, A., & Choudry, A. (2004). 'Boundary critique', community psychology and citizen participation. RIHSC occasional papers 5/04. Manchester, England: RIHSC. https://e-space.mmu.ac.uk/41847/.

Kagan, C., Duckett, P., Lawthom, R., & Burton, M. (2005). Community psychology and disabled people. In D. Goodley and R. Lawthom (Eds.), *Disability and psychology: Critical introductions and reflections.* London, England: Palgrave.

Kagan, C., Duggan, K., Richards, M., & Siddiquee, A. (2011). Community psychology. in P. Martin, F. Cheung, M. Kyrios, L. Littlefield, M. Knowles, B. Overmier & J.M. Prieto (Eds.). *The IAAP handbook of applied psychology* (Chapter 19). Oxford, England: Blackwell.

Kagan, C., Lawthom, R., Knowles, K., & Burton, M. (2000). *Community activism, participation and social capital on a peripheral housing estate.* Paper given at the European Community Psychology Conference, Bergen, Norway, September 2000.

Kagan, C., Lewis, S., Heaton, P., & McLean, I. (1999). *Community, work and family audit 1: Employing organisations*. IOD occasional papers 4/99. Manchester, England: IOD Research Group. https://e-space.mmu.ac.uk/41735/.

Kagan, C., McLean, T., Gathercole, C., & Austin, M. (1990). *Report on the work of the North Western Development Team for 1988–1990*. Whalley, England: North West Regional Health Authority.

Kagan, C., McLean, T., Gathercole, C., & Austin, M. (1988). *North Western Development Team annual report*. Whalley, England: North West Regional Health Authority. pp. 23.

Kagan, C., Lawthom, R., Siddiquee, A., Duckett, P., & Knowles, K. (2007). Community psychology through community action learning. In A. Bokszczanin (Ed.), *Community psychology: Social change in solidarity*. Opole, Poland: University Opole.

Kane, L. (2001). *Popular education and social change in Latin America*. London, England: Latin America Bureau.

Kawachi, I., & Berkman, L.F. (2001). Social ties and mental health. *Journal of Urban Health, 78*(3), 458–467.

Keenan, H.B. (2017). Unscripting curriculum: Toward a critical trans pedagogy. *Harvard Educational Review, 87*(4), 538–556. doi:10.17763/1943-5045-87.4.538.

Kelly, J.G. (2006). *Becoming ecological: An expedition into community psychology*. Oxford, England: Oxford University Press.

Kelvin, P. (1971). *The bases of social behaviour: An approach in term of order and value*. London, England: Holt, Rinehart and Winston.

Kessi, S. (2017). Community social psychologies for decoloniality: An African perspective on epistemic justice in higher education. *South African Journal of Psychology, 47*(4), 506–516.

Kilroy, A., Garner, C., Parkinson, C., Kagan, C., & Senior, P. (2007). *Towards transformation: Exploring the impact of culture, creativity and the arts on health and well-being. A consultation report for the Critical Friends event*. Manchester, England: RIHSC/Arts for Health. Available at https://e-space.mmu.ac.uk/24673/1/Critical_friends_report_final_amendments. pdf.

Klein, K., & D'Aunno, T. (1986). Psychological sense of community in the workplace. *Journal of Community Psychology, 14*, 365–377.

Klein, N. (2015). *This changes everything: Capitalism vs. the climate*. London, England: Penguin Books.

Klein, N. (2007). *The shock doctrine: The rise of disaster capitalism*. London, England: Penguin Books.

Knowles, K. (2001). *Evaluation of reorganisation of community psychiatric nursing services*. Unpublished PhD thesis, Manchester Metropolitan University, Manchester.

Knowles, K., & Kagan, C. (1995a). *Psychosocial rehabilitation in and with communities*. Paper presented to 1st International Conference of A.R.A.P.D.I.S.: Psychosocial Rehabilitation in and with Communities, Barcelona, Spain.

Knowles, K., & Kagan, C. (1995b). *Making your voice heard: Involving service users in the planning and development of services*. Paper presented to 1st International Conference of A.R.A.P.D.I.S.: Psychosocial Rehabilitation in and with Communities, Barcelona, Spain.

Knowles, M. (1980). *The modern practice of adult education: From pedagogy to andragogy* (2nd ed.). New York, NY: Cambridge Books.

Kolakowski, L. (1972). *Positivist philosophy: From Hume to the Vienna Circle*. Harmondsworth, England: Penguin.

Kolb, D.A. (1984). *Experiential learning: Experience as the source of learning and development*. New Jersey: Prentice-Hall.

Kothari, A., Demaria, F., & Acosta, A. (2014). Buen vivir, degrowth and ecological swaraj Alternatives to sustainable development and the green economy. *Development, 57*(3–4) 362–375.

Kowalsky, L.O., Verhoef, M.J., Thurston, W.E., & Rutherford, G.E. (1996). Guidelines for entr into an Aboriginal community. *The Canadian Journal of Native Studies 16*(2), 267–282.

Kropotkin, P.A. (1912). *Fields, factories, and workshops; Or, industry combined with agr culture and brain work with manual work* (new revised and enlarged ed.). New York, NY Thomas Nelson and Sons.

Kubler-Ross, E. (1969). *On death and dying*. New York, NY: Macmillan (Republished 1997 Touchstone).

Kundera, M. (1978). *The book of laughter and forgetting*. New York, NY: Columbia Univer sity Press.

Labra, I. (2001). *The development of power in grassroots groups. Skills and knowledge withi a self-managed production environment*. Paper presented to the conference on Work, Skill and Knowledge, Swiss Development Corporation, Interlaken Switzerland, September 2001

Lambert, S., & Hopkins, K. (1995). Occupational conditions and workers' sense of community Variations by gender and race. *American Journal of Community Psychology, 23*, 151–179.

Langer, E.J., & Rodin, J. (1976). The effects of choice and enhanced personal responsibilit for the aged: A field experiment in an institutional setting. *Journal of Personality and Socic Psychology, 34*, 191–198.

Lave, J., & Wenger, E. (1990). *Situated learning: Legitimate peripheral participation*. Can bridge, England: Cambridge University Press.

Lawthom, R. (2011). Developing learning communities: Using communities of practice withi community psychology. (Special edition: Inclusive communities). *International Journal c Inclusive Education 15*(1, February), 153–164.

Lawthom, R., Porretta, B., & Kagan, C. (2009). *Inclusion and integration through ESOL* Manchester, England: RIHSC.

Lawthom, R., Sixsmith, J., & Kagan, J. (2007). Interrogating power: The case of arts an mental health in community projects. *Journal of Community and Applied Social Psycholog 17*(4), 268–279.

Lawthom, R., Kagan, C., Baines, S., Lo, S., Sham, S., Mok, L., Greenwood, M., Gaule, S (2015). Experiences of forced labour amongst UK based Chinese migrant workers: Explo ing vulnerability and protection in times of empire. In L. Waite, G. Craig, H. Lewis, & K. Skrivankova (Eds.), *Vulnerability, exploitation and migrants* (pp. 174–186). Londor England: Palgrave Macmillan UK.

Lawthom, R., Kagan, C., Baines, S., Sham, S., Mok, L., Lo, S., Greenwood, M., & Gaule, S (2013). Experiences of forced labour amongst Chinese migrant workers: Emotional contair ment in a context of vulnerability and protection. *International Journal Work, Organisatio and Emotion, 5*(3), 261–280.

Lawthom, R., Woolrych, R., Fisher, J., Murray, M., Smith, H., Garcia-Ferrari, S., . . . Pereir G. (2018). Making methods age friendly: Methods, movement, and mapping. *Innovation i Aging, 2*(suppl_1), 242. doi:10.1093/geroni/igy023.906.

Lazarus, S., Bulbulia, S., Taliep, N., & Naidoo, A.V. (2015). Community-based participator research as a critical enactment of community psychology. *Journal of Community Psycho ogy, 43*(1), 87–98.

Leonard, P. (1984). *Personality and ideology: Towards a materialist understanding of the ind vidual*. London, England: Macmillan.

Leonard, P. (1975). Towards a paradigm for radical practice. In M. Bailey & M. Brake (Eds. *Radical social work*. London, England: Edward Arnold.

evin, M., & Greenwood, D. (2018). *Creating a new public university and reviving democracy. Action research in higher education.* New York, NY: Berghahn Books.

evine, M., & Perkins, D.V. (1997). *Principles of community psychology.* New York, NY: Oxford University Press.

evy, A., & Merry, U. (1986). *Organizational transformation: Approaches, strategies, theories.* New York, NY: Praeger.

ewin, K. (1997). *Resolving social conflicts and field theory in social science.* Washington, DC: American Psychological Association. (Reprints of books originally published in 1948 and 1951).

ewin, K. (1951). *Field theory in social science: Selected theoretical papers* (D. Cartwright, Ed.). New York, NY: Harper and Row. (Reprinted 1975 Greenwood Press and as Lewin, 1997).

ewin, K. (1943). Defining the field at a given time. *Psychological Review, 50,* 292–310. (Republished in Lewin, 1997).

ewis, S., Stumbitz, B., Miles, L., & Rouse, J. (2014). *Maternity protection in SMEs: An international review.* Geneva, Switzerland: International Labour Office.

ira, E. (2000). Psicología del miedo y conducta colectiva en Chile [The psychology of fear and collective behaviour in Chile]. In I. Martín-Baró (Ed.), *Psicología social de la guerra.* San Salvador, El Salvador: UCA Editores.

ira, E., & Castillo, M.I. (1991). *Psicología de la amenaza política y el miedo.* Santiago, Chile: ILAS.

ira, E., & Weinstein, E. (2000). La tortura. Conceptualización psicológica y proceso terapéutico. In I. Martín-Baró (Ed.), *Psicología social de la guerra* (3rd ed.). San Salvador, El Salvador: UCA Editores.

loyd, M. (2001). The politics of disability and feminism: Discord or synthesis? *Sociology, 35*(3), 715–728.

ocke, A., Lawthom, R., & Lyons, A. (2018). Social media platforms as complex and contradictory spaces for feminisms: Visibility, opportunity, power, resistance and activism. *Feminism & Psychology, 28*(1), 3–10. doi:10.1177/0959353517753973.

owndes, V. (2000). Women and social capital: A comment on Hall's 'social capital in Britain'. *British Journal of Political Science, 30,* 533–540.

uft, J. (1969). *Of human interaction.* Palo Alto, CA: National Press Books.

uger, A., & Massing, L. (2015). *Learning from our experience: A guide to participative systematisation. Horizon 3000.* Available at www.knowhow3000.org/wp/wp-content/files/ KM/KM%20public/Manuals%20%26%20Handbooks/ENG_MAN_Learning-From-Our-Experience-A-guide-to-participative-sistematisation_2015.pdf.

ukes, S. (1974). *Power: A radical view.* London, England: Macmillan.

uque-Ribelles, V., García-Ramírez, M., & Portillo, N. (2009). Gendering peace and liberation: A participatory-action approach to critical consciousness acquisition among women in a marginalized neighborhood. In M. Montero & C.C. Sonn (Eds.), *Psychology of liberation: Theory and applications.* New York, NY: Springer.

ykes, M.B., & Moane, G. (2009). Editors' introduction: Whither feminist liberation psychology? Critical explorations of feminist and liberation psychologies for a globalizing world. *Feminism and Psychology, 19*(3), 283–297.

ynd, R.S., & Lynd, H. (1929). *Middletown: A study of contemporary American culture.* New York, NY: Harcourt Brace.

MacGillivary, A., Weston, C., & Unsworth, C. (1998). *Communities count: A step by step guide to community sustainability indicators.* London, England: New Economics Foundation.

MacKay, T. (2008). Can psychology change the world? *The Psychologist, 21*(11), 928–931.

Mackenzie, D. (1981). Notes on the science and social relations debate. *Capital and Class* 14, 46–60.

Malm, A. (2016). *Fossil capital: The rise of steam-power and the roots of global warming* London, England: Verso.

Mantilla, G.E.V. (2010). Community systematization and learning: Project management for change. *Community Development Journal, 45*(3), 367–379.

Marcos, Subcomandante Insurgente. (2002). *Our word is our weapon: Selected writings of Subcomandante Insurgente Marcos*. New York, NY: Seven Stories.

Marcuse, H. (1965). Repressive tolerance. In R.P. Wolff, B. Moore & H. Marcuse (1969). *A critique of pure tolerance* (pp. 95–137). Boston, MA: Beacon Press. Available at www.marcuse.org/herbert/pubs/60spubs/65repressivetolerance.htm.

Martin, B. (1994). Plagiarism: A misplaced emphasis. *Journal of Information Ethics, 3*(2) 36–47. Available at: www.uow.edu.au/arts/sts/bmartin/pubs/94jie.html.

Martín-Baró, I. (1996). Toward a liberation psychology. In A. Aron & S. Corne (Eds.), *Writings for a liberation psychology*. New York, NY: Harvard University Press (Originally published as Hacia una psicología de la liberación. *Boletin de Psicología (UCA), 22,* 219–231, Available at www.uca.edu.sv/deptos/psicolog/hacia.htm.

Martín-Baró, I. (1989). *Sistema, grupo y poder: Psicología social desde Centroamérica II.* Sa Salvador, El Salvador: UCA Editores.

Martín-Baró, I. (1987). El latino indolente. Carácter ideológico del fatalismo latinoAmericano In M. Montero (Ed.), *Psicología política LatinoAmericana* (pp. 135–162). Caracas, Venezuela: Panapo. (Translated as The lazy Latino: The ideological nature of Latin America fatalism. Chapter 12 of Martín-Baró (1996)).

Martín-Baró, I. (1983). *Acción e ideología: Psicología social desde Centroamérica I.* San Salvador, El Salvador: UCA Editores.

Maton, K.I. (1989). Community settings as buffers of life stress? Highly supportive churches mutual help groups and senior centers. *American Journal of Community Psychology, 17* 203–232.

Mayer, C., & McKenzie, K. (2017). '. . . It shows that there's no limits': The psychological impact of co-production for experts by experience working in youth mental health. *Health & Social Care in the Community, 25*(3), 1181–1189.

Mayo, M. (1994). Community work. In Hanvey, C., & Philpot, T. (Eds.), *Practising social work*. London, England: Routledge.

Mayo, P. (1999). *Gramsci, Freire and adult education: Possibilities for transformative action* London, England: Zed Books.

McCarthy, J.D., & Zald, M.N. (1977). Resource mobilization and social movements: A partial theory *American Journal of Sociology, 82*(6), 1212.

McGill, I., & Brockbank, A. (2004). *The action learning handbook: Powerful techniques for education, professional development and training*. London, England: Routledge Falmer.

Mckenzie, L. (2015). *Getting by: Estates, class and culture in austerity Britain*. Bristol, England Policy Press.

McLaren, P. (2000). *Che Guevara, Paulo Freire and the pedagogy of revolution*. Lanham, MD Rowman and Littlefield.

McLaren, P., & Leonard, P. (Eds.). (1993). *Paulo Freire: A critical encounter*. London, England Routledge.

McLaughlin, J.A., & Jordan, G.B. (1999). Logic models: A tool for telling your program performance story. *Evaluation and Program Planning, 22*(1), 65–72.

McMillan, D.W., & Chavis, D.M. (1986). *Sense of community: Definition and theory*. London England: Routledge.

McNulty, D. (2005). *Dreams, dialogues and desires. Building a learning community in Blackburn with Darwen.* Leicester, England: NIACE.

Mead, M. (1978). *Culture and commitment.* New York, NY: Anchor Press.

Meadows, D.H. (2009). *Thinking in systems: A primer* (D. Wright, Ed.). London, England: Earthscan. Available at https://wtf.tw/ref/meadows.pdf.

Meari, L. (2015). Reconsidering trauma: Towards a Palestinian community psychology. *Journal of Community Psychology, 43*(1), 76–86.

Melluish, S., & Bulmer, D. (1999). Rebuilding solidarity: An account of a men's health action project. *Journal Community and Applied Social Psychology, 9*(2), 93–100.

Melucci, A. (1989). *Nomads of the present: Social movements and individual needs in contemporary society.* Philadelphia, PA: Temple University Press.

Merriam, S.B., Johnson-Bailey, J.; Lee, M-Y; Kee, Y., Ntseane, G., & Muhamad, M. (2001). Power and positionality: Negotiating insider/outsider status within and across cultures. *International Journal of Lifelong Education, 20*(5), 405–416.

Mewett, P.G. (1986). Boundaries and discourse in a Lewis crofting community. In A.P. Cohen (Ed.), *Symbolising community boundaries: Identity and diversity in British cultures.* Manchester, England: Manchester University Press.

Meyrowitz, J. (1986). *No sense of place: The impact of electronic media on social behaviour.* New York, NY: Oxford University Press.

Mezirow, J. (1983). A critical theory of adult learning and education. In M. Tight (Ed.), *Education for adults: Volume 1: Adult learning and education.* London, England: Croom Helm.

Michels, A., & De Graaf, L. (2010). Examining citizen participation: Local participatory policy making and democracy. *Local Government Studies, 36*(4), 477–491.

Mickelson, K.D., & Kubzansky, L.D. (2003). Social distribution of social support: The mediating role of life events. *American Journal of Community Psychology, 32*, 265–281.

Midgley, G. (2000). *Systemic intervention: Philosophy, methodology and practice.* New York, NY: Kluwer.

Midgley, G. (1992). Pluralism and the legitimation of systems science. *Systemic Practice and Action Research, 5*(2), 147–172.

Midgley, G., & Ochoa-Arias, A.E. (Eds.). (2004). *Community operational research: OR and systems thinking for community development.* New York, NY: Kluwer Academic/Plenum.

Midgley, G., Munlo, I., & Brown, M. (1998). The theory and practice of boundary critique: Developing housing services for older people. *Journal of the Operational Research Society, 49*, 467–478.

Milan, S., & van der Velden, L. (2016). The alternative epistemologies of data activism. *Digital Culture and Society, 2*(2), 57–74.

Miller, R.L. (2017). The practice of programme evaluation in community psychology. Intersections and opportunities for stimulating change. In M.A. Bond, I. García de Serrano, & C. Keys (Eds.), *APA handbook of community psychology* (1st ed., pp. 107–121). Washington, DC: American Psychological Association.

Mills, C.W. (1956). *The power elite.* New York, NY: Oxford University Press.

Moane, G. (2011). *Gender and colonialism: A psychological analysis of oppression and liberation.* Basingstoke, England: Palgrave Macmillan.

Moane, G. (2009). Reflections on liberation psychology in action in an Irish context. In M. Montero & C.C. Sonn (Eds.), *Psychology of liberation: Theory and applications.* New York, NY: Springer.

Moane, G. (2006). Exploring activism and change: Feminist psychology, liberation psychology, political psychology. *Feminism and Psychology, 16*(1), 73–78.

Moane, G. (2003). Bridging the personal and the political: Practices for a liberation psychology. *American Journal Community Psychology, 31*(1/2), 91–101.

Mollinson, B. (1988). *Permaculture: A designer's manual.* Tyalgum, Australia: Tagari.

Montero, M. (2013). Social consortium: A partnership of community agents. *Global Jour nal of Community Psychology Practice, 4*(2). Available at www.gjcpp.org/pdfs/Montero v4i2-20130531.pdf.

Montero, M. (2009). Methods for liberation: Critical consciousness in action. In M. Mon tero & C. Sonn (Eds.), *Psychology of liberation: Theory and applications.* New York, NY Springer.

Montero, M. (2006). *Hacer para transformar: El método en la psicología comunitaria.* [Actio for transformation: Method in community psychology]. Buenos Aires, Argentina: Ed. Paidós

Montero, M. (2004a). *Introducción a la psicología comunitaria: Desarrollo, conceptos y pro cesos* [Introduction to community psychology: development, concepts and processes]. Bue nos Aires, Argentina: Paidós.

Montero, M. (2004b). Relaciones entre psicología social comunitaria, psicología crítica y ps cología de la liberación: una respuesta latinoAmericana. *Psykhe (Chile), 13*(2), 17–28.

Montero, M. (2000a). Participation in action research. *Annual Review Critical Psycholog 2*, 131–143.

Montero, M. (2000b). Perspectivas y retos de la psicología de la liberación. In J.J. Vazque (Ed.), *Psicología social y liberación en América Latina* (pp. 9–26). Mexico City, Mexicc Universidad Autonoma de Mexico, Unidad de Iztapalapa.

Montero, M. (1998). Psychosocial community work as an alternative mode of political actio (the construction and critical transformation of society). *Community, Work and Famil, 1*(1), 65–78.

Montero, M. (1996). Parallel lives: Community psychology in Latin America and the Unite States. *American Journal of Community Psychology, 24*, 589–606.

Montero, M. (1994). Consciousness raising, conversion, and de-ideologization in communit psychosocial work. *Journal of Community Psychology, 22*(1), 3–11.

Montero, M. (1982). La psicología comunitaria: orígines, principios y fundamentos teóricc [Community psychology: origins, principles and theoretical foundations]. *Boletín de AVE PSO, 5*(1), 15–22.

Montero, M., & Montenegro, M. (2006). Critical Psychology in Venezuela. *Annuc Review of Critical Psychology, 5*, 257–268. Available at https://discourseunit.con annual-review/5-2006/.

Montero, M., & Varas-Díaz, N. (2007). Latin-American community psychology: Develo ment, implications and challenges within a social change agenda. In S. Reich, M. Rieme I. Prilleltensky & M. Montero (Eds.), *International community psychology: History an theories.* New York, NY: Springer.

Montero, M., Sonn, C., & Burton, M. (2016). Community psychology and liberation psy chology: Creative synergy for ethical and transformative praxis. In M.A. Bond, I. Garci de Serrano, & C. Keys (Eds.), *APA handbook of community psychology* (1st ed., Vol. 1 Washington, DC: American Psychological Association.

Moon, J.A. (2004). *A handbook of reflective and experiential learning: Theory and practic* Abingdon, England: Routledge and Falmer.

Morris, M. (2015). More than the Beatles: The legacy of a decade for community psycho ogy's contributions to evaluation ethics. *American Journal of Evaluation, 36*(1), 99–10 doi:10.1177/1098214014557808.

Moscovici, S., & Zavalloni, M. (1969). The group as a polarizer of attitudes. *Journal of Pe sonality and Social Psychology, 12*, 125–135.

Moscovici, S., Lage, E., & Naffrechoux, M. (1969). Influence of a consistent minority on th responses of a majority in a color perception task. *Sociometry, 32*, 365–380.

Murray, H., & Stewart, M. (2006). Who owns the theory of change? *Evaluation, 12*(2), 179–199.

Murtagh, B. (1999). Listening to communities: Locality research and planning. *Urban Studies, 36*(7), 1181–1193.

Napoleoni, L. (2008). *Rogue economics: Capitalism's new reality*. New York, NY: Seven Stories.

Natale, A., Di Martino, S., Procentese, F., & Arcidiacono, C. (2016). De-growth and critical community psychology: Contributions towards individual and social well-being. *Futures, 78–79*, 47–56. doi:10.1016/j.futures.2016.03.020.

New Economics Foundation (NEF). (2008a). *A green new deal. Joined-up policies to solve the triple crunch of the credit crisis, climate change and high oil prices: The first report of the Green New Deal Group*. London, England: New Economics Foundation.

New Economics Foundation (NEF). (2008b). *Co-production: A manifesto for growing the core economy*. London, England: New Economics Foundation.

New Economics Foundation (NEF). (1998). *Participation works! 21 techniques of community participation for the 21st century*. London, England: New Economics Foundation.

Nel, H. (2018). A comparison between the asset-oriented and needs-based community development approaches in terms of systems changes. *Practice, 30*(1), 33–52.

Nelson, G., & Prilleltensky, I. (Eds.). (2005). *Community psychology: In pursuit of liberation and well-being*. New York, NY: Palgrave/MacMillan.

Nelson, G., Poland, B., Murray, M., & Maticka-Tyndale, E. (2004). Building capacity in community health action research: Towards a praxis framework for graduate education. *Action Research, 2*, 389–408.

Neuwirth, R. (2006). *Shadow cities*, London, England: Routledge.

New Climate Economy. (2014). *Better growth, better climate*. New Climate Economy. Available at http://newclimateeconomy.report/2014/.

Nisbet, R.A. (1967). *The sociological tradition*. London, England: Heinemann.

North, P. (2010). Eco-localisation as a progressive response to peak oil and climate change: A sympathetic critique. *Geoforum 41*(4), 585–594. Published online at http://dx.doi.org/10.1016/j.geoforum.2009.04.013.

Odum, E.P. (1971). *Fundamentals of ecology* (3rd. ed.). Philadelphia, PA: Saunders Press.

Odum, H.T.O., & Odum, E.C. (2001). *A prosperous way down: Principles and policies*. Boulder: University Press of Colorado.

Office for National Statistics. (2018). *Labour market profile: Manchester* [Nomis: official labour market statistics]. Available at www.nomisweb.co.uk/reports/lmp/la/1946157083/report.aspx?town=Manchester#tabempunemp.

Oldenburg, R. (1989). *The great good place: Cafes, coffee shops, bookstores, bars, hair salons, and other hangouts at the heart of a community*. New York, NY: Marlowe and Company.

Oldenburg, R. (1997). Our vanishing third places. *Planning Commissioners Journal, 25*, 6–10.

Oldenburg, Ray (Ed.). (2001). *Celebrating the third place: Inspiring stories about the 'great good places' at the heart of our communities*. New York, NY: Marlowe & Co.

O'Leary, T., Burkett, I., Braithwaite, K., Carnegie United Kingdom Trust & IACD. (2011). *Appreciating assets*. Retrieved from https://d1ssu070pg2v9i.cloudfront.net/pex/carnegie_uk_trust/2011/06/14151707/pub1455011684.pdf.

O'Neil, J., & Marsick, V.J. (2007). *Understanding action learning*. New York, NY: Amacom.

Orford, J. (2008). *Community psychology: Challenges, controversies and emerging consensus* (2nd ed.). Chichester, England: Wiley.

Orford, J. (1998). Have we a theory of community psychology? *Clinical Psychology Forum 122*, 6–10.

Orford, J. (1992). *Community psychology: Theory and practice*. Chichester, England: Wiley.

Osterwalder, A., Pigneur, Y., & Clark, T. (2010). *Business model generation: A handbook fo* *visionaries, game changers, and challengers*. Hoboken, NJ: Wiley.

Packham, C. (1998). Community auditing as community development. *Community Develop* *ment Journal 33*(3), 249–259.

Pahl, K. (2004). Narratives, artefacts and cultural identities: An ethnographic study of com municative practices in homes. *Linguistics and Education. 15*(4), 339–358.

Pahl, R. (1970). *Patterns of urban life*. London, England: Longmans.

Painter, D., & Blanche, M.T. (2004). Critical psychology in South Africa: Looking back and looking forwards. *South African Journal of Psychology, 34*(4), 520–543 doi:10.1177/008124630403400402.

Painter, D., Terre Blanche, M., & Henderson, J. (2006). Critical psychology in South Africa Histories, themes and prospects. *Annual Review of Critical Psychology, 5*, 215–235.

Parker, I. (2007). *Revolution in psychology: Alienation to emancipation*. London, England Pluto.

Parker, I.A. (2005). *Qualitative psychology: Introducing radical research*. Maidenhead England: Open University Press.

Parker, I.A. (1999). *Deconstructing psychology*. London, England: Sage.

Parker, I., & Spears, R. (Eds.). (1996). *Psychology and society: Radical theory and practice* London, England: Pluto Press.

Parry, O., & Mauthner, N.S. (2004). Whose data are they anyway? Practical, legal and ethica issues in archiving qualitative research data. *Sociology, 38*(1), 139–152.

Parsons, T. (1957). The distribution of power in American Society. *World Politics, 10*(1 123–143.

Pawson, R., & Tilley, N. (2004). *Realist evaluation*. Available at www.communitymatters.com au/RE_chapter.pdf.

Pawson, R., & Tilley, N. (1997). *Realistic evaluation*. London, England: Sage.

Pearce, J. (2010). Co-producing knowledge: Critical reflections on researching participatior In J. Pearce (Ed.), *Participation and democracy in the twenty first century* (pp. 34–50). Bas ingstoke, England: Palgrave Macmillan.

Pearce, J., Raynard, P., & Zadek, S. (1996). *Social auditing for small organisations: The work book for trainers and practitioners*. London, England: New Economic Foundation.

Pearpoint, J., O'Brien, J., & Forest, M. (1993). *Path: A workbook for planning possible pos tive futures: Planning alternative tomorrows with hope for schools, organizations, bus nesses, families*. Toronto, Canada: Inclusion Press.

Pels, P. (1999). Professions of duplexity: A prehistory of ethical codes in anthropology. *Currer Anthropology, 40*, 101–136.

People's Plan. (2017). *People's Plan: Greater Manchester*. Manchester, England: People: PlanGM. Available at www.peoplesplangm.org.uk/wp-content/uploads/2017/04/PEOPLE PLAN-April-2017.pdf.

Perkins, D.D., García-Ramírez, M., Menezes, I., Serrano-García, I., & Stromopolis, M. (2016 Community psychology and public policy: Research, advocacy and training in internationa contexts. *Global Journal of Community Psychology Practice, 7*(1), *online*. Available at www gjcpp.org/en/article.php?issue=21&article=124.

Petras, J., & Veltmeyer, H. (2005). *Social movements and state power*. London, England: Plut Press.

Petras, J., & Veltmeyer, H. (2001). *Globalization unmasked: Imperialism in the 21st centur* London, England: Zed Books.

Pettigrew, A., Ferlie, E., & McKee, L. (1992). *Shaping strategic change*. London, England: Sag hythian, G. (2018). *Peterloo: Voices, sabres and silence*. Stroud, Gloucestershire, England: The History Press.

ortes, A., & Landolt, P. (1996). The downside of social capital. *American Prospect, 26*, 18–22.

otter, J. (2001). Wittgenstein and Austin. In M. Wetherell, S. Taylor & S. Yates (Eds.), *Discourse theory and practice*. London, England: Sage.

reskill, H., & Boyle, S. (2008). A multidisciplinary model of evaluation capacity building. *American Journal of Evaluation, 29*(4), 443–459.

retorius-Heuchert, J., & Ahmed, R. (2001). Community psychology: Past, present, and future. In M. Seedat, N. Duncan & S. Lazarus (Eds.), *Community psychology, theory, method, and practice. South African and other perspectives*. Cape Town, South Africa: Oxford.

riestley, M. (2006). Disability and old age: Or why it isn't all in the mind. In D. Goodley & R. Lawthom (Eds.), *Disability and psychology: Critical introductions and reflections*. Basingstoke, England: Palgrave Macmillan.

rilleltensky, I. (2008). The role of power in wellness, oppression, and liberation: The promise of psychopolitical validity. *Journal Community Psychology, 36*(2), 116–136.

rilleltensky, I., & Nelson, G. (1997). Community psychology: Reclaiming social justice. In I.D. Fox & I. Prilleltensky (Eds.), *Critical psychology: An introduction*. London, England: Sage. Psychologists Against Austerity (PAA). (2015). *The psychological impact of austerity* (p. 16). London, England: Psychologists for Social Change. Available at https://psychagain-stausterity.files.wordpress.com/2015/03/paa-briefing-paper.pdf.

sychologists for Social Change. (2017). *Universal basic income: A psychological impact assessment*. London, England: PSC. Available at www.psychchange.org/uploads/9/7/9/7/97971280/ubi_for_web_updated.pdf.

ublic Health England. (2018). Local authority health profiles. Available at https://fingertips.phe.org.uk/profile/health-profiles.

utnam, R.D. (1995). Bowling alone: America's declining social capital. *Journal of Democracy, 6*, 65–78.

Quijano, A. (2000). Coloniality of power, Eurocentrism, and Latin America. *Neplanta, 1*(3). Available at www.decolonialtranslation.com/english/quijano-coloniality-of-power.pdf.

adford, J. (2008). Psychology in its place. *Psychology Teaching Review, 14*, 38–50.

appaport, J., & Seidman, E. (Eds.). (2000). *Handbook of community psychology*. New York, NY: Kluwer/Plenum Publishers.

ashford, N.S., & Coghlan, D. (1989). Phases and levels of organisational change. *Journal of Managerial Psychology, 4*(3), 17–22.

avetz, J. (2000). *City region 2020: Integrated planning for a sustainable environment*. London, England: Earthscan.

ay, L.J. (1993). *Rethinking critical theory: Emancipation in the age of global social movements*. London, England: Sage.

aynes, N., Kagan, C., Varela-Raynes, A., & Bolt, B. (2013). *From generation to generation via Intergen: An intergenerational approach to active ageing*. Paper presented to International Initiative on Ageing, Istanbul. Available from http://fromgeneration2generation.org.uk/intergen-evidence-base/.

eason, P., & Bradbury, H. (2001). Introduction: Inquiry and participation in search of a world worthy of human aspiration. In P. Reason & H. Bradbury (Eds.), *Handbook of action research: Participative inquiry and practice*. London, England: Sage.

ebien, C.C. (1996). Participatory evaluation of development assistance: Dealing with power and facilitative learning. *Evaluation, 2*(2), 151–172.

eich, S., Riemer, M., Prilleltensky, I., & Montero, M. (Eds.). (2007). *International community psychology: History and theories*. New York, NY: Springer.

Revans, R. (1980). *Action learning: New techniques for management*. London, England: Blon‹ and Briggs, Ltd.

Revenson, T., D'Augelli, A., French, S., Hughes, D., Livert, D., Seidman, E., et al. (Eds.). (2002) *Ecological research to promote social change: Methodological advances from communit‹ psychology*. New York, NY: Kluwer Academic/Plenum Publishers.

Reyes Cruz, M., & Sonn, C.C. (2011). (De)colonizing culture in community psychology‹ Reflections from critical social science. *American Journal of Community Psychology, 47*(1‹ 2), 203–214.

Richards, M., Lawthom, R., & Runswick-Cole, K. (2018). Community-based arts researc‹ for people with learning disabilities: Challenging misconceptions about learning disabilitie‹ *Disability & Society*. 1–24, online.

Riley, V. (1998). Listening to caregivers: The community, work and family interface. *Commu‹ nity, Work and Family, 1*(1), 95–98.

Robertson, N., & Masters-Awatere, B. (2007). Community psychology in Aotearoa/New Zea‹ land. In S. Reich, M. Riemer, I. Prilleltensky & M. Montero (Eds.), *International communit‹ psychology: History and theories*. New York, NY: Springer.

Rockström, J., Steffen, W., Noone, K., Persson, Å., Chapin, F.S.I., Lambin, E., . . . Foley, ‹ (2009a). Planetary boundaries: Exploring the safe operating space for humanity. *Ecolog‹ and Society, 14*(2), art. 32, online. doi:10.5751/ES-03180–140232.

Rockström, J., Steffen, W., Noone, K., Persson, Å., Chapin, F.S., Lambin, E.F., . . . Foley, J.‹ (2009b). A safe operating space for humanity. *Nature, 461*(7263), 472–475.

Rogers, C. (1969). *Freedom to learn*. Ohio, OH: Merrill (Reprinted as Rogers & Frieberg, 1994

Rogers, C., & Frieberg, H.J. (1994). *Freedom to learn* (3rd ed.). Ohio, OH: Merrill/Macmilla‹

Runswick-Cole, K., Goodley, D., & Lawthom, R. (2018). Resilience in the lives of disable‹ children: A many splendoured thing. In K. Runswick-Cole, T. Curran, & K. Liddia‹ (Eds.), *The Palgrave handbook of disabled children's childhood studies* (pp. 425–442‹ doi:10.1057/978–1–137–54446–9_27.

Sacipa-Rodríguez, S., Tovar-Guerra, C., Villareal, L.F.G., & Bohórquez, V. (2009). Psycholog‹ cal accompaniment: Construction of cultures of peace among a community affected by wa‹ In M. Montero & C. Sonn (Eds.), *Psychology of liberation: Theory and applications*. Ne‹ York, NY: Springer.

Sale, K. (1985). *Dwellers in the land*. San Francisco, CA: Sierra Club.

Sampson, E.E. (2000). Reinterpreting individualism and collectivism: Their religious root‹ and monologic versus dialogic person-other relationship. *American Psychologist, 55*(12‹ 1425–1432.

Sánchez, E., Cronick, K., & Wiesenfeld, E. (1988). Psychosocial variables and participation: ‹ case study. In D. Canter, M. Kramping & D. Stea (Eds.), *New Directions in Environment‹ Participation* (Vol. 3). Aldershot, England: Avebury.

Sarason, S.B. (1988). *The psychological sense of community: Prospects for a community ps‹ chology* (2nd ed.). San Francisco, CA: Jossey-Bass.

Sarason, S.B. (1974). *The psychological sense of community: Prospects for a community ps‹ chology*. San Francisco, CA: Jossey-Bass.

Sarason, S.B. (1972). *The creation of settings and the future societies*. San Francisco, C‹ Jossey Bass.

Schön, D.A. (1983). *The reflective practitioner: How professionals think in action*. New Yor‹ NY: Basic Books.

Schrader McMillan, A., & Burton, M. (2009). From parent education to collective actio‹ 'Childrearing with love' in post-war Guatemala. *Journal of Community and Applied Ps‹ chology, 19*(3), 198–211.

eedat, M. (2015). Oral history as an enactment of critical community psychology: Oral history as critical enactment. *Journal of Community Psychology, 43*(1), 22–35.

eedat, M., Duncan, N., & Lazarus, S. (Eds.). (2001). *Community psychology: Theory, method and practice*. Cape Town, South Africa: Oxford University Press.

eidman, E. (1988). Back to the future, community psychology: Unfolding a theory of intervention. *American Journal Community Psychology, 16*(1), 3–24.

eidman, E. (1986). Justice, values and social science: Unexamined premises. In E. Seidman & J. Rapaport (Eds.), *Redefining social problems*. New York, NY: Plenum Press.

en, R., & Goldbart, J. (2005). Partnership in action: Introducing family-based intervention for children with disability in urban slums of Kolkata, India. *International Journal of Disability, Development and Education, 52*(4), 275–311.

errano-García, I. (2016). Social policy: The tightwire we walk (A commentary). *Global Journal of Community Psychology Practice, 4*(2), online. Available at www.gjcpp.org/pdfs/Serrano-Garcia-v4i2-20130613.pdf.

ève, L. (1975). *Marxism and the theory of human personality*. London, England: Lawrence and Wishart.

hankar, S., Dick, B., Passfield, R., & Swepson, P. (Eds.). (2002). *Effective change management using action learning and action research*. Lismore, Australia: Southern Cross Press.

haw, I., Greene, J., & Mark, M. (2006). *Sage handbook of evaluation*. London, England: Sage.

heldon, J.A., & Wolfe, S.M. (2015). The community psychology evaluation nexus. *American Journal of Evaluation, 36*(1), 86–89. doi:10.1177/1098214014558503.

hiell, A., & Riley, T. (2017). Methods and methodology of systems analysis. In M.A. Bond, I. Serrano-García, C.B. Keys, & M. Shinn (Eds.), *APA handbook of community psychology: Methods for community research and action for diverse groups and issues* (pp. 155–169). Washington, DC: American Psychological Association.

hore, C., & Wright, S. (1999). Audit culture and anthropology: Neo-liberalism in British higher education. *Journal of the Royal Anthropological Institute, 5*, 557–575.

iddiquee, A., & Kagan, C. (2006). The internet, empowerment, and identity: An exploration of participation by refugee women in a Community Internet Project (CIP) in the United Kingdom (UK). *Journal Community and Applied Social Psychology, 16*(2), 189–206.

ilverman, T. (2001). Expanding community: The internet and relational theory. *Community, Work and Family, 4*(2), 231–238.

ixsmith, J., & Kagan, C. (2005). *Pathways Project evaluation: Final report*. Manchester, England: RIHSC.

ixsmith, J., Callender, M., Hobbs, G., Corr, S., & Huber, J.W. (2014). Implementing the National Service Framework for long-term (neurological) conditions: Service user and service provider experiences. *Disability and Rehabilitation, 36*(7), 563–572. doi:10.3109/096 38288.2013.804594.

loan, T. (2005). Globalization, poverty and social justice. In G. Nelson & I. Prilleltensky (Eds.), *Community psychology: In pursuit of liberation and well-being*. Basingstoke, England: Palgrave Macmillan.

mail, D. (1999). *The origins of unhappiness*. London, England: Constable (Reproduced in *Power, responsibility and freedom*. Available at https://the-eye.eu/public/WorldTracker.org/Sociology/David%20Smail%20-%20Power%2C%20Responsibility%20and%20Freedom%20-%20 Internet%20Publication%20%282005%29.pdf.

mail, D. (1993). Putting our mouths where our money is. *Clinical Psychology Forum, 61*, 11–14.

mith, M.K. (2002). 'Paulo Freire and informal education', *Encyclopaedia of informal education*. http://infed.org/mobi/paulo-freire-dialogue-praxis-and-education.

Smith, N.L. (2007). Empowerment evaluation as evaluation ideology. *American Journal c Evaluation, 28*(2), 169–178.

Smithers, R. (2017, January 10). UK throwing away £13bn of food each yea: *Guardian.* Available at www.theguardian.com/environment/2017/jan/1C uk-throwing-away-13bn-of-food-each-year-latest-figures-show.

Smits, P.A., & Champagne, F. (2008). An assessment of the theoretical underpinnings of pract cal participatory evaluation. *American Journal of Evaluation, 29*(4), 427–442.

Social Value UK. (n.d.). *What is social value?* Available at www.socialvalueuk.org what-is-social-value/.

Society for Community Research and Action (SCRA). (2012). Competencies for communit psychology practice: Draft August 15, 2012. *The Community Psychologist, 45*(4), 7–14.

Society for Community Research and Action (SCRA). (n.d.). *An evidence informed commu nity psychology value proposition.* Available at www.scra27.org/files/4513/9007/7333/Ev dence_based_CP_Value_Proposition__Final_20110829.pdf.

Spangler, B. (2003). Coalition building. In G. Burgess & H. Burgess (Eds.), *Beyond intracta bility.* Boulder: Conflict Research Consortium, University of Colorado. Available at www beyondintractability.org/essay/coalition_building.

Sprigings, N., & Allen, C. (2005). The communities we are regaining but need to lose. A crit cal commentary on community building in beyond-place societies. *Community, Work an Family, 8*(4), 389–411. doi:10.1080/13668800500263032.

Stake, R.E. (1980). Program evaluation, particularly responsive evaluation. In W.B. Dockerell & D. Hamilton (Eds.), *Rethinking educational research.* London, England: Hodder and Stoughtor

Standing, G. (2018). *The precariat: Today's transformative class.* Available at www.greattrans tion.org/publication/precariat-transformative-class.

Steffen, W., Richardson, K., Rockström, J., Cornell, S.E., Fetzer, I., Bennett, E.M., . . . Sorlin, ! (2015). Planetary boundaries: Guiding human development on a changing planet. *Scienc 347*(6223), 1259855–1259855. doi:10.1126/science.1259855.

Stewart, A., & Kagan, C. (2008). *The 'In Bloom' competition: Gardening work as a commu nity involvement strategy.* Manchester, England: RIHSC. Available at https://e-space.mmu ac.uk/41941/1/978-1-900139-24-3.pdf.

Stiegler, B. (2006). The disaffected individual in the process of psychic and collective disind viduation. Extract from the 3rd chapter of *Mécréance et Discrédit: Tome 2. Les sociéte incontrôlables d'individus désaffectés* (Paris, France: Editions Galilée, 2006), published as working paper for the Ars Industrialis seminar, 'Suffering and consumption', February 2: 2006, translated by Patrick Crogan & Daniel Ross. Available at http://tinyurl.com/yjregfv

Streck, D.R., & Jara, O. (2015). Research, participation and social transformation: Groundin systematization of experiences in Latin American perspectives. In Hilary Bradbury (Ed. *The SAGE handbook of action research* (3rd ed., pp. 472–480). London, England: SAG Publications Ltd.

Stringer, E. (1999). *Action research* (2nd ed.). Palo Alto, CA: Sage.

Suárez-Herrara, J.C., Springett, J., & Kagan, C. (2009). Critical connections between partic patory evaluation, organizational learning and intentional change in pluralistic organiza tion. *Evaluation, 15*(30), 321–342.

Suffla, S., Seedat, M., & Bawa, U. (2015). Reflexivity as enactment of critical community ps chologies: Dilemmas of voice and positionality in a multi-country photovoice study. *Journ of Community Psychology, 43*(1), 9–21.

Sultana, F. (2007). Reflexivity, positionality and participatory ethics: Negotiating fieldwor dilemmas in international research. *ACME: An International E-Journal for Critical Geo raphies, 6*(3), 374–385.

utherland, W.J., Spiegelhalter, D., & Bergman, M.A. (2013). Twenty tips for interpreting scientific claims. *Nature, 503*, 335.

windells, R., Lawthom, R., Rowley, K., Siddiquee, A., Kilroy, A., & Kagan, C. (2013). Eudaimonic well-being and community arts participation. *Perspectives in Public Health, 133*(1), 60–65.

ynnot, B., & Fitzgerald, R. (2007). *The toolbox for change: A practical approach.* Brisbane, Australia: Danjugah.

zreter, S. (2002). The state of social capital: Bringing back in power, politics, and history. *Theory and Society, 31*, 573–621.

aket, A., & White, L. (2000). *Partnership and participation. Decision making in the multiagency setting.* Chichester, England: John Wiley.

anguay, J. (2012). *Well-being in Vanuatu.* Vanuatu: VKS Studios. Available at www.youtube. com/watch?v=jtnLl1Jp0K0.

awney, R.H. (1938). *Religion and the rise of capitalism: A historical study.* Harmondsworth, England: Pelican.

aylor, M., & Burns, D. (2000). *Auditing community participation: An assessment handbook.* Bristol, England: Policy Press.

aylor, M., Purdue, D., Wilson, M., & Wilde, P. (2005). *Evaluating community projects: A practical guide.* Available at www.jrf.org.uk/sites/files/jrf/1859354157.pdf.

aylor-Gooby, P., & Dale, J. (1981). *Social theory and social welfare.* London, Edward Arnold.

herborn, G. (2009). The killing fields of inequality. *Soundings, 42*, 20–32.

herborn, G. (1980). *What does the ruling class do when it rules? State apparatuses and state power under feudalism, capitalism and socialism.* London, England: Verso.

homas, D., & Veno, A. (1992). *Psychology and social change: Creating an international agenda.* Palmerston North, New Zealand: Dunmore Press.

homas, D.R., & Robertson, N. (1992). A conceptual framework for the analysis of social policies. In D. Thomas & A. Veno. (1992). *Psychology and social change: Creating an international agenda.* Palmerston North, New Zealand: Dunmore Press.

hompson, J.B. (1990). *Ideology and modern culture: Critical social theory in the era of mass communication.* Cambridge, England: Polity Press.

hompson, S., & Thompson, N. (2008). *The critically reflective practitioner.* Basingstoke, England: Palgrave Macmillan.

iffany, G. (2009). *Community philosophy: A project report.* York, England: Joseph Rowntree Foundation.

ilakaratna, S. (1990). *A short note on participatory research.* Paper presented to a seminar of Sri Lankan social scientists and community specialists in January 1990. www.caledonia. org.uk/research.htm.

önnies, F. (1887/2002). *Community and society.* Newton Abbott, England: David and Charles (First published in 1887 as *Gemeinschaft und Gesellschaft*, Leipzig, Germany: Fues's Verlag).

opping, A. (2008, March 12). Communalist revolution. *Society Guardian.* Available at www. guardian.co.uk/society/2008/mar/12/regeneration.communities.

ouraine, A. (1988). *The return of the actor: Social theory in post-industrial society.* Minneapolis: University of Minnesota Press.

ouraine, A. (1981). *The voice and the eye: An analysis of social movements.* Cambridge, England: Cambridge University Press.

oval Guerra, C. (2014). Personal resources and empowerment in a psychosocial accompaniment process. In S. Sacipa-Rodríguez & M. Montero (Eds.), *Psychosocial approaches to peace-building in Colombia* (pp. 75–87). Cham, Switzerland: Springer.

Trades Union Congress (1995). *Britain divided: Insecurity at work*. London, England: TUC.

Trickett, E.J., Barone, C., & Watts, R.J. (2000). Contextual influences in mental health consultation: Toward an ecological perspective on radiating change. In J. Rapaport & E. Seidma (Eds.), *Hand-book of community psychology*. New York, NY: Kluwer Academic/Plenur Publishers.

Tyler, C. (2013, December 2). Top 20 things scientists need to know about policy making. *Guardian*. Available at www.theguardian.com/science/2013/dec/02 scientists-policy-governments-science.

UK Community Psychology Network. (2007). *York Statement on Poverty – September 2007* Available from www.compsy.org.uk.

UK Government. (2015). *The English Indices of Deprivation: Statistical release*. Londor England: Ministry of Housing Communities and Local Government. Available at https: assets.publishing.service.gov.uk/government/uploads/system/uploads/attachment_data file/465791/English_Indices_of_Deprivation_2015_-_Statistical_Release.pdf.

Ulrich, W. (2005). *A brief introduction to critical systems heuristics (CSH)*. ECOSENSUS project website, The Open University, Milton Keynes, England, October 14, 2005. Available a http://projects.kmi.open.ac.uk/ecosensus/publications/ulrich_csh_intro.pdf.

Ulrich, W., & Reynolds, M. (2010). Critical systems heuristics. In M. Reynolds & S. Holwe (Eds.), *Systems approaches to managing change: A practical guide*. (pp. 243–292). Londor England: Springer.

Veno, A., & Thomas, D.R. (1992). Psychology and the process of social change. In D.R. Thoma & A. Veno. (1992). *Psychology and social change: Creating an international agenda*. Palm erston North, New Zealand: Dunmore Press.

Vergara-Camus, L. (2014). *Land and freedom: The MST, the Zapatistas and peasant alterna tives to neoliberalism*. London, England: Zed Books.

Vidales, R. (2014). Memory, narrative and the social transformation of reality. In S. Sacipa Rodríguez & M. Montero (Eds.), *Psychosocial approaches to peace-building in Colombi* (pp. 89–110). Cham, Switzerland: Springer.

Wainwright, H. (2009). *Reclaim the state: Experiments in popular democracy*. Londor England: Seagull Books.

Walker, C. (2017). *Attacking the neoliberal university from 'within' – Statactivism, critica praxis and the National Senior Managers Survey*. Presented at the 3rd UK community Psy chology Festival, Bristol, England: UWE//BPS Community Psychology Section. Available a http://eprints.uwe.ac.uk/33503/6/CPF%20Book%20of%20Abstracts.pdf.

Walker, C., Hart, A., & Hanna, P. (2017). *Building a new community psychology of ment health: Spaces, places, people and activities*. London, England: Palgrave Macmillan.

Walker, I., & Smith, H.J. (eds). (2002). *Relative deprivation: Specification, development, an integration*. Cambridge, England: Cambridge University Press.

Wallerstein, I. (2004). *World systems analysis*. Durham, NC: Duke University Press.

Wallerstein, I. (1996a). *Historical capitalism, with capitalist civilization*. London, Englanc Verso.

Wallerstein, I. (1996b). *World-systems analysis: An introduction*. Durham, NC: Duke Unive sity Press.

Wandersman, A., Snell-Johns, J., Lentz, B.E., Fetterman, D.M., Keener, D.C., Livet, M., Imn P.S., Flaspohler, P. (2005). The principles of empowerment evaluation. In Fetterman, D., & Wandersman, A. (Eds.), *Empowerment evaluation principles in practice*. New York, N\ Guildford Press.

Watkins, M. (2015). Psychosocial accompaniment. *Journal of Social and Political Psycholog* 3(1), 324–341.

Watson, B. (2005). *Bread and roses: Mills, migrants, and the struggle for the American dream.* New York, NY: Viking.

Watson, E.R., & Foster-Fishman, P.G. (2013). The exchange boundary framework: Understanding the evolution of power within collaborative decision-making settings. *American Journal of Community Psychology, 51*(1–2), 151–163.

Weber, M. (1946). *From Max Weber: Essay in sociology* (Hans H. Gerth & C. Wright Mills, Trans. & Ed.). New York, NY: Oxford University Press.

Weber, M. (1904/1930). *The Protestant ethic and the spirit of capitalism.* London, England: George Allen and Unwin University Books. (Ethik und der Geist des Kapitalismus, Archiv für Sozialwissen-schaft und Sozialpolitik, 20.).

Weil, S.W., & McGill, I. (Eds.). (1989). *Making sense of experiential learning. Diversity in theory and practice.* Milton Keynes, England: Open University Press.

Wenger, E. (1998). *Communities of practice: Learning meaning and identity.* New York, NY: Cambridge University Press.

Wenger, E.C., McDermott, R., & Snyder, W.C. (2002). *Cultivating communities of practice: A guide to managing knowledge.* Cambridge, MA: Harvard Business School Press.

Wertsch, J. (1990). The voice of rationality in a sociocultural approach to mind. In Moll, L.C. (Ed.), *Vygotsky and education.* New York, NY: Cambridge University Press.

Whelan, P. & Lawthom, R. (2009). Transdisciplinary learning. Exploring pedagogical links between feminism and community psychology. Special Issue of *Feminism and Psychology, 19*(3), 414–418.

Whyte, W.F. (1943). *Street corner society* (4th ed., 1993). Chicago, IL: University of Chicago Press.

Wilcox, D. (1994). *Guide to effective participation.* York, England: Joseph Rowntree Foundation. Available at http://partnerships.org.uk/guide/.

Wilkinson, R. (2005). *The impact of inequality: How to make sick societies healthier.* London, England: Routledge.

Wilkinson, R.G. (1996). *Unhealthy societies: The afflictions of inequality.* London, England: Routledge.

Wilkinson, R., & Pickett, K. (2009). *The spirit level: Why more equal societies almost always do better.* Harmondsworth, England: Penguin.

Wilkinson, R.G., Kawachi, I., & Kennedy, B.P. (1998). Mortality, the social environment, crime and violence. *Sociology of Health and Illness, 20*(5), 578–597.

Williams, C.C., Aldridge, T., Lee, R., Leyshon, A., Thrift, N., & Tooke, J. (2001). Local exchange and trading schemes (LETS): A tool for community renewal? *Community, Work and Family, 4*(3), 355–361.

Williams, R. (1980). *Problems in materialism and culture: Selected essays.* London, England: Verso. (Reissued as *Culture and materialism*, Verso radical thinkers series, 2005).

Williams, R. (1976). *Keywords: A vocabulary of culture and society.* Glasgow, Scotland: Collins Fontana.

Willmott, P. (1989). *Community initiatives. Patterns and prospects.* London, England: Policy Studies Institute.

Wittgenstein, L. (1953). *Philosophical investigations.* Oxford, England: Blackwell.

Wolff, T. (2001a). Community coalition building: Contemporary practice and research: Introduction. *American Journal Community Psychology, 29*(2), 165–172.

Wolff, T. (2001b). A practitioner's guide to successful coalitions. *American Journal Community Psychology, 29*(2), 173–191.

Woolrych, R.D., & Sixsmith, J.A. (2008). *Final report: Understanding health and well-being in the context of urban regeneration.* Manchester case study for HEFCE: Urban Regeneration – Making a Difference Project. Manchester, England: RIHSC.

Woolrych, R., Sixsmith, J., & Kagan, C. (2007). *The impact of regeneration on the well-being of local residents: The case of East Manchester*. Manchester, England: RIHSC. Available at https://e-space.mmu.ac.uk/41939/.

Worley, C. (2005). It's not about race. It's about the community: New Labour and community cohesion. *Critical Social Policy, 25*(4), 483–496.

Wrong, D.H. (1979). *Power: Its forms, bases and uses*. Oxford, England: Blackwell.

Yeo, S., & Evans, S. (2016). *The 35 countries cutting the link between economic growth and emissions*. Carbon Brief Website. Available at www.carbonbrief.org the-35-countries-cutting-the-link-between-economic-growth-and-emissions.

Zacharzewski, A. (2011). *Democracy for new radicals*. Available at www.demsoc.org blog/2011/05/03/democracy-for-new-radicals.

Zald, M.N., & McCarthy, J.D. (1988). *The dynamics of social movements: Resource mobilization, social control, and tactics*. Lanham, MD: University Press of America.

Zambrano, A.C. (2007). Participación y empoderamiento comunitario: Role de las methodology's implicativas. In A.C. Zambrano, G.O. Rozas, I.F. Magaña, D.S. Asún & R.A. Pérez-Luco (Eds.), *Psicología comunitaria en Chile: Evolución, perspectivas y proyecciones* [Community psychology in Chile: Development, perspectives and projections]. Santiago d Chile: RIL editores.

Zúñiga, R. (1975). The experimenting society and radical social reform: The role of the social scientist in Chile's Unidad Popular experience. *American Psychologist, 30*(2), 99–115.

Chapter 4
Social status and disadvantage

Catherine Haslam, Jolanda Jetten, Tegan Cruwys,
Genevieve Dingle and S. Alexander Haslam

Wherever people live together, hierarchies quickly develop. Because of their income, wealth, education, living conditions, skills, gender, ethnicity, geographical location, or social standing more generally, some individuals and some groups find themselves at the top of the hierarchy while others occupy lower-status positions. The rank that people have in society or in particular groups also affects important outcomes in life: access to resources, education, housing, quality of employment, and the extent to which they can exert power and social influence over others.

Even though social status, social rank, social class, and socio-economic status (SES) are not identical concepts and all refer to different divisions in society, in this chapter, we will refer to them as 'social status' for short. Importantly for our current purposes, this general social status concept is also a major determinant of health and well-being. Typically, we find that people at the bottom of a particular status hierarchy have the poorest health and those at the top have the best health. This so-called "*health gradient*" (Marmot, 2004, 2015) is not only found when examining various health risk factors (such as smoking, obesity, high blood pressure, or lack of exercise), but also is strongly associated with the prevalence of illnesses (such as depression, heart disease, diabetes, and cancer). Notably too, SES is a powerful predictor of mortality (for reviews see Braveman, Cubbin, Egerter, Williams, & Pamuk, 2010; Marmot, 2004, 2015; Putnam, 2000; Syme & Berkman, 1976; Wilkinson & Pickett, 2009). As Figure 3.1 shows, the statistics are stark. In Australia, for example, the richest 20% of the population live on average six years longer than the poorest 20% (Friel, 2014).

In this chapter we will focus on the reasons why social status (and in particular the lack of social status that is associated with social disadvantage) has such a profound effect on health and well-being. Even though the root causes of social disadvantage are many (including low levels of education, adverse early-life experiences, disability, stigma, and discrimination), in this chapter we will home in on the health-related effects of disadvantage (e.g., those relating to living in a deprived community, poor housing, or housing instability). In that sense, social disadvantage is more than a lack of access to financial and economic resources and involves multiple forms of social exclusion (see Cruwys et al., 2013a; Saunders, 2008). The negative health effects of stigma and discrimination will then be the focus of the next chapter.

An astute reader may ask why we would be interested in attempting to develop psychosocial explanations of the health gradient (see Figure 3.2). Is it not the case that there are straightforward non-psychosocial explanations for this relationship? For example, might it not be explained simply by the fact that poor people have less access to the health system and so do not get appropriate help for their mental and physical health conditions? Likewise, might it not simply be the case that those with lower education have poorer health than their more educated counterparts because they lack knowledge about how to live a healthy life and/or are more likely to engage in risky health behaviour (e.g., excessive alcohol consumption, drug taking)?

Although there is some logic to this reasoning (see Compton & Shim, 2015), findings from a range of studies suggest that these economic factors do not fully account for the health gradient (see Marmot, 2015; Sapolsky, 2004; Wilkinson & Pickett, 2009). This is for a number of reasons. First, the gradient can be found in all countries, and it is unaffected by the extent to which health care is affordable and accessible to all citizens. Second, the gradient exists even for diseases where preventative health or quality of health care is less relevant (e.g., juvenile diabetes; see Sapolsky, 2004). A health gradient is also present in mental illnesses (e.g., depression, schizophrenia, anxiety) – conditions where it is

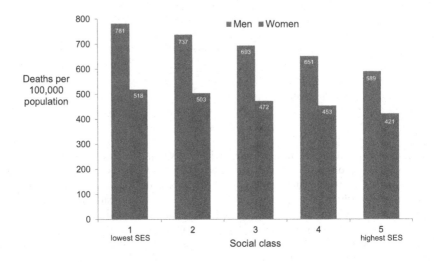

Figure 3.1 The health gradient

Note: This graph plots death rates among 15- to 64 year-old Australians between 2009 and 2011 as a function of socio-economic status (SES). This shows two clear main effects: men and members of low SES groups are much more likely to die than women and members of high SES groups.

Source: Australian Institute of Health and Welfare (2014)

clear that there is not a straightforward biological or genetic cause (Syme & Berkman, 1976; e.g., see Chapters 8 and 13). Third, and perhaps more intriguingly, data suggest that worse health is not only observed for those below a particular poverty line or education level. Instead, the health gradient is linear: with every increment of wealth and education, health improves. As we will explain further, this means that the health of people in the top 5% income bracket is better than that of those in the 5% income bracket just below them. And their health in turn is better than that of those in the 5% income bracket just below them, and so on. Put differently, even for those groups for whom all basic economic and financial needs are well met and where it is unlikely that there are substantial differences in education or key health services, we find that differences in wealth and income matter for health and well-being. This suggests that social disadvantage is about a lot more than just "having enough money".

In an attempt to better understand the psychosocial determinants of the health gradient, we start this chapter with a review of the biological and social determinants of health. Building on work by social scientists who have highlighted the important role that social capital and control play in determining our health, we explain how this is linked to a social identity analysis of health. In particular, we will outline how our social group memberships are integral to the development of social capital and a sense of control. Indeed, we argue that how we manage our social group memberships (and the social identities associated with them) holds the key to a better understanding of these processes.

One of the key insights of this chapter is that the way social status affects health may be quite different depending on whether people find themselves in a stable versus more unstable situation. Instability in particular threatens health, but it does so differently for people of high and low status. For

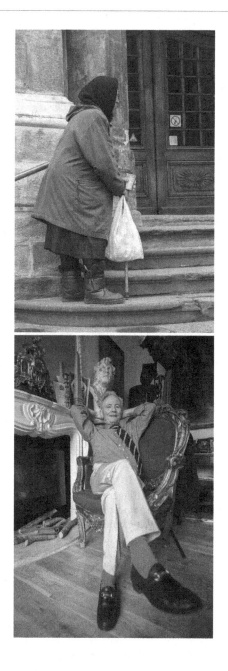

Figure 3.2 Wealth inequality: a cause of ill health for both the poor and the rich

Note: A large body of evidence shows that wealth inequality has a significant negative impact on the health of all members of a given society (e.g., see Wilkinson & Pickett, 2009). It is easy to understand why this is the case for those who are poor, but it is less obvious why this is also true for those who are wealthy.

Source: Pixabay

high-status groups, health declines when their social status is threatened; whereas for low-status groups health declines when there are insufficient resources or opportunities to improve their status. We will start to unpack this issue by first exploring different forms of status threats (in particular, related to situations where status is unstable, illegitimate, or when group boundaries are not permeable). After this, we will explore how status affects our health when we are going through major life changes such as moving countries or entering university. More specifically, we present research which shows that health disparities come to the fore when people undergo important life transitions that involve identity change. To integrate and elaborate these points, we then introduce the *social identity model of identity change* (SIMIC) – a model that has broad relevance to the themes of this book.

Current approaches to the health effects of social status

Physiological models

In an attempt to gain insight into the biological aspects of the relationship between social status and health, we first need to look at animal studies. According to this research, there is a very basic reason why status affects health: low status in a particular hierarchy evokes a strong biological stress response. Across numerous animal species, research has shown that subordinate animals both secrete more stress hormones and can show a lack of, or a blunted, stress response (e.g., in rats; Blanchard et al., 1995, guinea pigs; Sachser & Prove, 1986, and in squirrel monkeys; Manogue, Leshner, & Candland, 1975). Moreover, if the stressor is not dealt with effectively and the stress response remains chronically high, health is negatively affected, resulting in – amongst other things – immune suppression, gastric ulcers, loss of muscle mass, and reproductive suppression (Creel, 2001).

Interestingly, however, this work suggests that the heightened stress response for subordinate animals compared to dominant animals is not straightforward. It depends on which type of physiological stress response is examined, the type of stressor that the animal is exposed to, and importantly, the situation in which the animal finds themselves when stress responses are recorded (see Creel, 2001). For example, at baseline levels (in situations that do not evoke stress), dominant squirrel monkeys have lower levels of cortisol (a stress hormone) than subordinate animals. However, a study of squirrel monkeys by Kirk Manogue and colleagues showed that after exposure to different types of stressors (e.g., a live snake, physical restraint), dominant male squirrel monkeys showed greater reactivity to stress than subordinate male monkeys – with the latter showing a more sluggish physical response after exposure to a stressor (Manogue, Leshner, & Candland, 1975). This physical reactivity is likely to be adaptive when confronted with a stressor: the stressor triggers a rapid response among dominant animals, and this is arguably functional because it is aimed at resolving the stressful situation.

Findings are more straightforward when examining cardiovascular responses to stress among subordinate and dominant animals. Although stress has been found to negatively affect cardiovascular function among many different types of animals, subordinate status amplifies these effects. Among a range of different animals, subordinate status is associated with elevated resting blood pressure, higher levels of cholesterol, and more vascular damage than found in dominant animals (for a review see Sapolsky, 2004).

Even though the negative relationship between subordinate status and health among animals is well established, the challenge lies in explaining this relationship. There is some indirect evidence of the mechanisms that might be at work here. In particular, classic work suggests that poor health among subordinate animals appears to result from low predictability and lack of control, lack of other outlets for frustration and aggression, and lack of social support (Weiss, 1970). Indeed, each of these factors has been found to be related to a biological stress response (see Creel, 2001; Sapolsky, 2004).

Importantly, however, social context matters here. For depending on the nature of the animal group and the circumstances the group finds itself in, both lower- and higher-ranked animals may experience low predictability, control, and lack of social support. This in turn has a negative impact

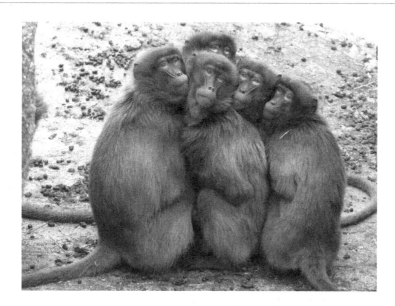

Figure 3.3 Social support can attenuate the heath-threatening effects of low status

Note: Studies of monkeys show that although subordinate animals tend to have higher cortisol levels than dominant ones, this difference is attenuated when members of the subordinate group provide each other with social support (Abbott et al., 2003).

Source: Pixabay

on their health (Goymann & Wingfield, 2004). For example, when dominant status is insecure (e.g., because ranks within a group change on a regular basis), dominant animals in the group experience the least control and predictability and they constantly need to compete to defend their position. It has been repeatedly observed that in such contexts, dominant status is no longer associated with health benefits. For example, Deborah Gust and her colleagues studied the formation of a new group among nine rhesus monkeys that were housed together after being relocated from elsewhere (Gust et al., 1991). They found that although all animals showed a stress response in the initial stages, once the dominance structure was established, the stress response remained high for the dominant group and continued to be higher for this group than for the subordinate animals nine weeks later.

There is also evidence that the higher stress response (leading to poorer health) among subordinate or more vulnerable animals is not found when there are high levels of social support among the subordinate group (Boccia et al., 1997). This was demonstrated by David Abbott and his colleagues in a comparative analysis of various primates living in captivity (rhesus, cynomolgus, talapoins, squirrel monkeys, and olive baboons; Abbott et al., 2003). Here subordinates only showed higher concentrations of the stress hormone cortisol than dominant animals when they had lower opportunities for social support (see Figure 3.3).

Although there are always issues when seeking to generalise from animal models (Shapiro, 1998), there are two important lessons for our understanding of status and disadvantage that we can take from this biological research. First, it suggests that the health-related problems that flow from low status are not inevitable. Second, it suggests that improving one's status is not the only way to address those problems. In particular, this is because it appears that the harmful health effects of stress can be remediated through social solidarity. This is a point that resonates with evidence relating to the role of group processes in ameliorating stress more generally that we discuss in greater depth in Chapter 5.

Human biological models

Although the animal research is instructive, it cannot fully capture the health effects of social status in humans. Recently, researchers have started to do this. Some of the trailblazing work in this regard was conducted by Jim Blascovich (2008) in work on the *bio-psychosocial model of challenge and threat* (BPM-CT). Focusing on the measurement of threat, Blascovich proposed that people are more likely to experience threat when the demands of the situation they face outweigh the resources that they bring to the situation to deal with these demands. For example, giving a speech is more threatening when facing a tough audience (i.e., a highly demanding situation) and one does not have much time to prepare (i.e., having limited resources). In contrast, when resources match or exceed demands (e.g., if a person has had days to prepare for a speech and the audience is friendly and encouraging), then the person is more likely merely to feel challenged rather than threatened. Importantly, threat and challenge are associated with different types of physiological response – with "unhealthier" responses (associated with higher blood pressure, slower heart rate recovery) more likely when a situation evokes threat rather than challenge.

Important for our current purposes, Daan Scheepers and Naomi Ellemers (2005) provided the first evidence of differences – albeit complex ones – in the physiological responses of members of high- and low-status groups. This study used a minimal group paradigm in which participants were randomly allocated to one of two groups, ostensibly on the basis of their perceptual style, and told that one group (detailed perceivers) had higher status than the other (holistic perceivers; see Chapter 2 for a discussion of this paradigm). Blood pressure (which tends to be elevated in response to threat; Blascovich & Mendes, 2000) was measured multiple times. The first time was when participants were initially told that their group had high or low status and, here, those in the low-status group had higher blood pressure than those in the high-status group. Blood pressure was measured a second time when participants were told that they were going to engage in a range of tasks that would define their status for the rest of the experiment. Now blood pressure was higher for those in the high-status group. Consistent with findings from animal studies, then, it appears that when high-status group members become aware that they may lose their social standing, they have a stronger stress response than their low-status counterparts. In contrast, as we will discuss in more detail later, for low-status group members, the possibility that status relations might improve was appraised more positively, and here their status was associated with a challenge rather than a threat response (i.e., lower blood pressure; see also Scheepers, Ellemers, & Sintemaartensdijk, 2009).

These findings make it clear that there is more to health disparities between groups of different status than merely physiological differences between subordinates and dominants. In other words, there is no genetic or biological difference between subordinate and dominant groups (in either animals or humans) that makes either group healthier or fitter for survival at birth. Moreover, it appears that biological stress responses that are associated with poor health are not simply a function of differences in social status. Instead, studies that have examined changing status hierarchies indicate that the relationship between social status and health is shaped in important ways by social context and, in particular, reflects the dynamics of *experienced and anticipated intergroup relations*.

This in turn suggests that to explain physiological responses to social status, we need to move beyond biology and focus on the environment and social inequality. Interestingly, when we do, we find corroborating evidence that many of the factors that were identified above (notably, the predictability of the environment, control, and social support) play an important role in producing the health gradient. It is this literature that we review next.

Sociological and epidemiological models

A vast body of work by sociologists and epidemiologists has documented the capacity for status inequalities to produce the health gradient in a range of different societies and populations. The following statistics are illustrative of the findings from this work and are presented by Michael Marmot (2015) in his best-selling book *The Health Gap:*

- In the poorest parts of Baltimore (where there have been many riots in recent years), life expectancy for men is currently 63 years. In the richest part of Baltimore it is 83 years.
- In the poorest parts of Tottenham in North London (one of the places where the 2011 London riots started) the life expectancy for men is 17 years lower than it is for men living in affluent suburbs such as Kensington and Chelsea. In Glasgow between 1998 and 2002 life-expectancy gaps for men were even more pronounced; whereas men's life expectancy was 82 in upmarket Lenzie, it was only 54 in the poor parts of Calton. This difference has reduced from 28 years to around 20 years in 2015, yet remains stark for residents in a single city.
- In Australia today, middle-aged people with fewer than 12 years of education have a 70% higher mortality risk than the most educated Australians. Meanwhile, the difference in the life expectancy of Indigenous and non-Indigenous people in Australia is 11 years. A 2012 report by Australia's National Centre for Social and Economic Modelling concluded that "Australia suffers the effects of a major differential in the prevalence of long-term health conditions. Those who are most socio-economically disadvantaged are twice as likely to have a long-term health condition as those who are the least disadvantaged" (Brown, Thurecht, & Nepal, 2012, p. vii).

Although the magnitude of these effects is stark, as we noted earlier, one might still explain them away by arguing that they all involve extreme comparisons: between the poorest and the wealthiest in a particular location or the least educated and the highest educated. Moreover, because there are many differences between these groups, aside from those that involve social status, other explanations for these differences cannot easily be ruled out. For example, they could reflect the influence of different lifestyles, cultures, or family structures.

One very influential research programme that sought to address some of these concerns was conducted by Marmot with British civil servants in Whitehall (2004; 2015; see Figure 3.4). The first study was a large prospective examination of 18,000 male civil servants between the ages of 20 and 64, assessed over a period of ten years starting in 1967. Starting two decades later, a second study focused on the health of 10,308 civil servants aged 35 to 55 of whom around two-thirds were men. Clearly the public servants who were participants in these studies had much in common (e.g., they were all employed, not poor, and had comparable social backgrounds). Nevertheless, in the first study, Marmot found clear evidence of a health gradient such that the higher their employment grade, the longer employees lived. Indeed, men at the bottom of the hierarchy were more than four times more likely to die in the course of the study than the men at the top.

Importantly too, for all men, data were collected on a range of health behaviours, and this allowed the researchers to control for risk factors such as obesity, smoking, reduced leisure time, physical activity, prevalence of underlying illness, and blood pressure. These risk factors are important to control for because men with lower status generally score worse on these factors, and each is associated with poorer health in its own right. Inclusion of these risk factors in the analysis accounted for 40% of the variance in health outcomes, so they were clearly important. However, even after controlling for these factors, there was still a substantial health gradient. For example, the risk of cardiovascular disease was still 2.1 times higher for those in the lowest employment grade than for those in the highest.

There is one further important point that these data drive home. This is that when we talk about the implications of social status for health, we should not simply be concerned about *absolute* level of disadvantage. Instead, we should be looking at the degree of inequality between those who are

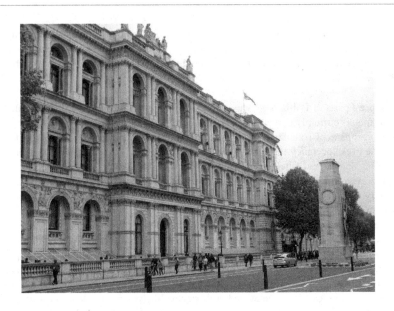

Figure 3.4 Civil service buildings in Whitehall, London

Note: Michael Marmot's (2004, 2015) studies of British civil servants showed that even in this relatively advantaged and homogeneous group there was a substantial health gradient such that higher-ranking employees had far better health outcomes than lower-ranking ones.

Source: Pixabay

most disadvantaged and those who are the most advantaged within a particular community or society (also known as *relative* disadvantage). This observation accords with a classic social identity principle that we discussed in Chapter 2: social disadvantage cannot be objectively established, but depends largely on comparisons with others in the immediate context (Tajfel & Turner, 1979). In other words, *regardless of how large objective differences in status or wealth actually are, to the extent that they are perceived to be large, they will have an adverse impact on the perceiver's health.*

So how, then, are we to explain the Whitehall findings? Interestingly, Marmot's explanation for the results is quite similar to the one provided to explain findings from the animal studies that we reviewed earlier (see Sapolsky, 2004). Specifically, he suggests that workers in lower employment grades had lower predictability and control in their work and in their lives more generally than their higher employment grade counterparts and that it was this lack of control and predictability that was the source of their poor health (Marmot, 2004; 2015; Vaananen et al., 2008; see also Martin, 2016).

Other researchers interested in the social determinants of health have argued that the health gradient can be explained by the amount of *social capital* in a particular group or society. Based on work by the Organization for Economic Co-operation and Development (OECD), Robert Putnam (2000, p. 41) defines social capital as "networks together with shared norms, values and understandings that facilitate co-operation within or among groups". The key idea here is that membership in groups affects individuals because it confers benefits (Hawe & Shiel, 2000). Social capital is often measured in terms of trust and the number of ties within a particular group or society. It is higher when individuals are more likely to trust each other and when ties between members in a community are tighter and when there are more frequent interactions between them (i.e., when there are high levels of social cohesion; Helliwell, 2006; Helliwell & Barrington-Leigh, 2012; Oh, Chung, & Labianca, 2004).

Consistent with our hypothesis that group memberships are important psychological resources (the multiple identities hypothesis, H11), researchers in the social capital tradition have highlighted a number of ways in which social capital promotes health and well-being. Of particular importance here is the distinction that is often made between *bonding* and *bridging* capital. Bonding capital relates to relationships between people. It reflects trust and social cohesion, and also resembles shared social identity (as defined in Chapter 2). High bonding capital is often also seen as a pre-requisite for the development of bridging capital – which is defined as the ability of an individual to take on new group memberships and/or their ability to maintain their memberships in important groups (Johnstone, Jetten, Dingle, Parsell, & Walter, 2016, see also Kim, Subramanian, & Kawachi, 2006).

Importantly, the distinction between bonding and bridging capital is useful in helping us understand the health gradient. This is because people with higher status in groups typically have more bonding capital in being better able to sustain an active social life and more opportunities to develop a network of group memberships (Ball, Reay, & David, 2003; Bourdieu, 1979/1984). Moreover, the more social capital one has, the easier it is to extend social capital (because strong group memberships are a good platform for developing further strong group memberships; Hawe & Shiel, 2000), and this means that individuals with high bonding capital also tend to develop more bridging capital. Speaking to this point, a large body of evidence suggests that the more social groups a person belongs, to the happier and healthier they tend to be (Cohen & Janicki-Deverts, 2009; see also Haslam, Holme, et al., 2008; Iyer, Jetten, Tsivrikos, Postmes, & Haslam, 2009; see Jetten, Haslam, Iyer, & Haslam, 2010a, for an overview).

Yet even though this account sheds light on the processes underlying the health gradient, it has also been argued that because the concept of social capital has tended to be used both broadly and loosely, its explanatory power has been weakened (Hawe & Shiel, 2000). A key part of the problem here is that it is quite difficult to specify precisely what social capital is, and hence to measure it (Whiteley, 1999). This is a challenge that we will return to in the second part of this chapter.

Despite these conceptual and measurement concerns, research into the social determinants of health has been important for several reasons. Not only has it shown that social status, poverty, and disadvantage are profound predictors of health, but it has also helped to drive a growing recognition among policy makers that these social factors matter and need to be addressed. It has also led to changes in the type of recommendations that are provided to the general public about how to stay healthy and well. So whereas standard formulations – in particular, those informed by the biomedical model that we discussed in Chapter 1 – have focused on behaviours that individuals should engage in to improve their health (e.g., of the form identified in the "ten traditional tips for better health" presented in Table 3.1), research on social determinants has led us to focus more on the ways in which individuals' social environment needs to be improved (see the somewhat tongue-in-cheek "ten alternative tips for better health" in Table 3.1).

Such insights present a radical departure from traditional health models and fit well with the social identity approach to health that we present in this book. The social determinants approach also aligns well with the policy implications that emerge from the social cure approach (e.g., see Haslam, Jetten, & Haslam, 2012; Jetten, Haslam, Haslam, Dingle, & Jones, 2014). For when health is understood as being determined in large part by the social environment in which a person finds themselves, then responsibility for that person's health lies not with them alone but also with the groups, communities, and societies to which they belong. Although very simple, this is a point that has enormous policy implications (e.g., see Agich, 1982; World Health Organization & United Nations Children's Fund, 1978).

Table 3.1 Two different lists of top ten tips for health

Ten traditional tips for better health

1. Don't smoke. If you can, stop. If you can't, cut down.
2. Follow a balanced diet with plenty of fruit and vegetables.
3. Keep physically active.
4. Manage stress by, for example, talking things through and making time to relax.
5. If you drink alcohol, do so in moderation.
6. Cover up in the sun, and protect children from sunburn.
7. Practice safer sex.
8. Take up cancer-screening opportunities.
9. Be safe on the roads: follow the Highway Code.
10. Learn the first aid ABCs: airways, breathing, circulation.

Ten alternative tips for better health

1. Don't be poor. If you can, stop. If you can't, try not to be poor for long.
2. Don't live in a deprived area. If you do, move.
3. Don't be disabled or have a disabled child.
4. Don't work in a stressful, low-paid manual job.
5. Don't live in damp, low-quality housing or be homeless.
6. Be able to afford to pay for social activities and annual holidays.
7. Don't be a lone parent.
8. Claim all the benefits to which you are entitled.
9. Be able to afford your own car.
10. Use education to improve your socio-economic position.

Note: The first of these lists was developed by England's chief medical officer, the second was developed by researchers interested in social determinants of health at the Townsend Centre for International Poverty Research (cited in Raphael, 2000, p. 403).

The social identity approach to social status and health

As suggested in the previous section, social identity theorising (e.g., as outlined in Chapter 2) is well placed to build upon work into the social determinants of health. Not only can it help us to better understand some of the findings in this literature, it can also help us more precisely target efforts to flatten the health gradient that this work identifies. For instance, having recognised that lack of control is at the core of the health gradient, a social identity analysis can help us understand what makes disadvantage so disempowering and how control can be increased through strategies that build social identification (e.g., after Greenaway et al., 2015). It can also shed light on when those who are socially disadvantaged are most likely to feel disempowered (e.g., after Drury & Reicher, 2009).

These are ideas that the remainder of this chapter will now explore in greater detail. As we noted in the previous chapter, our approach starts from the assumption that groups can differ in many ways, but that the differences that are probably most consequential are those that relate to social status (Mullen, Brown, & Smith, 1992; Otten, Mummendey, & Blanz, 1996; Sachdev & Bourhis, 1987). This was certainly an understanding that informed the development of social identity theory, as it sought to explain the general behavioural consequences of psychological group membership (Tajfel & Turner, 1979) and it has proved no less important in understanding the implications of social identities for health and well-being (e.g., as suggested by Haslam et al., 2009).

Social identities are important determinants of social status

Within social identity theory, status is defined as the position of a group in the social hierarchy of a given society or culture *relative* to other groups (i.e., relevant outgroups). Status is thus not fixed, but always determined in comparison to other groups. This is an important point because it helps us appreciate the complexities of the health gradient. For example, a person in a poor suburb of Baltimore may be objectively wealthier and more educated than a relatively advantaged person in Bangladesh, but *compared to others in their city or in their country*, they are likely to be disadvantaged on these dimensions, and it is this *relative standing* that will determine their health outcomes. This, then, helps to explain why, on some indicators, their health is actually worse than that of the average person in Bangladesh (see Marmot, 2015).

Status can be achieved on different dimensions. For example, high status can reflect a group's superior skill, knowledge, physical strength, or power. But of particular relevance here, high status often reflects a group's superior wealth, education, and social standing more generally. And because our personal identity is defined in important ways by the groups to which we belong, the status of those groups not only affects the self-esteem and well-being we derive as a *group member* (e.g., collective self-esteem; Crocker & Luhtanen, 1990; Luhtanen & Crocker, 1991) but also our *personal* self-esteem and well-being (Jetten et al., 2015). In line with the identification hypothesis (H2), this is especially true if individuals identify highly with their social group such that it is internalised as an important aspect of self (i.e., so that this *self-categorization* furnishes them with a sense of *social identity*; Turner, Hogg, Oakes, Reicher, & Wetherell, 1987).

A key premise of the social identity approach is that group members strive to compare themselves positively with other groups on relevant dimensions of comparison (Turner, 1975). If the comparison with other groups is favourable, they achieve or maintain a positive identity, and this has positive implications for their well-being and self-esteem (in line with the group circumstance hypothesis, H3a). However, when the comparison is negative and emphasises their ingroup's lower standing, it is more difficult to achieve a positive identity, and this will tend to compromise well-being and self-esteem (H3b). Consistent with these hypotheses, there is now an abundance of evidence that higher (perceived) group status is beneficial for individuals' well-being and health. In particular, it is associated with higher self-esteem, life satisfaction, and general well-being and lower levels of anxiety and depressive symptoms (Anderson, Kraus, Galinsky, & Keltner, 2012; Begeny & Huo, 2016; Sani, Magrin, Scrignaro, & McCollum, 2010; Singh-Manoux, Marmot, & Adler, 2005; Smith, Tyler, & Huo, 2003).

Evidence for the processes underlying this effect is provided by the research of Fabio Sani and his colleagues. They studied two populations: prison guards in Italy and families in Scotland (Sani, Magrin, Scrignaro, & McCollum, 2010). Drawing on social identity theorising, the researchers reasoned first that people should identify more strongly with high- (rather than low-) status groups because these are more likely to provide them with a sense of positive identity. Second, they argued that because identification generally promotes health and well-being (due to it being a psychological resource that people can fall back on when facing challenges in their life, as outlined in the previous chapter), then health and well-being should be higher among members of high-status groups. In line with this reasoning, in both populations higher subjective ingroup status was associated with greater psychological health (in the form of lower perceived stress, lower depression, and greater satisfaction with life). And in both cases this effect was explained by higher identification with ingroups that were perceived to be of high status.

Features of socio-structural context determine responses to group disadvantage

Important as social status is, a key insight from social identity theory is that low social status or disadvantage will not *always* be associated with lower self-esteem. Indeed, even though self-categorization as a member of a socially disadvantaged group will tend to compromise self-esteem – and hence have negative consequences for well-being – this does not mean that people who have low status will simply resign themselves to their dismal fate and give up on the search for a positive identity. On the contrary, and consistent with the identity restoration hypothesis (H4), in such situations social identity theory predicts that people will continue to be motivated to engage in identity management strategies that help them achieve the best possible outcomes for themselves and/or for their group. Indeed, it is precisely because members of low-status groups will search (and often therefore find) avenues to improve their fate that there are no straightforward relationships between social status and well-being (measured as self-esteem, see Martiny & Rubin, 2016; Rubin & Hewstone, 1998). To see why this is the case, we can explore a few of these avenues and see how they lead to different outcomes.

Resisting identification with disadvantaged groups

One way for members of socially disadvantaged groups to protect their well-being is to deny that they belong to the group in question. To illustrate how this might work, consider the case of someone who is homeless. In light of their perilous position in society, it is not surprising that people experiencing homelessness have mental and physical health problems that are considerably more pronounced than those of the rest of the general population (Chamberlain & McKenzie, 2006; Johnson & Chamberlain, 2011). Indeed, poor health is sometimes the reason why people become homeless and it is certainly exacerbated by the experience of becoming and being homeless (Busch-Geertsma, Edgar, O'Sullivan, & Pleace, 2010; Johnson & Chamberlain, 2008).

When Zoe Walter and colleagues (Walter, Jetten, Parsell, & Dingle, 2015b) interviewed a large number of people who met the definitional criteria for homelessness, many (55%) described themselves as homeless. More surprising was the fact that nearly a third of respondents (31%) refused to describe themselves in this way. Some of the reasons they gave for this refusal are presented in Table 3.2.

Importantly for our argument, those who rejected the 'homeless' self-categorization reported higher personal well-being and better mood than those who accepted the label, independent of the duration of their homelessness (Walter et al., 2015b). These findings point to the importance of how one self-defines, or self-categorizes, for well-being and also show that people do not passively accept labels that might seem to describe their situation objectively. Instead, for some of these participants at least, self-categorization was an active process of identity negotiation in which they *resisted* externally imposed labels, presumably in an attempt to protect their self-worth and well-being (see also Parsell, 2011).

There are also other ways in which members of low-status groups can escape the negative well-being consequences of their group membership, at least psychologically, without actually leaving the group. In three studies with naturally occurring and laboratory-created groups, Sonja Roccas (2003) showed that group members tend to identify more with a group if a different group (to which they also belonged) is both salient and lower in status. One can interpret these findings as showing that because most of us belong to multiple groups, we can strategically emphasise our membership of those particular groups that are higher in status. Belonging to this higher-status group not only gives us a *relatively* positive identity (and remember that relativities matter here), but at the same time it reduces

Table 3.2 Examples of alternative self-categorizations in the face of homelessness

Defining homelessness as different from, and worse than, one's current situation

"*To me homeless is on the street. This is a hostel, it's a refuge, it's a roof over your head, a shower, food, so I wouldn't say I was homeless. I've got somewhere to go everyday to sleep, so I wouldn't say I'm homeless*" (male, age 44).

"*I did a little bit of time on the streets. Compared to that no. Struggling yeah, but not homeless*" (male, age 24).

Rejecting a homeless self-categorization because one has alternative housing options

"*I could have some options if I really want them but no, I'm not really homeless . . . but I choose to live here because it's the safest place to be*" (female, age 43).

Rejecting a homeless self-categorization because one has found a "home" in the homeless shelter

"*It might be a homeless shelter, but it doesn't feel like one. . . . So, basically I'm not homeless, I feel like this is my home*" (female, age 19).

Note: The table identifies the different ways in which respondents who met criteria for homelessness negotiated their self-categorization.

Source: Based on Walter et al. (2015b)

---

the negative effects that belonging to lower-status groups has on health and well-being. Indeed, even though well-being was not measured in these studies, Roccas speculated that because people had other social groups to which they could turn to achieve a positive identity, this might be one reason why there is not an overwhelmingly negative relationship between group status and self-esteem (see also Diener & Diener, 1996). At the same time, we can also see that the capacity for alternative group memberships to afford opportunities for strategic self-enhancement is one further reason why there is a reliable relationship between multiple group memberships and psychological health (as noted earlier; e.g., see Jetten et al., 2010a, for an overview).

Leaving disadvantaged groups

Of course, a more direct way of dealing with the esteem- (and, thus, health-) related threats associated with belonging to a low-status group is simply to leave it (Ellemers, 1993; Tajfel & Turner, 1979). However, an obvious reason why people do not always take this route is that it is not always open. In particular, this is because the likely success of this strategy depends very much on the extent to which boundaries between groups are *permeable*, and thereby allow for *individual mobility* (as suggested by the mobility hypothesis, H5; Ellemers & van Rijswijk, 1997; Ellemers, van Knippenberg, & Wilke, 1990; Lalonde & Silverman, 1994; Wright, Taylor, & Moghaddam, 1990).

But even if individual mobility *is* an option, it often turns out to be a double-edged sword. For even though the health of those who are able to cross boundaries and join a higher-status group may increase, costs are associated with going down this path. For instance, those who engage in individual mobility and decide to leave the disadvantaged group may be penalised by the group for being disloyal (Branscombe, Wann, Noel, & Coleman, 1993), for being a traitor to the cause, or even for being an impostor because they claim to be something they are not (Warner, Hornsey, & Jetten, 2007). Moreover, the high-status group they join may not treat them especially well (e.g., looking upon them as an upstart, a 'Johnny-come-lately', or a 'blow in'; De Nooy, 2016) and they may only be allowed to occupy a 'token' position in the group (Branscombe & Ellemers, 1998). In both these scenarios, a person's personal standing will be diminished, and this is likely to have negative implications for their health and well-being.

A study by Tom Postmes and Nyla Branscombe (2002) of African Americans in the United States who were living and working in predominantly White communities provides powerful insights into these dynamics. On the basis of social identity theory, these researchers hypothesised that minority group members who attempt individual mobility in this way may suffer from the dual handicap of being rejected both (1) by their new ingroup (Whites) on grounds that they are 'different' and (2) by their former ingroup (Blacks) on grounds that they are 'deserters' or 'traitors'. Moreover, they reasoned that this latter response might be accentuated by the fact that, in seeking acceptance from their new ingroup, members of minorities feel obliged to denounce their former group membership. In short, as suggested by the mobility hypothesis (H5) when members of minority groups attempt to become part of the majority by engaging in an individual mobility strategy, they may gain social status by moving up the social hierarchy, but also in the process be cut off from their former group and, importantly, the health benefits that this group can provide (e.g., in the form of social support).

When boundaries between groups are more impermeable (e.g., if group membership is based on ethnicity), the strategies that members of low-status groups engage in to achieve a more positive identity (and thus higher well-being) are likely to be quite different – again in ways predicted by social identity theory (Tajfel & Turner, 1979). In this situation it is not easy (and it may in fact be impossible) to improve one's status by leaving the low-status group behind, but this does not always lead to disempowerment (and hence a reduction in well-being). If they share a strong sense of social identity with one another, members of low-status groups are likely to provide each other with social support and solidarity, and this will help to buffer them from the negative consequences of their social status for well-being.

This is a finding that emerges from the animal studies that we reviewed earlier (e.g., Abbott et al., 2003, see Figure 3.3), but there is now considerable evidence of the same process in other branches of psychological research. For instance, Jetten and colleagues (2015; see also Walter, Jetten, Dingle, Parsell, & Johnstone, 2015a) found that former residents of a homeless shelter who went on to belong to multiple important groups showed increased personal self-esteem and well-being as they were tracked over time. In this study, all the participants were asked to list their friends and close others by name (i.e., to list their interpersonal ties) and to list the important groups they belonged to (i.e., the ones they identified with) when they first moved into a homeless shelter (Time 1). They were also asked to do the same three months later (Time 2) and then again nine months after that (Time 3). Interestingly, participants' self-esteem was not predicted by the number of interpersonal ties that they had at Time 1 nor by any increase in number of interpersonal ties over time. Rather, the best predictor of self-esteem 12 months after leaving the shelter was the number of important *groups* that people belonged to at Time 1. Clearly then, important groups matter as they have unique powers to protect us from the health-disrupting ravages of low status.

The aforementioned research by Postmes and Branscombe (2002) also provides evidence of the specific role that group-based social support plays in countering the negative health effects of social disadvantage. For whereas African Americans who had engaged in individual mobility had poorer health outcomes because they had lost social support by leaving their minority group behind, those who continued to live and work in Black communities reported receiving more social support, being more accepted by their ingroup, and having enhanced levels of psychological well-being. From this we can see that the positive effects of group membership are most apparent when members of minorities are not forced to discard their group membership and assimilate to the majority, but are able to simultaneously maintain their social identity as members of that minority in systems that are pluralist (Berry 1997; Hornsey & Hogg, 2000). This is because under such conditions – where individuals are not required to relinquish valued social identities –they are best placed to benefit from the social support that groups provide (as proposed by H14, see also Chapter 5).

In this regard, one of the most comprehensive explorations of responses to low social status was provided by the BBC Prison Study (Reicher & Haslam, 2006a; see Figure 3.5). In this, 15 men were randomly assigned to either a high- or a low-status group – Guards or Prisoners – within a simulated

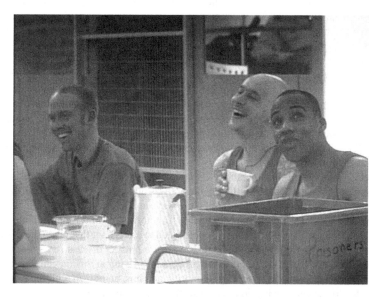

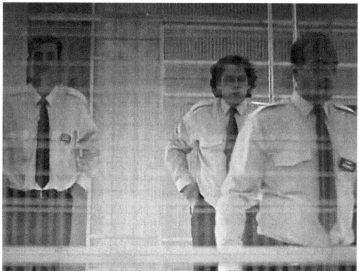

Figure 3.5 Prisoners and Guards in the BBC Prison Study

Note: At the start of the study the high-status Guards had better mental health than the low-status Prisoners. However, as the Prisoners' sense of shared social identity increased (after promotion was no longer possible and group boundaries were impermeable), they started working together to improve their situation, and their psychological health and well-being improved markedly. At the same time, the Prisoners' actions contributed to a reduced sense of shared social identity among the Guards and, as a result, their health and well-being declined.

Source: Reicher and Haslam (2006a); see also www.bbcprisonstudy.org

prison environment and their behaviour was then studied closely over a period of 8 days. Informed by the principles of social identity theory, the design of the study involved manipulating factors that were expected to have an impact on the Prisoners' degree of social identification and examining the impact of this on both groups' behaviour as well as on the functioning of the prison system as a whole. At the study's outset, participants were led to believe that the boundaries between the two groups were permeable and hence that it was possible to be promoted from Prisoner to Guard. At this stage it was expected that Prisoners would adopt an individual mobility strategy and pursue a self-enhancement strategy of working individually to gain favour with the Guards (in line with the mobility hypothesis, H5). However, after one seemingly fortunate prisoner had been promoted in this way, group boundaries were made impermeable by ruling out further opportunities for promotion. It was expected that this would increase Prisoners' social identification and encourage collective responses to their situation (in line with the competition hypothesis, H7).

As predicted, social identification among the low-status group (Prisoners) increased once group boundaries were impermeable. Importantly too, once it was no longer possible for individuals to transition between groups, the Prisoners started to explore ways to improve their status collectively. In particular, they worked together to undermine the Guards' authority and to formulate plans to overthrow their regime. Indeed, ultimately this resistance contributed to a breakout that made the Guards' regime unworkable and brought the study to a premature end (for a broader discussion of the psychology of resistance, see Haslam & Reicher, 2012). In the process of arriving at this outcome, the Guards also became increasingly apprehensive about their authority, and this, combined with the Prisoners' insurgency, contributed to a steady decline in their sense of shared social identity.

As we will explore later in Chapters 5 and 13, these processes also had a significant bearing on the participants' health and well-being. Most particularly, as the Prisoners' sense of shared identity increased, they became less stressed, less depressed, and less paranoid. On the other hand, as the Guards' sense of shared identity declined, they became more stressed, more depressed, and more paranoid. So, whereas at the start of the study the Prisoners' low status had negative implications for their health and well-being, as they came together to improve their status collectively, things improved markedly, and it was now the high-status Guards whose health and well-being were threatened.

Social identification is beneficial for well-being even in disadvantaged groups

Whereas the BBC study showed that group identification provides important resources to respond to devaluation and thereby improve psychological health, one could argue that it is also the case that these benefits for well-being came to the fore at a time in the study when the Prisoners were resisting the Guards' power and authority. Were the Prisoners still seeing themselves as a low-status group at this point? Perhaps not, and by the time they were breaking out of their cells, status relations may, in their own mind, have effectively reversed so that it was the Guards who were now in the low-status position.

If this is true, then it leaves unanswered the question of whether it is generally the case that when low-status members turn to their group for social support this will prove to be good for their psychological health. The significance of this question arises from the fact that there is something quite ironic about turning to a low-status group for support when membership of that group was itself the cause of the original threat to health and well-being. As Niamh McNamara, Clifford Stevenson, and Orla Muldoon (2013) observe:

> The paradox of community deprivation is therefore that although the community identity can provide resources to cope with the daily challenges and stresses faced by disadvantaged communities, the stigmatisation of disadvantage itself can undermine this resource by reducing collective support and cooperation as well as inhibiting engagement with external services and other communities.

(p. 393)

Indeed, bearing this in mind, one might well ask why members of disadvantaged groups do not simply disengage from them and turn to *other* groups to help them cope with the threats to well-being that they face?

Even though this might be an intuitively appealing strategy (and one that people certainly pursue sometimes; see Roccas, 2003), there is now a growing body of evidence that group identification delivers health benefits *even in disadvantaged communities which offer limited social resources*. For example, in a study of immigrants in Switzerland, Mouna Bakouri and Christian Staerklé (2015) found that higher perceived disadvantage was associated with feeling there were more barriers to taking control of one's life and that this predicted lower self-esteem. However, it was also clear that bonding identities (consisting of existing social relationships in the form of interpersonal connections and group memberships) buffered this relationship. That is, the negative effect of perceived barriers to control was less pronounced for people who reported having more bonding identities. Looking to explain this relationship, the researchers found that this was because bonding identities increased the immigrants' sense of self-efficacy (rather than their sense of being supported). This is again consistent with our argument that one of the reasons why social identities are important psychological resources is that they serve to empower otherwise disadvantaged groups (in line with the agency hypothesis, H15).

In a similar vein, in a household survey conducted in disadvantaged areas of Limerick in Ireland, Niamh McNamara and her colleagues (2013) found positive effects of identifying with the community on well-being. Further analyses showed that this relationship was accounted for by the greater perceived collective efficacy of those who identified more strongly with the community. Respondents' better well-being was thus explained by a sense that they were coping collectively with challenges that their community as a whole were facing.

Other work has also reinforced this point that identifying with others who are similarly devalued can enhance efficacy and empowerment in disadvantaged groups. In a study of African Americans, it was found that higher identification with one's racial ingroup was associated with a greater sense that its members would provide social support (Outten, Schmitt, Garcia, & Branscombe, 2009). Higher group identification also predicted a stronger belief that the group could cope effectively with disadvantage, and again it was these perceptions of collective efficacy (rather than perceptions of social support) that predicted self-esteem and life satisfaction.

In sum, despite the fact that devaluation is an obvious stress factor in and of itself, those who turn to the devalued group generally appear to experience (1) higher levels of collective efficacy (believing that their groups can counter some of the challenges it faces) and (2) higher social support. Both of these factors have been found to boost health and well-being – although which is the most potent resource appears to vary from group to group.

As a final thought, it is also important to bear in mind that although membership in higher-status groups usually confers more health benefits than membership in lower-status groups, this is not true in all circumstances. Consistent with some of the animal research that we reviewed earlier in this chapter, it appears that those who are privileged, powerful, and wealthy are likely to become less healthy if their status position is threatened and becomes unstable. This was seen among the Guards in the BBC Prison Study, and it was also seen in the research of Scheepers and colleagues (2009) that we discussed earlier in which only high-status groups who feared losing their status displayed a physiological stress response (see also Scheepers & Ellemers, 2005). As the Prisoner who was promoted to be a Guard in the BBC Prison Study found out, even if one were to try to join a more advantaged group with a view to improving one's health and well-being, this would not always have the desired results.

Social identity resources facilitate adjustment to life transitions

Ironically, despite the fact that those who are socially disadvantaged are often most motivated to acquire a more positive identity, it is also this group that tends to struggle most whenever they face life transitions and changes. Indeed, members of low-status groups experience their disadvantage most profoundly when they are undergoing life transitions (Bakouri & Staerklé, 2015). Before we outline why this is the case, we first review a large body of research in the social identity tradition that has examined how social identity is implicated in life transitions and changes more generally.

The social identity model of identity change (SIMIC)

Life transitions can have both positive and negative outcomes. Transitions can be positive when they provide individuals with new opportunities and experiences. For example, a promotion at work may mean an increase in salary, job responsibilities, and overall prestige. Similarly, entering university provides students with an opportunity to extend their knowledge and develop critical thinking skills. On the other hand, life transitions can be a negative experience when they involve such things as becoming unemployed, being forced into early retirement, or being diagnosed with a life-threatening illness.

When an important social identity is threatened or changed, this has a range of negative conse-quences for well-being, and these are well-documented in the literature (e.g., see Breakwell, 1986; Haunschild, Moreland, & Murrell, 1994). Amongst other things, when we can no longer retain mem-bership in a valued group – either because we change or the group does – this tends to be disorienting and stressful (e.g., Jetten, O'Brien, & Trindall, 2002). Indeed, as we will see in later chapters (e.g., Chapters 7 and 8) the social identity loss that this entails can precipitate significant cognitive decline and depression.

Yet despite the recognition that identity change and/or loss tends to have negative consequences for health and well-being, it turns out that group identification also plays a key role in protecting people against these negative consequences. In particular, this is because the negative consequences of identity change will generally be limited when individuals are able to join a new group and thereby take on a *new* social identity. Here the new sense of identification that this affords – and the various positive consequences that flow from this (as discussed in Chapter 2) – will tend to counteract the sense of identification that has been lost. For instance, threats to well-being will be minimised if employees quickly take on the identity of a new work team when their old work team is disbanded, or if university students quickly identify as a university student after losing their secondary-school identity. More generally, an important way in which people protect long-term well-being in the face of identity loss is by joining groups to help them adjust to and 'get over' the loss. Speaking to this point, and as we will discuss in later chapters, *support groups* are widely recognised as helping people cope effectively with such things as bereavement, injury, illness, and trauma (Wuthnow, 1994).

Over the course of the last decade, these processes of adjustment to social identity change have been theorised and integrated within the *social identity model of identity change* (SIMIC; Haslam, Holme et al., 2008; Jetten, Haslam, Haslam, & Branscombe, 2009). As we outlined in the previous chapter, because the self is defined in important ways by our membership in social groups, losing an identity or experiencing a permanent change in the meaning of the identity is likely to affect our sense of self in important ways (Hopkins & Reicher, 1996). Moreover, regardless of whether it leads to desired or undesired outcomes, change itself may adversely affect well-being because it requires adjustment on the part of those who undergo it (Ethier & Deaux, 1994; Hopkins & Reicher, 1996; Jetten et al., 2002). Change, then, is associated with uncertainty and often requires the individual to reorient themselves to the world.

Another reason why identity change is challenging is that those who undergo it need to start defining themselves as members of the new group that they have joined. Indeed, changes to social identities often require a redefinition of the meaning of identity for the self as well as a reformulation of the relationship between oneself and others in the group. As represented schematically in Figure 3.6 SIMIC identifies a number of processes that hinder or facilitate this process of adjustment in the face of major life events and transitions (Haslam, Holme et al., 2008; Jetten et al., 2009).

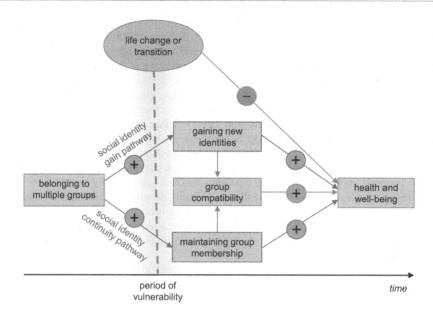

Figure 3.6 The social identity model of identity change (SIMIC)

Note: SIMIC identifies two key pathways that help people cope with identity change in the face of major life transitions and events. The first is a *social identity gain* pathway associated with the acquisition of new group memberships; the second is a *social identity continuity* pathway associated with the maintenance of pre-existing group memberships. Both pathways are more likely to be accessible the more group memberships a person had prior to the life transition. The impact of the two pathways on health and well-being also depends on the compatibility of the social identities they involve.

Source: Based on Jetten et al. (2009)

First, the adverse impact of change will be minimised when individuals are able to *maintain* valued social identities (the *social identity continuity pathway*). However, this is not always possible, and change may require individuals to give up or move away from old group memberships ('unfreezing'; Lewin, 1948). This is often a difficult process because, even if those old identities are negative and problematic (e.g., being an addict or unemployed), people are often unwilling to give up identities that have been important in defining themselves in the past. Indeed, losing one's grounding is stressful in part because it is associated with a break from that which we know best. Indeed, when the connection between the past and the present becomes interrupted, this loss of *self-continuity* in itself presents a threat to individuals' well-being (Sani, 2008; Sani, Bowe, & Herrera, 2008).

Second, adjustment will also depend on a person's ability and willingness to take on a *new* social identity in the new situation that they find themselves (the *social identity gain pathway*). Taking on a new identity not only provides a new sense of grounding and belonging, but it also forms the basis for receiving and benefiting from new sources of social support (Haslam, O'Brien, Jetten, Vormedal, & Penna, 2005; Iyer et al., 2009). More generally, joining new groups after important life transitions can protect and sometimes even reverse the negative effects of change because, to the extent that those groups provide a basis for self-definition, the resources they provide access to are likely to make the experience of entering a new phase in life a positive opportunity for personal growth, rather than a stressful experience of loss (see Haslam, Jetten, Haslam, & Postmes, 2009).

Third, successful adaptation to identity change depends very much on the features of a person's pre-change social identity network. Previous research has shown that two aspects of this identity network are particularly important in determining the way that identities promote successful adjustment to important life transitions (Iyer et al., 2009; Jetten, Haslam, Pugliese, Tonks, & Haslam, 2010b). First, the extent of a person's social connections before the life transition are likely to be an important predictor of their ability to cope successfully with identity change (see Iyer, Jetten, & Tsivrikos, 2008; Jetten & Pachana, 2012; Jetten et al., 2015). In particular, we have argued that *multiple group memberships* provide people with more *social identity capital* and that this protects well-being in times of change because when people belong to multiple groups, this increases the likelihood of them being able (1) to maintain some group memberships post-transition (and thereby benefit from the social identity continuity pathway) and (2) to use their old identity network as a platform for building new identities (and thereby benefit from the social identity gain pathway). Second, when predicting adjustment to change, it is not just the number of identities that matters, but also the relationships among them. In particular, this is because identity change can strain relationships – and therefore compromise well-being – when new identities are not *compatible*.

A large body of research now provides strong support for various components of SIMIC. In particular, there is abundant evidence that maintaining strong social identities helps to protect health and well-being in the context of significant life changes (Haslam, Holme et al., 2008; Iyer & Jetten, 2011; Sani et al., 2008). For example, a study of people who had recently had a stroke found that life satisfaction *after* the stroke was appreciably higher for those who had belonged to more social groups *before* their stroke (Haslam, Holme et al., 2008). Other studies have reported similar effects on well-being among students transitioning to university (Iyer et al., 2009), women becoming mothers (Seymour-Smith, Cruwys, Haslam, & Brodribb, 2017), and older adults retiring from work (Steffens et al., 2016). We will discuss many of these studies in more detail in later chapters (e.g., Chapter 7 on ageing and Chapter 8 on depression), but in all these cases, belonging to multiple groups is observed to predict increased resilience and better mental health (see also Linville, 1985, 1987; Thoits, 1983). Importantly too, effects are not limited to measures of psychological well-being, but are also found on indices of physical health and mortality.

There is now also considerable evidence that health and well-being are enhanced by the *acquisition* of new social identities in times of change. For example, longitudinal studies that we will discuss next and in later chapters show that joining new groups is beneficial in helping people to overcome depression (Cruwys et al., 2013b; Cruwys, Haslam, Dingle, Haslam, & Jetten, 2014b, see also Chapter 8) or to recover from acquired brain injury (Jones, Williams et al., 2012; see Chapter 11).

The ability to gain new group memberships is particularly important when individuals embark on life changes where they aim to lose problematic social identities. This is the case, for example, if they belong to groups defined by drug or alcohol addiction (Dingle, Stark, Cruwys, & Best, 2015) or by violence (Williams et al., 2010). Here developing new social networks and joining new groups that promote recovery and avoid violence is found to be crucial for recovery from substance dependence and avoiding serious injury. As we will discuss further in Chapter 9, when it comes to substance abuse it is also apparent that when individuals form new social networks with non-users, the chances of them staying clean are far higher.

But it is not only those who struggle with serious negative life changes who benefit from acquiring new group memberships in the context of life transitions. In longitudinal research studying students entering a British university, Aarti Iyer and her colleagues found that the more groups that students belonged to before they moved, the more likely it was that they would quickly adopt and start to identify with their new student identity (Iyer et al., 2009). This in turn was associated with higher well-being and lower depression. Likewise, Katharine Greenaway and colleagues found that university students who gained group memberships in their final (and most challenging) year of study were more likely to report having their global needs for control, belonging, self-esteem, and meaning in life satisfied (Greenaway, Cruwys, Haslam, & Jetten, 2016). And as with all the other studies we have discussed in this section, in both these cases, these patterns remained statistically reliable when controlling for other potentially relevant factors (e.g., a person's financial circumstances).

In sum, then, it appears that the two key pathways identified within SIMIC – the social identity gain pathway and the social identity continuity pathway – delineate two very effective ways in which people can tackle the challenges of major life transitions. At the same time, though, in a final twist to our story, it is also the case that these two pathways are not equally accessible to everyone. On the contrary, it turns out that one of the main factors that stops people accessing them is social disadvantage. We will draw this chapter to a close by considering the reasons for this – and thereby also bring our analysis full circle.

Disadvantage can be a barrier to successful social identity change

Why then is identity change particularly hard for members of lower-status groups? There are a number of reasons for this. First, classic developmental research shows that well-being is determined in important ways by a person's feelings of control over the goals and events in their life, including the sense that they are in a position to shape their own environment (Bandura, 1982). As discussed earlier in this chapter, this is where those in higher-status positions have an advantage over their lower-status counterparts: for their access to various social and material resources means that they have more control over their lives and are in a better position to determine their own fate than those at the bottom of the social ladder. Members of lower-status groups are also more likely to face barriers and constraints in the course of pursuing their goals for a better future, and they are less likely to find themselves in the optimal environment for realising those goals.

Moreover, as a number of researchers have observed, these fundamental differences in control are most likely to come to the fore and to have the effect of reproducing inequalities in the context of important life transitions (Bakouri & Staerklé, 2015; Heinz, 2009). For example, in a classic study of people with cancer in Boston, 1- and 3-year survival rates were found to be much lower for low-income than for higher-income groups even after controlling for type of tumour, stage of cancer at diagnosis, age, or type of treatment received (Lipworth, Abelin, & Conelly, 1970). In what follows, we will explore the dynamics that contribute to these steeper health gradients for members of disadvantaged groups in three different transitional contexts: (1) in education as people move between institutions, (2) in housing as people endeavour to break out of homelessness, and (3) in whole communities that undergo major upheaval.

Education contexts

Education is one domain in which the health gradient is particularly pronounced. In particular, this is seen when students enter university. As George Akerlof and Rachel Kranton (2000) observe, even though "individuals may – more or less consciously – choose who they want to be . . . the limits on his choice may also be the most important determinant of an individual's economic well-being" (p. 3).

This point is well illustrated by the work of Iyer and colleagues (2009) that we referred to in the previous section. This study surveyed British undergraduate students entering university and found that, before they came to university, students from lower SES backgrounds reported belonging to significantly fewer social groups than their higher SES counterparts. This finding accords with other research which has found that people from higher-class backgrounds are more likely to develop rich social networks composed of multiple groups (Ball et al., 2003; Bourdieu, 1979/1984).

In line with SIMIC, this difference proved important once the students had entered university. For as we noted earlier, those students with fewer group memberships were less adept at managing this transition successfully. In particular, because they had belonged to fewer groups previously, low SES students were less well placed to take on the new identity as a university student, and this was associated with substantially lower well-being (see also Jetten, Haslam, & Barlow, 2013).

Entering university is more difficult for students from disadvantaged backgrounds for other reasons too. In particular, and consistent with SIMIC, even though gaining an education represents a good investment in one's future (as suggested by research into the social determinants of health; e.g., see Table 3.1), it is more likely to be incompatible with the previous identities of low SES students than is the case for their more affluent counterparts. Unsurprisingly, then, students from disadvantaged backgrounds tend to feel less comfortable in educational institutions and they are more likely to drop out (Friel, 2014; Rubin, 2012). Moreover, as we noted earlier, those who strive to enhance their personal status through individual mobility may encounter double discrimination when new and old groups are incompatible – for they may be rejected both by the group they try to leave behind and by the group they try to join (Postmes & Branscombe, 2002). Furthermore, in this case the self-*dis*continuity between the past (as a member of groups for whom universities are foreign places) and the present (as a university student) is more marked, and this also stands in the way of taking on the new identity as a university student.

Consistent with this reasoning, in a study of young people aspiring to go to university, Jetten and colleagues found that the more entering university was perceived by respondents to be incompatible with their SES background, the less prepared for university they reported being and the lower their expected level of identification was (Jetten, Iyer, Tsivrikos, & Young, 2008; Jetten, Iyer, & Zhang, 2017). A second study showed that this story was not any different for those who had recently entered university. Individuals identified more highly with the university when their social background was compatible with the new context that they were entering. There was also evidence that the less willing students were to take on the new identity in the long run, the less likely they were to endorse the belief that a university degree is an effective individual mobility strategy. These findings are somewhat depressing, in that they suggest that individual mobility strategies appear most costly to those who stand to gain the most from them.

Related findings emerge from a longitudinal study of the transition of Hispanic students into two Ivy League American universities conducted by Kathleen Ethier and Kay Deaux (1994). This examined the way that university entry affected these minority group students' ethnic identity over their first year at university. From this, the researchers identified two paths of identity negotiation, each with quite different implications for well-being.

The first pathway was more typical for those students who started with lower initial ethnic identification but also did not come to identify with the university (i.e., who did not go down SIMIC's identity gain pathway). As with the students in Jetten and colleagues' (2008) study, these students perceived entry into university as more of a threat to their ethnic identity (presumably because their Hispanic identity was incompatible with a university student identity), and they were more stressed during the transition. This resulted in even lower ethnic identification and lower self-esteem.

The second pathway had more positive outcomes. Consistent with the social identity continuity pathway of SIMIC, some of the students chose to engage in ethnic activities at university, thereby establishing continuity between their past and present identities. This type of behaviour was associated with stronger ethnic identification at the end of their first year at university. Notably though, this pathway was more likely to be chosen by students who had high ethnic identification initially. Interestingly too Ethier and Deaux (1994) point out that the ethnic identity of these students *did* change over the course of this year. For example, although before entering university many students' ethnic identity was shaped by interactions with their family and the communities in which they lived, once they were at university they sought out people and took part in activities that were consistent with a Hispanic identity on campus. Nevertheless, because these students were able to 'remoor' (i.e., re-attach) their old identity, add new meaning to it, and connect it to supportive elements in the new environment, positive effects of identity continuity ensued. In other words, because they experienced identity continuity during the change, the students felt less threatened by the transition and adjusted better to it.

Whatever path they take, though, it is clear that the barriers for lower SES or minority group students entering mainstream educational institutions are substantial. The irony here is that getting a good education (e.g., by going to university) is widely recognised as a way to improve one's life conditions and, by extension, one's health and well-being (Marmot, 2004; Putnam, 2000; Siegrist & Marmot, 2006). Accordingly, it would appear that this *upward mobility* function is least accessible to the people who need it most. In this way too, we see that barriers to education have a disproportionately negative impact (e.g., in terms of health and well-being) on those who are disadvantaged (see also Jetten et al., 2017).

Again, though, while students from lower SES backgrounds typically need to negotiate multiple obstacles on their path to a good education, there are also reasons to believe that this does not have to be the case. In particular, this is because these obstacles can be addressed through various forms of structural change (e.g., to student funding; see Rubin & Wright, 2017). An example of how this can work is provided by research with the children of rural workers in China. Historically, these children were an extremely disadvantaged group within the Chinese educational system – having little or no access to resources that would make higher education possible. In particular, this was because they were forced to attend schools that were under-resourced and provided only basic schooling relative to the facilities enjoyed by children of city workers (Huang & Xu, 2006). However, in 2011 the government introduced legislation that outlawed segregation in education and required urban authorities to provide rural workers' children with access to mainstream public schools.

For a while during this transition, segregated schools and integrated schools continued to exist alongside each other. Airong Zhang and colleagues (Zhang, Jetten, Iyer, & Cui, 2013) saw this as an opportunity to compare the self-esteem of children in different school systems. As one would expect, in both the old (segregated) and the new (integrated) schools, rural workers' children reported lower self-esteem than city children (i.e., the advantaged group). However, the self-esteem of rural workers' children in integrated schools was significantly higher than that of rural workers' children in segregated schools. Knowing that one's group might be able to engage in collective mobility was thus heartening for the lower-status children in the integrated schools, and their well-being clearly benefitted from the availability of "*cognitive alternatives*" to the status quo (Tajfel, 1978, p. 93). These same ideas were tested more formally in two further studies in which these perceptions of cognitive alternatives were measured (Study 1) and manipulated (Study 2). Both studies showed that students had higher self-esteem to the extent that they perceived there to be cognitive alternatives to the educational status quo.

Together, then, these lines of research show that although it may be more difficult for students from lower SES backgrounds to take advantage of life transitions than it is for their higher SES peers, the gap in their educational experience – and hence in their health and well-being outcomes – can be narrowed by appropriately targeted socio-structural change. If one is interested in narrowing this gap, the big questions for any given society are thus how willing its leaders are to devise, defend, and deliver such changes (Marmot, 2015). More generally too, we see that the primary obstacles to improvement in the health and well-being of those who are disadvantaged are not psychological but political.

Housing contexts

The barriers that the most disadvantaged people in society encounter when they undergo change are also apparent when it comes to housing. Whereas having a roof over one's head is a given for most of us, it again turns out that those who are most in need of this basic necessity are also least equipped to acquire it. Again, though, looking at this life challenge through the lens of identity change is useful because it helps explain who is most likely to escape homelessness and who is not. In particular, work by Walter and her colleagues has documented the profound benefits of social connectedness not just to the physical and mental well-being of homeless people, but also to their ability to break the cycle of homelessness (Walter et al., 2015a).

Although no-one disputes that this is a complex and difficult process, it is generally the case that individuals who are homeless are not in the best position to join groups. This is because they tend to have fewer social connections than those who are not homeless and relatively few opportunities to develop new group memberships by building on existing social networks (i.e., to develop bonding capital). Nevertheless, in a study of 119 clients of homelessness services in Australia, Walter and colleagues found that group-based social support still played a critical role in people's ability to transition out of homeless shelters and into secure housing (Walter et al., 2015a). In particular, the more that people came to identify with the service that provided the homeless shelter (i.e., the more bridging identity capital that they built), the more they were able to benefit from the support that that service provided and ultimately to remain in stable housing.

This finding is all the more remarkable given that research suggests that shelters can be hotbeds for the development of negative social relationships as well as relationships that undermine people's efforts to escape homelessness (e.g., because some residents engage in drug use or criminal activities; Auerswald & Eyre, 2002; Snow & Anderson, 1993). This means that staying in shelters can sometimes be more dangerous than sleeping in public places (Fitzpatrick & Jones, 2005).

In this context, it is thus important to distinguish between positive and negative sources of social support and to recognise that whereas some forms of social identification will have positive implications for health and well-being, others will not (see also Chapter 9). This conclusion is consistent with a recent study that examined resilience among women living in trailer parks in the United States (Notter, MacTavish, & Shamah, 2008). Here the researchers found that positive turning points were related to residents' ability to build effectively on support from positive groups while also distancing themselves from negative group influences. Consistent with this, Walter and colleagues' research found that these interactional patterns were associated with residents perceiving there to be, and using, more opportunities at the service. This in turn fed into better well-being when they came to leave (Walter et al., 2015b).

Here again, then, we see that social identity capital proves critical to the process of successfully negotiating change in ways predicted by SIMIC. And while again we see that members of disadvantaged groups (in this case homeless people) start with a profound disadvantage – because they have poorer initial networks and hence a limited social support base – social identity processes nevertheless play a key role either in cementing these disadvantages or in helping their most pernicious effects to be ameliorated. Critically though, we also need to acknowledge the role that *other groups* – and the support they provide (or do not provide) – play in this process. This reinforces the point that the fate of disadvantaged groups is never entirely in their own hands. In particular, it is determined in no small part by the treatment they receive from those who are more advantaged.

Community contexts

Disadvantage does not just hamper the attempts of particular subgroups in society to come to grips with change. It also affects whole communities. Speaking to this point, influential research by Michael Chandler and Christopher Lalonde (1998) examined youth suicide rates in Indigenous communities in Canada and showed that rather than being a simple reflection of poverty and disadvantage, these were powerfully determined by the group culture of the communities and, in particular, by the way that this had been shaped by governmental authorities.

Of course, given the fact that these Indigenous communities are the poorest group in North America, poverty is an important contributor to the high rates of youth suicide rates that are seen in these communities relative to those in the general population. However, Chandler and Lalonde's (1998) research also makes it clear that this is not the full explanation of the problem. In particular, this is because while all the communities that they examined were poor, there was very substantial variation in their rates of reported youth suicide. Indeed, 90% of suicides occurred in just 12% of the communities, whereas in about half of the 111 communities that were studied there had been no suicides for

5 years. Many Indigenous communities were therefore doing just as well as the most affluent non-Indigenous communities in terms of this particular health statistic. What, though, was going on in the communities where youth suicide was a particular problem?

According to Chandler and Lalonde (1998, 2008), the answer to this question is found by looking at the extent to which these communities had been able to maintain a sense of *collective continuity* (see also Chandler, Lalonde, Sokol, & Hallett, 2003). As they argue, this sense of collective continuity is particularly important for young people transitioning from childhood to adulthood. To support their claims, the researchers examined the prevalence of six markers of collective continuity in each of these communities (e.g., participation in land claims, self-governance, establishment of cultural facilities, community control over education). They found that suicide rates within Indigenous communities were dramatically increased when these communities had been managed in a way that disrupted the connection with the past and when they had not been able to hold on to their cultural history. In fact, the observed 5-year suicide rate fell to zero when all six of these protective factors were in place in any particular community.

This is an important point with which to draw this chapter to a close, speaking as it does to the importance of the social identity continuity pathway that is central to SIMIC. Indeed, consistent with our analysis, the authors themselves conclude by observing that:

> Where all of this leaves us is with a deep conviction that a better understanding of the problem of suicide in First Nations communities can only be had by focusing attention on the interface between personal and cultural change.
>
> (Chandler & Lalonde, 1998, p. 19)

Conclusion

There is a growing recognition that when it comes to the negative effects of social status on health and well-being "it does not have to be like this" (see Friel, 2014; Marmot, 2015). Precisely because there are no biological or genetic reasons for systematic differences in health and well-being on the basis of social status, these differences also are increasingly seen as unfair and unacceptable. In the words of Sharon Friel (2014, p. 161):

> Pursuit of health equity recognises the need to redress the inequitable distribution of these resources. Creating a fairer distribution of the resources relates to freedoms and empowerment at the individual, community, and whole country level. Empowerment is affected by three core things: basic material requisites for a decent life, control over our lives, and voice and participation in the policy decisions that affect the conditions in which people are born, grow, live, work, age and die.

She goes on to note that "these dimensions of empowerment are influenced by public policy and the way in which society, at the international, national and local level, chooses to run its affairs" (p. 161, see also Marmot, 2015).

Moreover, as Leonard Syme and Lisa Berkman first noted in 1976, the health gradient cannot be tackled by individuals on their own. Instead, these researchers argue that it requires large-scale action that targets whole communities. We agree, and our analysis is consistent with this conclusion. Moreover, the consensus that is emerging on this point is important because recognising that social status and disadvantage *do not need* to affect our health and well-being should encourage us all to participate in efforts to flatten the health gradient.

Importantly, though, we think that understanding the important role that group memberships and social identities play in creating this gradient is also critical to these efforts. The reason for this is that just as multiple group memberships and social identity capital are the key psychological resources that are conferred by wealth and privilege, so, too, they are key resources that are compromised by poverty and disadvantage. Accordingly, investment that focuses on (re)building these resources is likely to be particularly well targeted and peculiarly beneficial.

Points for practice

The key insight of this chapter is that for members of disadvantaged communities, their group membership is both the problem and a resource that they can draw from to counter negative effects on health and well-being. Given this, the following three points can assist those working with members of these groups.

1. *Avoid the need for the individual to self-categorize as belonging to a disadvantaged group.* When members of disadvantaged communities do not feel forced to categorize as members of a disadvantaged group they do not want to belong to (e.g., as homeless), the very fact that they can negotiate their identity the way they want contributes not only to health and well-being, but also empowers them when interacting with services.

2. *Do not assume a person's health and well-being status on the basis of their 'objective' social status.* Because *relative* disadvantage, the permeability of boundaries between status groups, and inequality within a particular society are such important predictors of health and well-being, an individual's objective social status (as determined by income, occupation, and education) should always be judged in context. What is more, because social status is relative, it is not fixed and determined by birth, but open to change (e.g., via interventions from health care workers).

3. *It is essential to recognise the identity-related barriers that members of disadvantaged groups encounter when they undergo important life transitions.* For example, recognising that a person belonged to very few groups before they faced an important life change (e.g., illness, retirement) or that they belong to a disadvantaged group and have limited group resources to fall back on to help manage such a change is likely to be very important in working out how best to support them.

Resources

Further reading

The following provide a good introduction to work that explores the links between social status and health.

① Marmot, M. (2015). *The health gap: The challenge of an unequal world.* London, UK: Bloomsbury.

This book represents a comprehensive, accessible, and well-written overview of research on the health gradient.

② Iyer, A., Jetten, J., & Tsivrikos, D. (2008). Torn between identities: Predictors of adjustment to identity change. In Sani, F. (Ed.). *Self-continuity: Individual and collective perspectives* (pp. 187–197). New York: Psychology Press.

This chapter provides an overview of predictions derived from the social identity model of identity change (SIMIC). It shows that social identity processes have an essential role to play in adjustment to life changes.

③ Sani, F. (2008). *Self-continuity: Individual and collective perspectives*. New York: Psychology Press.

This edited book brings together work by researchers in a wide range of fields – all of which speak to the important contribution of personal and collective-level continuity to health and well-being.

Audio and video

① Search for "Marmot Boyer Lectures" to listen to the 2016 lecture by Prof. Michael Marmot on "Health inequality and the causes of the causes". www.abc.net.au/radionational/programs/boyer-lectures/boyer-lecture-health-inequality-and-the-causes-of-the-causes/7763106. (57 minutes)
② Search for "Wilkinson Spirit Level Ted talk" to watch a 2011 TED talk by Richard Wilkinson on "How economic inequality harms societies". This provides an overview of ideas presented in more detail in the influential book *The Spirit Level* that he wrote with Kate Pickett in 2009. www.ted.com/talks/richard_wilkinson (17 minutes)

Websites

① www.who.int/social_determinants/thecommission/finalreport/key_concepts/en/. This World Health Organization site provides a rich resource for anyone interested in the social determinants of health. It contains publications, evidence for the social gradient of health, and training tools on how to implement insights to practice.
② www.bbcprisonstudy.org This is the official website for the BBC Prison Study. It contains a range of materials and resources that are relevant to the issues explored in this chapter.

References

Abbott, D. H., Keverne, E. B., Bercovitch, F. B., Shively, C. A., Mendoza, S. P., Salzman, W., . . . Sapolsky, R. M. (2003). Are subordinates always stressed? A comparative analysis of rank differences in cortisol levels among primates. *Hormones and Behavior, 43*, 67–82.

Agich, G. J. (Ed.). (1982). *Responsibility in health care*. Hingham, MA: Reidel.

Akerlof, G. A., & Kranton, R. E. (2000). Economics and identity. *Quarterly Journal of Economics, 105*, 715–753.

Anderson, C., Kraus, M. W., Galinsky, A. D., & Keltner, D. (2012). The local ladder effect: Social status and subjective well-being. *Psychological Science, 23*, 764–771.

Auerswald, C. L., & Eyre, S. L. (2002). Youth homelessness in San Francisco: A life cycle approach. *Social Science and Medicine, 54*, 1497–1512.

Australian Institute of Health and Welfare. (2014). *Mortality inequalities in Australia 2009–2011*. AIHW, Bulletin, 124. Retrieved from www.aihw.gov.au/WorkArea/DownloadAsset.aspx?id=60129548364

Bakouri, M., & Staerklé, C. (2015). Coping with structural disadvantage: Overcoming negative effects of perceived barriers through bonding identities. *British Journal of Social Psychology, 54*, 648–670.

Ball, S. J., Reay, D., & David, M. (2003). Ethnic choosing: Minority ethnic students, social class, and higher education choice. *Race, Ethnicity, and Education, 5*, 333–357.

Bandura, A. (1982). Self-efficacy mechanism in human agency. *American Psychologist, 37,* 122–147.

Begeny, C. T., & Huo, Y. J. (2016). Is it always good to feel valued? The psychological benefits and costs of higher perceived status in one's ethnic minority group. *Group Processes & Intergroup Relations.* Advance online publication. doi:10.1177/1368430216656922

Berry, J. W. (1997). Immigration, acculturation, and adaptation. *Applied Psychology: An International Review, 46,* 5–34.

Blanchard, D. C., Spencer, R. L., Weiss, S. M., Blanchard, R. J., McEwen, B., & Sakai, R. R. (1995). Visible burrow system as a model of chronic social stress: Behavioural and neuroendocrine correlates. *Psychoneuroendocrinology, 20,* 117–134.

Blascovich, J. (2008). Challenge, threat, and health. In J. Y. Shah & W. L. Gardner (Eds.), *Handbook of motivation science* (pp. 481–493). New York, NY: Guilford Press.

Blascovich, J., & Mendes, W. B. (2000). Challenge and threat appraisals: The role of affective cues. In J. Forgas (Ed.), *Feeling and thinking: The role of affect in social cognition* (pp. 59–82). Cambridge, UK: Cambridge University Press.

Boccia, M. L., Scanlan, J. M., Laudenslager, M. L., Berger, C. L., Hijazi, A. S., & Reite, M. L. (1997). Juvenile friends, behaviour, and immune responses to separation in bonnet marque infants. *Physiology and Behavior, 61,* 191–198.

Bourdieu, P. (1979/1984). *Distinction: A social critique of the judgment of taste* (R. Nice, Trans.). Cambridge, MA: Harvard University Press.

Branscombe, N. R., & Ellemers, N. (1998). Coping with group-based discrimination: Individualistic versus group-level strategies. In J. K. Swim & C. Stangor (Eds.), *Prejudice: The target's perspective* (pp. 243–266). New York, NY: Academic Press.

Branscombe, N. R., Wann, D. L., Noel, J. G., & Coleman, J. (1993). Ingroup or outgroup extremity Importance of the threatened identity. *Personality and Social Psychology Bulletin, 19,* 381–388.

Braveman, P. A., Cubbin, C., Egerter, S., Williams, D. R., & Pamuk, E. (2010). Socio-economic disparities in health in the United States: What the patterns tell us. *American Journal of Public Health, 100,* 186–196.

Breakwell, G. M. (1986). *Coping with threatened identities.* London: Methuen.

Brown, L., Thurecht, L., & Nepal, B. (2012). *The cost of inaction on the social determinants of health* University of Canberra: National Centre for Social and Economic Modelling (NATSEM).

Busch-Geertsema, V., Edgar, W., O'Sullivan, E., & Pleace, N. (2010). *Homelessness and homeless policies in Europe: Lessons from research.* Brussels: FEANTSA.

Chamberlain, C., & MacKenzie, D. (2006). Homeless careers: A framework for intervention. *Australian Social Work, 59,* 198–212.

Chandler, M. J., & Lalonde, C. E. (1998). Cultural continuity as a hedge against suicide in Canada's First Nations. *Transnational Psychiatry, 35,* 191–219.

Chandler, M. J., & Lalonde, C. E. (2008). Cultural continuity as a protective factor against suicide in First Nations youth. *Horizons, 10,* 68–72.

Chandler, M. J., Lalonde, C. E., Sokol, B. W., & Hallett, D. (2003). Personal persistence, identity development, and suicide: A study of native and non-native North American adolescents. *Monographs of the Society for Research in Child Development, 68,* 1–138.

Cohen, S., & Janicki-Deverts, D. (2009). Can we improve our physical health by altering our social networks? *Perspectives on Psychological Science, 4,* 375–378.

Compton, M. T., & Shim, R. S. (2015). *The social determinants of mental health.* Arlington, VA: American Psychiatric Association Publishing.

Creel, S. (2001). Social dominance and stress hormones. *Trends in Ecology and Evolution, 16,* 491–497

Crocker, J., & Luhtanen, R. (1990). Collective self-esteem and ingroup bias. *Journal of Personality and Social Psychology, 58,* 60–67.

Cruwys, T., Berry, H. L., Cassells, R., Duncan, A., O'Brien, L., Sage, B., & D'Souza, G. (2013a). *Marginalised Australians: Characteristics and predictors of exit over ten years 2001–2010*. Canberra: University of Canberra.

Cruwys, T., Dingle, G. A., Haslam, C., Haslam, S. A., Jetten, J., & Morton, T. A. (2013b). Social group memberships protect against future depression, alleviate depression symptoms and prevent depression relapse. *Social Science and Medicine, 98*, 179–186.

Cruwys, T., Haslam, S. A., Dingle, G. A., Haslam, C., & Jetten, J., (2014). Depression and Social Identity: An integrative review. *Personality and Social Psychology Review, 18*, 215–238.

De Nooy, J. (2016). Distant (be)longings: Contemporary Australian memoirs of life in France. *Australian Journal of French Studies, 53*, 39–52.

Diener, E., & Diener, C. (1996). Most people are happy. *Psychological Science, 7*, 181–185.

Dingle, G. A., Stark, C., Cruwys, T., & Best, D. (2015) Breaking good: breaking ties with social groups may be good for recovery from substance misuse. *British Journal of Social Psychology, 54*, 236–254.

Drury, J., & Reicher, S. D. (2009). Collective psychological empowerment as a model of social change: Researching crowds and power. *Journal of Social Issues, 65*, 707–725.

Ellemers, N. (1993). The influence of socio-structural variables on identity enhancement strategies. *European Review of Social Psychology, 4*, 27–57.

Ellemers, N., Van Knippenberg, A., & Wilke, H. (1990). The influence of permeability of group boundaries and stability of group status on strategies of individual mobility and social change. *British Journal of Social Psychology, 29*, 233–246.

Ethier, K. A., & Deaux, K. (1994). Negotiating social identity when contexts change: Maintaining identification and responding to threat. *Journal of Personality and Social Psychology, 67*, 243–251.

Fitzpatrick, S., & Jones, A. (2005). Pursuing social justice or social cohesion? Coercion in street homelessness policies in England. *Journal of Social Policy, 34*, 389–406.

Friel, S. (2014). Inequities in the freedom to lead a flourishing and healthy life: Issues for healthy public policy. *International Journal of Health Policy and Management, 3*, 161–163.

Goymann, W., & Wingfield, J. C. (2004). Allostatic load, social status and stress hormones: The costs of social status matter. *Animal Behaviour, 67*, 591–602.

Greenaway, K. H., Cruwys, T., Haslam, S. A., & Jetten, J. (2016). Social identities promote well-being because they satisfy global psychological needs. *European Journal of Social Psychology, 46*, 294–307.

Greenaway, K. H., Haslam, S. A., Branscombe, N. R., Cruwys, T., Ysseldyk, R., & Heldreth, C. (2015). From "we" to "me": Group identification enhances perceived personal control with consequences for health and well-being. *Journal of Personality and Social Psychology, 109*, 53–74.

Gust, D. A., Gordon, T. P., Wilson, M. E., Ahmed-Ansari, A., Brodie, A. R., & McClure, H. M. (1991). Formation of a new social group of unfamiliar female rhesus monkeys affects the immune and pituitary adrenocortical systems. *Brain, Behavior, and Immunity, 5*, 296–307.

Haslam, S. A., & Reicher, S. D. (2012). When prisoners take over the prison: A social psychology of resistance. *Personality and Social Psychology Review, 16*, 152–179.

Haslam, S. A., Jetten, J., Postmes, T., & Haslam, C. (2009). Social identity, health and well-being: An emerging agenda for applied psychology. *Applied Psychology: An International Review, 58*, 1–23.

Haslam, C., Holme, A., Haslam, S. A., Iyer, A., Jetten, J., & Williams, W. H. (2008). Maintaining group memberships: Social identity continuity predicts well-being after stroke. *Neuropsychological Rehabilitation, 18*, 671–691.

Haslam, C. Jetten, J., & Haslam, S. A. (2012). Advancing the social cure: Implications for theory, practice and policy. In J. Jetten, C. Haslam, & S. A. Haslam (Eds.), *The social cure: Identity, health, and well-being* (pp. 319–343). Hove, UK: Psychology Press.

Haslam, S. A., O'Brien, A., Jetten, J., Vormedal, K., & Penna, S. (2005). Taking the strain: Social identity, social support and the experience of stress. *British Journal of Social Psychology, 44,* 355–370.

Haunschild, P. R., Moreland, R. L., & Murrell, A. J. (1994). Sources of resistance to mergers between groups. *Journal of Applied Social Psychology, 24,* 1150–1178.

Heinz, W. R. W. (2009). Structure and agency in transition research. *Journal of Education and Work, 22,* 391–404.

Helliwell, J. F. (2006). Well-being, social capital and public policy. *The Economic Journal, 116,* 34–45.

Helliwell, J. F., & Barrington-Leigh, C. P. (2012). How much is social capital worth? In J. Jetten, C. Haslam, & S. A. Haslam (Eds.), *The social cure: Identity, health and well-being* (pp. 55–71). Hove, UK: Psychology Press.

Hopkins, N., & Reicher, S. D. (1996). The construction of social categories and processes of social change: Arguing about national identity. In G. M. Breakwell & E. Lyons (Eds.), *Changing European identities: Social psychological analyses of social change* (pp. 69–93). Oxford: Butterworth-Heinemann.

Hornsey, M. J., & Hogg, M. A. (2000). Intergroup similarity and subgroup relations: Some implications for assimilation. *Personality and Social Psychology Bulletin, 26,* 948–958.

Huang, Z., & Xu, K. (2006). Education of migrant workers and their children and its solutions. *Journal of Zhejiang University (Humanities and Social Sciences), 36,* 108–114.

Iyer, A., & Jetten, J. (2011). What's left behind: Identity continuity moderates the effect of nostalgia on well-being and life choices. *Journal of Personality and Social Psychology, 101,* 94–108.

Iyer, A., Jetten, J., Tsvrikos, D., Postmes, T., & Haslam, S. A. (2009). The more (and the more compatible) the merrier: Multiple group memberships and identity compatibility as predictors of adjustment after life transitions. *British Journal of Social Psychology, 48,* 707–733.

Jetten, J., & Pachana, N. A. (2012). Not wanting to grow old: A social identity model of identity change (SIMIC) analysis of driving cessation among older adults. In J. Jetten, C. Haslam, & S. A. Haslam (Eds.), *The social cure: Identity, health and well-being* (pp. 97–113). Hove, UK: Psychology Press.

Jetten, J., Branscombe, N. R., Haslam, S. A., Haslam, C., Cruwys, T., Jones, J. M., . . . Zhang, A. (2015). Having a lot of a good thing: Multiple important group memberships as a source of self-esteem. *PLoS ONE, 10*(6), e0131035.

Jetten, J., O'Brien, A., & Trindall, N. (2002). Changing identity: Predicting adjustment to organizational restructure as a function of subgroup and superordinate identification. *British Journal of Social Psychology, 41,* 281–298.

Jetten, J., Haslam, C., Haslam, S. A., & Branscombe, N. (2009). The social cure. *Scientific American Mind, 20,* 26–33.

Jetten, J., Haslam, S. A., Iyer, A., & Haslam, C. (2010a). Turning to others in times of change: Social identity and coping with stress. In S. Stürmer & M. Snyder (Eds.), *The psychology of prosocial behavior: Group processes, intergroup relations, and helping* (pp. 139–156). Oxford, UK: Blackwell.

Jetten, J., Haslam, S. A., Cruwys, T., Greenaway, K., Haslam, S. A., & Steffens, N. R. (2017). Advancing the social identity approach to health and well-being: Progressing the social cure research agenda. *European Journal of Social Psychology, 47,* 789–802.

Jetten, J., Haslam, S. A., & Barlow, F. (2013). Bringing back the system: One reason why conservatives are happier than liberals is that higher socio-economic status gives them access to more group memberships. *Social Psychological and Personality Science, 4,* 6–13.

Jetten, J., Haslam, C., Haslam, S. A., Dingle, G. A., & Jones, J. M. (2014). How groups affect our health and well-being: The path from theory to policy. *Social Issues and Policy Review, 8,* 103–130.

Jetten, J., Haslam, C., Pugliese, C., Tonks, J., & Haslam, S. A. (2010b). Declining autobiographical memory and the loss of identity: Effects on well-being. *Journal of Clinical and Experimental Neuropsychology*, *32*, 408–416.

Jetten, J., Iyer, A., & Zhang, A. (2017). The educational experience of low SES background students. In K. Mavor, M. Platow, & B. Bizumic (Eds.), *Self, social identity and education* (pp. 112–125). London: Routledge.

Jetten, J., Iyer, A., Tsivrikos, D., & Young, B. M. (2008). When is individual mobility costly? The role of economic and social identity factors. *European Journal of Social Psychology*, *38*, 866–879.

Johnstone, M., Jetten, J., Dingle, G. A., Parsell, C., & Walter, Z. C. (2015). Discrimination and well-being amongst the homeless: The role of multiple group membership. *Frontiers in Psychology*, *6*. doi:10.3389/fpsyg.2015.00739

Jones, J. M., Williams, W. H., Jetten, J., Haslam, S. A., Harris, A., & Gleibs, I. H. (2012). The role of psychological symptoms and social group memberships in the development of post-traumatic stress after traumatic injury. *British Journal of Health Psychology*, *17*, 798–811.

Kim, D., Subramanian, S. V., & Kawachi, I. (2006). Bonding versus bridging social capital and their associations with self rated health: a multilevel analysis of 40 US communities. *Journal of Epidemiological Community Health*, *60*, 116–122.

Lalonde, R. N., & Silverman, R. A. (1994). Behavioral preference in response to social injustice: The effects of group permeability and social identity salience. *Journal of Personality and Social Psychology*, *66*, 78–85.

Linville, P. W. (1985). Self-complexity and affective extremity: Don't put all of your eggs in one cognitive basket. *Social Cognition*, *3*, 94–120.

Linville, P. W. (1987). Self-complexity as a cognitive buffer against stress-related illness and depression. *Journal of Personality and Social Psychology*, *52*, 663–676.

Lipworth, L., Abelin, T., & Conelly, R. R. (1970). Socio-economic factors in the prognosis of cancer patients. *Journal of Chronic Disability*, *23*, 105–116.

Luhtanen, R., & Crocker, J. (1991). Self-esteem and intergroup comparison: Toward a theory of collective self-esteem. In J. Suls & T. A. Wills (Eds.), *Social comparison: Contemporary theory and research* (pp. 211–234). Hillsdale, NJ: Lawrence Erlbaum.

Manogue, K. R., Leshner, A. I., & Candland, D. K. (1975). Dominance status and adrenocortical reactivity to stress in squirrel monkeys, *Primates*, *16*, 457–463.

Marmot, M. (2004). *Status syndrome: How our social standing affects your health and life expectancy*. London, UK: Bloomsbury Publishing.

Marmot, M. (2005). Social determinants of health inequalities. *Lancet*, *365*, 1099–1104.

Martiny, S. E., & Rubin, M. (2016). Towards a clearer understanding of social identity theory's self-esteem hypothesis. In S. McKeown, R. Haji, & N. Ferguson (Eds.), *Understanding peace and conflict through social identity theory: Contemporary global perspectives* (pp. 19–32). New York, NY: Springer.

McNamara, N., Stevenson, C., & Muldoon, O. T. (2013). Community identity as resource and context: A mixed method investigation of coping and collective action in a disadvantaged community. *European Journal of Social Psychology*, *43*, 393–403.

Muldoon, O. T. (2013). Understanding the impact of political violence in childhood: A theoretical review using a social identity approach. *Clinical Psychology Review*, *33*, 929–939.

Mullen, B., Brown, R., & Smith, C. (1992). Ingroup bias as a function of salience, relevance, and status: An integration. *European Journal of Social Psychology*, *22*, 103–122.

Notter, M. L., MacTavish, K. A., & Shamah, D. (2008), Pathways toward resilience among women in rural trailer parks. *Family Relations*, *57*, 613–624.

Oh, H., Chung, M. H., & Labianca, G. (2004). Group social capital and group effectiveness: The role of informal socializing ties. *Academy of Management Journal, 47*, 860–875.

Otten, S., Mummendey, A., & Blanz, M. (1996). Intergroup discrimination in positive and negative outcome allocations: Impact of stimulus valence, relative group status, and relative group size. *Personality and Social Psychology Bulletin, 22*, 568–581.

Outten, H. R., Schmitt, M. T., Garcia, D. M., & Branscombe, N. R. (2009). Coping options: Missing links between minority group identification and psychological well-being. *Applied Psychology, 58*, 146–170.

Parsell, C. (2011). Homeless identities: Enacted and ascribed. *British Journal of Sociology, 62*, 442–461.

Postmes, T., & Branscombe, N. R. (2002). Influence of long-term racial environmental composition on subjective well-being in African Americans. *Journal of Personality and Social Psychology, 83*, 735–751.

Raphael, D. (2000). Health inequities in the United States: Prospects and solutions. *Journal of Public Health Policy, 21*, 394–427.

Reicher, S. D. (1987). Crowd behaviour as social action. In J. C. Turner, M. A. Hogg, P. J. Oakes, S. D. Reicher, & M. S. Wetherell (Eds.), *Rediscovering the social group: A self-categorization theory* (pp. 171–202). Oxford: Blackwell.

Reicher, S. D., & Haslam, S. A. (2006a). Rethinking the psychology of tyranny: The BBC Prison Study. *British Journal of Social Psychology, 45*, 1–40.

Roccas, S. (2003). The effects of status on identification with multiple groups. *European Journal of Social Psychology, 33*, 351–366.

Rubin, M. (2012). Social class differences in social integration among students in higher education: A meta-analysis and recommendations for future research. *Journal of Diversity in Higher Education, 5*, 22–38.

Rubin, M., & Hewstone, M. (1998). Social identity theory's self-esteem hypothesis: A review and some suggestions for clarification. *Personality and Social Psychology Review, 2*, 40–62.

Rubin, M., & Wright, C. L. (2017). Time and money explain social class differences in students' social integration at university. *Studies in Higher Education, 42*, 315–330.

Sachdev, I., & Bourhis, R. Y. (1987). Status differentials and intergroup behaviour. *European Journal of Social Psychology, 17*, 277–293.

Sani, F. (2008). *Self continuity: Individual and collective perspectives*. New York, NY: Psychology Press.

Sani, F., Bowe, M., & Herrera, M. (2008). Perceived collective continuity and social well-being: Exploring the connections. *European Journal of Social Psychology, 38*, 365–374.

Sani, F., Magrin, M. E., Scrignaro, M., & McCollum, R. (2010). Ingroup identification mediates the effects of subjective ingroup status on mental health. *British Journal of Social Psychology, 49*, 883–893.

Sapolsky, R. M. (2004). Social status and health in humans and other animals. *Annual Review of Anthropology, 33*, 393–418.

Saunders, P. (2008). Measuring wellbeing using non-monetary indicators: Deprivation and social exclusion. *Family Matters, 78*, 8–17.

Scheepers, D. T., & Ellemers, N. (2005). When the pressure is up: The assessment of social identity threat in low and high status groups. *Journal of Experimental Social Psychology, 41*, 192–200.

Scheepers, D. T., Ellemers, N., & Sintemaartensdijk, N. (2009). Suffering from the possibility of status loss: Physiological responses to social identity threat in high status groups. *European Journal of Social Psychology, 39*, 1075–1092.

Seymour-Smith, M., Cruwys, T., Haslam, S. A., & Brodribb, W. (2017). Loss of group membership predicts depression in postpartum mothers. *Social Psychiatry and Psychiatric Epidemiology, 52*, 201–210.

Shapiro, K. J. (1998). *Animal models of human psychology*. Seattle, WA: Hogrefe & Huber.

Siegrist, J., & Marmot, M. (2006). *Social inequalities in health: New evidence and policy implications*. Oxford, UK: Oxford University Press.

Singh-Manoux, A., Marmot, M., & Adler, N. E. (2005). Does subjective social status predict health and change in health status better than objective status? *Psychosomatic Medicine, 67*, 855–861.

Smith, H. J., Tyler, T. R., & Huo, Y. J. (2003). Interpersonal treatment, social identity and organizational behavior. In S. A. Haslam, D. van Knippenberg, M. J. Platow, & N. Ellemers (Eds.), *Social identity at work: Developing theory for organizational practice* (pp. 155–171). Philadelphia, PA: Psychology Press.

Snow, D. A., & Anderson, L. (1993). *Down on their luck: A study of homeless street people*. Berkeley, CA: University of California Press.

Steffens, N. K., Cruwys, T., Haslam, C., Jetten, J., & Haslam, S. A. (2016). Social group memberships in retirement are associated with reduced risk of premature death: Evidence from a longitudinal cohort study. *BMJ Open, 6*, e010164. doi: 10.1136/bmjopen-2015–010164

Syme, S. L., & Berkman, L. F. (1976). Social class, susceptibility and sickness. *American Journal of Epidemiology, 104*, 1–8.

Tajfel, H. (Ed.). (1978). *Differentiation between social groups: Studies in the social psychology of inter-group relations*. London: Academic Press.

Tajfel, H., & Turner, J. C. (1979). An integrative theory of intergroup conflict. In W. G. Austin & S. Worchel (Eds.), *The social psychology of intergroup relations* (pp. 33–47). Monterey, CA: Brooks/Cole.

Thoits, P. (2013). Dimensions of life events that influence psychological distress: An evaluation and synthesis of the literature. In H. B. Kaplan (Ed.), *Psychosocial stress: Trends in theory and research* (pp. 33–106). New York, NY: Academic Press.

Turner, J. C. (1975). Social comparison and social identity: Some prospects for intergroup behaviour. *European Journal of Social Psychology, 5*, 5–34.

Turner, J. C., Hogg, M. A., Oakes, P. J., Reicher, S. D., & Wetherell, M. S. (1987). *Rediscovering the social group: A self-categorization theory*. Oxford, UK: Blackwell.

Vaananen, A., Koskinen, A., Joensuu, M., Kivimak, M., Vahtera, J., Kouvonen, A., & Jappinen, P. (2008). Lack of predictability at work and risk of acute myocardial infarction: An 18-year prospective study of industrial employees. *American Journal of Public Health, 98*, 2264–2271.

Walter, Z. C., Jetten, J., Dingle, G. A., Parsell, C., & Johnstone, M. (2015a). Two pathways through adversity: Predicting well-being and housing outcomes among homeless service users. *British Journal of Social Psychology, 55*, 357–374.

Walter, Z. C., Jetten, J., Parsell, C., & Dingle, G. A. (2015b). The impact of self-categorizing as "homeless" on well-being and service use. *Analyses of Social Issues and Public Policy, 15*, 333–356.

Warner, R., Hornsey, M. J., & Jetten, J. (2007). Why minority group members resent impostors. *European Journal of Social Psychology. 37*, 1–18.

Weiss, J. (1970). Somatic effects of predictable and unpredictable shock. *Psychosomatic Medicine, 32*, 397–414.

Whiteley, P. F. (1999). The origins of social capital. In J. W. van Deth, M. Maraffi, K. Newton, & P. F. Whiteley (Eds.), *Social capital and European democracy* (pp. 25–44). Abingdon, UK: Routledge.

Wilkinson, R., & Pickett, K. (2009). *The spirit level: Why more equal societies almost always do better*. London, UK: Allen Lane.

Williams, W. H., Mewse, A. J., Tonks, J., Mills, S., Burgess, C. N., & Cordan, G. (2010). Traumatic brain injury in a prison population: Prevalence and risk for re-offending. *Brain Injury, 24*, 1184–1188.

World Health Organization, & United Nations Children's Fund. (1978). *Primary health care: A joint report*. Geneva: WHO.

Wright, S. C., Taylor, D. M., & Moghaddam, F. M. (1990). Responding to membership in a disadvantaged group: From acceptance to collective protest. *Journal of Personality and Social Psychology*, *58*, 994–1003.

Wuthnow, R. (1994). *Sharing the journey: Support groups and America's new quest for community*. New York, NY: Simon and Schuster.

Zhang, A., Jetten, J., Iyer, A., & Cui, L. (2013). "It will not always be this way": Cognitive alternatives improve self-esteem in contexts of segregation. *Social Psychological and Personality Science, 4*, 159–166.

CHAPTER 5

Human welfare

Wendy Stainton Rogers

This chapter talks about welfare rather than health, because of all the complicated baggage attached to our contemporary concept 'health' – the way it has become moralised; the domination of biomedicine; and that it health is seen as an individual state rather than something that operates communally. The initial sections of this chapter challenge all of these, arguing for a much broader and more contextualised approach to physical illness and mental distress. Next follows a section on issues of governmentality and identity and the ways in which health services are inequitably distributed. Attention is then directed to the concept of human welfare and its emphasis on improving the social and community support available to promote human wellbeing. It takes up the themes of social connectedness, community resilience and social capital and their role in enabling people to 'live well' – and what that means. It looks too at the roles that public health measures (like proper housing and sewage), religion and legislation all play.

> A new popular health consciousness pervades our culture. The concern with personal health has become a national preoccupation. Ever increasing personal effort, political attention, and consumer dollars are being expanded in the name of health.
>
> (Crawford, 1980: 365)

Healthism

Crawford defined this new consciousness as 'healthism'. Notice that this was published in 1980! I think it is even more extreme today – a worldview that assumes that being healthy is a matter of preeminent importance, and sees it mainly in terms of personal 'choice' and 'lifestyle' (see, for example, Lewis, 2009) where people *choose* what and how much to eat, how much to exercise and whether to indulge in risky behaviour such as smoking or in extreme sports.

However, this worldview has its critics who argue that we have become subject to 'neo-liberal ideologies of healthism, active living and consumership' (Silk and Andrews, 2006: 1–13). The fundamental assumption underpinning healthism is that

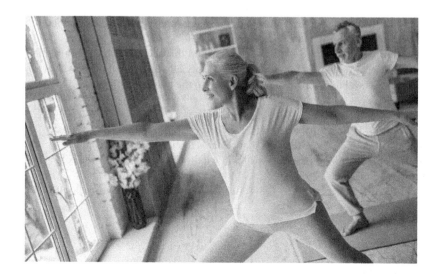

individuals not only have control over their own health but are, more fundamentally, *responsible* for it: 'To be a citizen in the new public health . . . one has to be dutiful and governable, and one has to take responsibility for one's own health and physical activity' (Fusco, 2006: 58). It is a worldview that has, according to Barbara Ehrenreich, made the lives of people who are growing old a burden, rather than something to be enjoyed for all the joys and satisfactions it can bring (as evidenced by Pheonix and Orr, 2014, as discussed in Chapter 3):

> You can think of death bitterly or with resignation, as a tragic interruption to your life, and take every possible measure to postpone it. Or, more realistically, you can think of life as an interruption of an eternity of personal nonexistence, and seize it as a brief opportunity to observe, and interact with the living, ever surprising world around us.
>
> (Ehrenreich, 2018: XV)

In her recent polemic against healthism – the worldview that has, she says, (within in the American insurance-based healthcare system), come to dominate the understandings and beliefs people have about health, the lifestyles they adopt (or try to) and the moral judgements they make – Ehrenreich laments the way in which, these days, people (especially older people) are vilified if they fail to 'look after their health' and, more than that, if they do not actively pursue a lifestyle of personal and medical surveillance. She argues instead for growing old with panache, verve and optimism (as does, very eloquently, Jayne Raisbrough, 2018).

Human welfare, not health

I will admit that this chapter has an awful lot about health in it – and yet I've entitled it 'Human Welfare'. My reason for that is that, progressively, 'health' has become an increasingly problematic word in itself, a concept carrying an awful lot of emotional and moralising baggage – for me and many other critical psychologists. This 'troubling' of health makes it difficult to talk about it (or even think about it) very clearly. Almost universally 'health' has become such a 'hurrah word', a word that signifies everything good and desirable (as opposed by 'boo words' that stand for everything bad and horrid). To say something is 'healthy' is to claim that only good can come of it, and that it is something to which all sensible people should aspire. Doing something – almost anything – that will make you healthier is heavily sold to us as both an entitlement and an investment.

My word swap, therefore, is part of the way that this chapter directs our attention away from the pressure to act in healthy ways, especially the kind of pressure that Ehrenreich was seeking to avoid – not to give in to the normal bodily decay that inevitably happens in later life.

> Not only do I reject the torment of a medicalized death, but I refuse to accept a medicalized life. . . . As the time that remains to me shrinks, each month and day becomes too precious to spend in windowless rooms under the cold scrutiny of machines.
>
> (Ehrenreich, 2018: 13)

Like her, instead of concentrating on the imperative to be healthy, this chapter will focus on the pursuit of human welfare – a much broader and less ideologically dubious aspiration. In particular, I will challenge 'healthism' and its neoliberal mission, disparage mainstream health psychology's collusion in this enterprise, and explore the ways in which critical health psychology enables us to offer a more human alternative; and look more widely at concepts and ideas that are more human in their approach.

Challenging biomedicine's claims to superior knowledge

Not only is there a fixation with healthism, science-based biomedicine tends to dominate the way that people make sense of healthiness and illness. Its whole enterprise is based on the assumption that it – and only it – can tell us how to plan and provide healthcare services – heal the sick, care for the infirm, improve health and promote it. All other explanatory frameworks are viewed as an 'ignorant lack of understanding', 'superstitious nonsense' or worse. Even established forms of traditional medicine (such as Chinese Herbal and Ayurvedic) tend to be seen as having limited effectiveness and to act only as placebos. Medical science very much sees itself as a *superior* form of knowledge – science being the only means to provide sound empirical knowledge about what makes us healthy or ill. The sociologist Eliot Friedson (1970) wrote of the medical profession as the 'architects of medical knowledge' (accorded the power to determine what constitutes 'real illness', as opposed, say, to hysteria, hypochondria or malingering) and, these days, what constitutes a 'healthy lifestyle', 'a healthy diet' and 'a healthy state of mind').

Looked at from a human psychology perspective, however, the practice of biomedicine is more a matter of exercising power than necessarily having superior expertise. The anthropologist Michael Taussig (1980) made this point explicitly – talking of biomedicine as 'reproducing a political ideology in the guise of a science of (apparently) "real things"' (19). I would take it further, arguing that it is strongly influenced, these days, by a highly politicised neoliberal ideology that has been appropriated by food companies, gyms, spas and so on as a way to add value to their products and services and of making them more desirable.

The term 'illness' and its discontents

There are two main ways in which the term 'illness' is problematic – first its reification, and second the way biomedicine's dualism raises all sorts of issues.

Illness is a social construction

We often treat illnesses as if they were actual, real phenomena ('real things' as Taussig calls them), but they are not. They are created by human 'effort after meaning'. You may find this a strange idea, but bear with me. Patrick Sedgewick (1982) put it rather poetically when he wrote:

> The fracture of a septuagenarian's [70-year-old's] femur has, within the world of nature, no more significance than the snapping of an autumn leaf from its twig: the invasion of a human organism by cholera carries no more the stamp of 'illness' than does the souring of milk by other forms of bacteria.

(30)

Illnesses are 'made up' by the way humans think about the world – their 'reality' reflects the human concerns of the time and in the location of their use. A good example is an illness with a gloriously florid title – drapetomania. It was coined by Samuel Cartwright in 1851, a slave owner in the 'Deep South' of America, to describe the imprudent propensity of slaves to run away from their owners, against the will of God. As a 'medical condition', he argued, it needed 'medical treatment' – his recommendation was a thorough whipping! To be fair, his idea was severely mocked and lampooned in the Northern states at the time. But perhaps, today, with the benefit of hindsight, we can fully recognise not only that it was utter rubbish, but how incredibly self-serving it was.

Reflection 10.1

Can you think of other 'made up' illnesses – or ones you think are so, at least?

For me the most groan-inducing made-up illness is 'ageing actress syndrome', apparently suffered by women who were beautiful in their youth but suffer as they age because they don't get the attention they are used to. Remember that 'homosexuality' was treated as an illness (Chapter 1) up until the 1960s, and that it was not until 2008 that 'gender identity disorder' was recognised by the APA as to do with prejudice, rather than being a mental condition (Chapter 5). There are a whole panoply of 'female sicknesses' that we now recognise as serving patriarchal purposes – 'hysteria' (womb sickness) being the most blatant. I have my concerns too about PTSD (post-traumatic stress disorder), as it is so very general and highly pathologising in its implications for the sufferer. Would it not be better not to name it at all, but rather to focus on the nature of the distress and what is the best way, for the person concerned, to deal with the consequences they have suffered from the trauma? However, I do recognise that in the world in which we live 'getting a diagnosis' can be a relief – an explanation of why a whole bundle of emotions and effects are happening, offering the hope that the distress can be tackled. Increasingly, too, the only way to get services provided is to get a diagnosis, in a world where health care is increasingly rationed. So we live with terms like 'diabetes' and 'post-natal depression' even though it is far from simple to define what they 'are'.

The body/mind problem

Biomedicine also creates conceptual distortions in our thinking by its separation of 'mind' from 'body'. This distinction causes all sorts of problems for the practice of medicine, as was spelled out in Chapter 8. The notion of 'psychosomatic illness' creates very real difficulties within traditional biomedical settings – both for its sufferers and for those seeking to treat it. Patients in particular face a tricky contradiction. Normally, calling a certain condition an 'illness' provides a powerful justification for absolving the sufferer from any responsibility. Yet the very idea that what is wrong is 'all in the mind' generally invalidates the dispensation – any hint of mental illness is stigmatising.

But the problem is so very much broader. Healthcare systems based on biomedicine, in today's minority world, have come to define pretty well all expressions and experiences of human distress as 'illness' (albeit a mental illness). As such, it is seen to be in need of the medical procedures of diagnosis, treatment and, potentially, cure. In this way a whole bunch of negative emotions – sadness, grief, loneliness and mental anguish; feeling troubled, threatened and worried – can get medicalised in ways that can undermine the kinds of caring and support that can be provided in other more powerful, more appropriate (and often more successful) ways. Examples include 'forest therapy' from Japan, based on getting involved in outdoor activities in woodlands and other places of spiritual solace, or, more informally, joining walking groups and other collective activities like craft, which promote social connectedness.

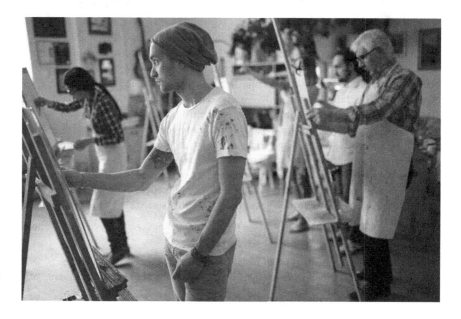

I am not for one moment suggesting we should simply abandon medical treatment for anyone with mental distress. But if this is the *only* approach we consider, we fail to recognise the serious risks that arise from medicalising feelings like hopelessness and insecurity. Doing so inherently locates the problem within an individual's illness, and therefore requires the sufferer to seek a solution through biomedical means (such as taking anti-depressants or having eye-movement desensitisation therapy). Yet if we locate the problem in the *circumstances* that the person is having to deal with – such as the impact of zero-hours work contracts, sleeping in doorways or being unable to feed their children – then a serious amount of 'mental illness' can be dealt with much more effectively by tackling problems like these at source. Examples include making changes to employment law, investing in social housing and providing state benefits directed towards children's healthy development or at least ensuring that food banks are welcoming to families with children. In other words, the solution often lies in providing welfare services of various kinds as well as providing it with kindness and respect.

It is worth adding that being referred to as 'suffering from mental illness', can, in itself, be highly traumatising, likely to add to feelings of despair, hopelessness and self-doubt. The English language is littered with abusive ways to describe people classified as 'mentally ill' which is one of the reasons why I studiously avoid the term. For all of these reasons, both concepts, 'health' and 'illness', are relatively unhelpful in knowing what to do when life gets tough for people, or, especially for children, they are failing to flourish and meet their full potential.

Individualising health

This individualising concept of health decontextualises it. Opinions within the medical profession have loosened up a bit since I first got involved in this argument, getting on for 30 years ago (Stainton Rogers, 1991). But biomedicine still continues to view human suffering as primarily determined by things going wrong in the operation of the body – itself seen as a mechanistic, biological system, wherein 'body' and 'mind' are separate from each other. As we saw in Chapter 8, biomedicine finds it hard to tolerate the very possibility that body and mind can intersect, such as when someone experiences psychosomatic conditions. Furthermore, within the practice of medical diagnosis, treatment (especially for chronic conditions) and the support given in recovery, there is still insufficient consideration of, for example, the emotional turmoil people experience when they receive 'bad news' or when they have to undergo invasive and destructive forms of treatment.

Māori health care

Contrast the biomedical worldview with, for example, Māori understandings about health, as described by Darren Powell (2018) in his blog entry on the issue of childhood obesity:

> In the New Zealand context, for instance, a unidimensional focus on *tinana* (physical dimension) as a main indicator of healthy food and healthy bodies does not align well with Māori perspectives of health and wellbeing that may also encompass *wairua* (spiritual), *hinengaro* (mental and emotional), and *whānau* (close and wider family), as well as *te whenua* (the land, identity and belonging), *te reo* (language), *te taiao* (the environment) and *whanaungatanga* (extended family and relationships).

In response to this set of beliefs, in bi-cultural Aotearoa/New Zealand, the health service now provides, for instance, dedicated midwife care for Māori who choose it. It operates around the more collective, *whanau*-focused understanding of giving birth, which reflects the Māori beliefs about how to manage the child's entry into the family. For example, the midwife is trained to work together with the

Kaiwhakawhanau (the person chosen to assist the mother in childbirth, rather like a doula in the minority world, but with much greater spiritual significance and cultural knowledge) to ensure that not only is the birth as medically safe as possible for the mother and her child, but also that the right rituals are performed and the right people are involved.

Failing to look at situation and context

The Māori understanding of health offers a brilliant contrast with the way that biomedicine tends to look at it as a closed system, separate from the contexts and settings in which, say, illness is experienced. In particular, in practice, biomedicine makes a lot of false distinctions – between, for example, the different organs of the body to fit in with different medical specialisms. Decontextualising health tends to set it apart from the myriad other things that are going on in people's life-worlds at the time, and is the very much the poorer for it.

Treating context as unimportant inevitably creates tensions around how to tackle 'social problems' such as drug addiction, homelessness, theft and knife crime that pose threats not just to the individuals concerned, but also those around them and society as a whole. The question is – should they be seen as matters of individual failures and misbehaviours – criminality (to be strenuously 'rooted out' by the police and punished by the law), or fecklessness (that can be blamed on a lack of character and dismissed as 'not our problem')? Or are they better conceived of at a more collective level, as the consequences of inequality, economic and social ills? Increasingly we are seeing calls for treating such conditions as matters of public health – requiring interventions that seek to prevent and ameliorate human suffering that have little, if anything, to do with biomedicine.

Treating criminal behaviour as located solely within the individual obscures the influence on crime of factors like poverty, unemployment and ghettoisation and institutional racism whereby black youths, in particular, are more likely to be subjected to scrutiny and penalties. And there is a growing consensus that tackling these aspects of criminality can be considerably more effective than treating it solely as a matter of criminal behaviour. A good example is Glasgow's Violence Reduction Unit.

Glasgow's Violence Reduction Unit

From about 2005, rising concerns about the horrific levels of knife crime among young people in Glasgow led the Scottish Government to set up a Violence Reduction Unit (VRU). At first it simply concentrated on traditional police action, which soon proved unable to make much difference. In 2005 Karyn McCluskey, an analyst for Strathclyde police, suggested 'doing something different' – not expecting anything to happen. But it did.

She identified the main drivers of violence as poverty, inequality, toxic masculinity and alcohol use, none of which policing could do much about. Supported by local organisations like Medics against Violence, led by Christine Goodall, the VRU put in place a range of interventions based both in hospitals, where young men came into A&E suffering from knife wounds; and in the community, working with victims of knife crime in the aftermath of the attack. In 2017, of the 35 under-18s who were killed by knife wounds in Britain, none were from Scotland.

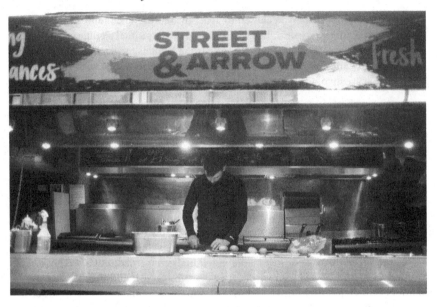

Street & Arrow i
enterprise cafe r
the Scottish Viol
duction Unit in C
offering employ
mentoring to pe
convictions for v

There are a number of reasons why this kind of intervention – where police, medical staff and social services worked together – was effective in Glasgow. For a start, there isn't the same level of hostility towards the police in Scotland as there is, say, in London. Also the politics of the Scottish Government tends to favour approaches like this one. So applying this strategy in other situations will not be easy. But there are lessons to learn and reasons to hope from this example of treating knife crime as a public health matter rather than a criminal one.

The evidence from Scotland suggests that while knife crime, like most crimes, can never be eradicated, it need not be understood as an intractable, cultural feature of urban life. To successfully tackle it, however, there needs to be a shift in understanding of the root causes of the problem and, therefore, what a durable solution might look like.

(Younge and Barr, 2017)

Reflection 10.2

It is well worth discovering how schemes like this function – growing numbers are being set up across the world. Do an Internet search to find, if you can, a project like this operating near where you live. Or take a different tack by looking at several different countries. Play around with terminology around 'violence reduction' and look at government sites, charities, hospitals and journalism. After you have got an overall impression of how and whether they seem to 'work', write some notes for yourself on the benefits they offer, the hurdles they must overcome and the potential they may have to cause harm of some kind.

Blaming and stigmatising

According to a more recent paper by Robert Crawford (2006), mainstream approaches to health need to be understood through an appreciation of the lingering influence of eugenic ideas. Initiated by Francis Galton, the eugenics movement was based on the evolutionary theory of the 'survival of the fittest' and argued that welfare provision undermines this process and allows many – such as the 'feeble-minded' – to reproduce and thus 'weaken the race'.

> Eugenics projected a nightmare vision of an epidemic of genetically transmitted degeneration – a reproductive triumph of lower types who would physically, mentally and morally weaken and eventually destroy the social body.
>
> (Crawford, 2006: 406)

According to Crawford, because of the lingering effect of eugenic thinking, even into the 21st century, health continues to use 'strategies of classification and stigmatisation'. This lingers on still in many people's minds, as evident in the way Donald Trump talks about 'low IQ people', based on eugenic thinking that persists within some popularist worldviews.

Misattributing responsibility

My main concern is that mainstream health psychology – alongside many other health professions – ends up (often unwittingly) blaming certain individuals and groups for the poor health they suffer. They assume they are responsible because of their careless and chaotic life-styles and lack of self-control. This aspect of 'healthism' makes the fundamental attribution error, attributing responsibility to the individual and, in so doing, obscuring and denying the considerable influence of external factors that lead to ill health and distress. It draws attention (and therefore blame) away from the impact of not only exploitation in the workplace, failure to provide adequate and affordable housing, but also things like pollution and environmental damage. It barely even acknowledges the profound effects of poverty, inequality and exclusion on people's capacity to live a healthy lifestyle or eat a healthy diet.

In so doing, mainstream health psychology has the effect of profoundly moralising health – twisting and distorting our understanding of it and failing to recognise the ideological nature of the assumptions made. This has a damaging impact on how medical services and support for healthy living get planned, delivered and funded. Rather than having any clear moral and practical framework to drive them, these processes operate within dense webs of judgement-making, scapegoating and self-justification. In this way, health care gets politicised – planned, delivered and funded according to the public's perception of who is 'deserving' and who is not. The powerful ideology of personal responsibility justifies the commodification of health care – something that can be bought and sold, sometimes in really inhuman ways.

Governmentality, identity and health

Here I am inspired by the work of Anne Scott, an academic who is also a user of mental health services herself. Together with her colleague, Lynere Wilson, she published a very powerful paper on the ways in which neoliberalism creates different identities in relation to health. They write about the Wellness Recovery Action Planning (WRAP) programme, introduced into Aotearoa/New Zealand as a more 'respectful' and user-friendly approach to tackling mental distress – which, on the surface, looks pretty benign. However, Scott and Wilson's research uncovers the extent to which WRAP acts in a powerfully governmental way. They begin by spelling out very clearly the valued identity (you may recognise these characters from Chapter 2) of a *healthy* user of health services:

> a neo-liberal subject of health policy and practice who is active, autonomous, informed and a maker of rational health decisions within a field characterised by calculations of risk. The ideal health consumer takes individualised responsibility for maintenance of their own health rather than depending on medical professionals and health services to do this for them.
>
> (Scott and Wilson, 2011: 8)

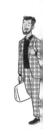

The clever choo valued identity.

By contrast, someone who has a mental *illness* is seen as unable to exercise choice because their mental state makes them incapable of doing so. The ideal user of mental health services is, therefore:

> a prudent, responsible subject who plans ahead, maintains control, is constantly engaged in self-surveillance and works incessantly to sustain a healthy lifestyle. Mental health consumers using this form of self-management must construct themselves as always being 'at risk' of becoming unwell, and strive to forestall these risks.
>
> (Scott and Wilson, 2011: 9)

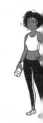

The mindful sel monitor – or se saint on a slippe

Scott and Wilson's paper also depicts the 'feckless wastrels' of mental health programmes – they suggest these people have deficit identities and do not have the capacity to choose nor the self-discipline to comply. They are:

> mental health consumers who are unwilling or unable to commit to maintaining the healthy lifestyle . . . can be easily coded as passive, irresponsible, or otherwise lacking in moral qualities.
>
> (Scott and Wilson, 2011: 10)

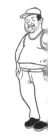

The feckless wa a deficit identit

Depicted in this way, WRAP can be seen as an iron-fist-in-a-velvet-glove approach, one that wields power subversively. It is not intended to stigmatise, but stigmatise it does, by claiming that people who experience mental distress cannot make choices, and that non-compliant service users 'lack moral qualities'.

Critical health psychology

Those of us who built the critical health psychology community mostly came to it through critical psychology more generally. My own journey was inspired by the work of Claudine Herzlich, who demonstrated how psychology could, using qualitative research, pursue issues like the ones outlined so far in this chapter. I read her book on sick-leave when I was trying to make sense of why I had become so ill that I needed emergency surgery followed by three months of recovery.

Early beginnings

Critical health psychology can be traced back to social representations theory, drawing on the work developed by Serge Moscovici. His PhD, completed at the Sorbonne in 1961, was '*La psychanalyse, son image, son public*' (*Psychoanalysis: Its Image and Its Public*, 2008). It investigated the way that ideas and terminology from psychoanalytic theory percolated out from the local mental hospital into the community around it. The hospital had a policy of placing its patients in local families to help their recovery. Very soon terms like 'complex', 'defence mechanism' and 'ego', used in their psychoanalytic senses, began to seep into village gossip.

Moscovici was interested in how information gets transmitted in this way, and can go from being strictly expert knowledge to 'what everybody knows'. But, coming from a French background, Moscovici's big move in the 1960s was to address this question outside of the scientific mould so dominant in the English-speaking world at that time. He defined social representations as organised rather like theories, but more fluid, made up of a kind of 'network of ideas, metaphors and images' (Moscovici, 1961, 1985: 243). There is a clear resonance here with the term 'discourse' adopted somewhat later by Foucault and subsequently by Potter and Wetherell. Both approaches presented a fundamental shift towards what I am calling here, a human psychology.

Even more influential on me was the social representations work of another French psychologist, Claudine Herzlich, in her book, *Health and Illness*, not published in English until 1973 (Herzlich, 1974). She also took a more eclectic approach to her work (see Santiago-Delefosse and del Rio Carral, 2018), including collecting qualitative data by talking to a range of people about their beliefs about what constituted 'health' and their reports about what being ill was like and how it made them feel. Based on an open-ended, data-driven scrutiny of what these people said, she came up with, for example, what she called three alternative metaphors for illness:

Illness as a destroyer	Getting ill destroys you – it stops you being who you are, and meeting your responsibilities. It has to be fought as hard as you can.
Illness as an occupation	Getting ill is something you must take in your stride – you must be a good patient, follow your doctor's orders and do your best to recover.
Illness as liberation	Getting ill sets you free – it means you don't have to meet your responsibilities, and can just take life easy.

What was so very different from the emergent mainstream psychology of the time is that it drew its conclusions *from* the data she collected – she *interpreted* it rather than categorised it using content analysis based on a prior hypothesis. Herzlich effectively used what we now call 'grounded theory' – she painstakingly drew insights from how certain assertions clustered together to give a sense of 'what is going on'. In this way she extracted just these three dominant metaphors for illness – each one different but also recognisable and plausible. She worked from the assumption that people *collectively* make sense (in the form of gossip and conversations) of what happens and what it feels like – in this case when illness strikes.

For me and many others, Herzlich revealed a very new and inspirational approach to psychology. She clearly drew upon the methods being developed at that time by medical anthropologists and sociologists, operating in a transdisciplinary manner in which she sought to transcend disciplinary boundaries beyond the limitations of scientific psychology. She has recently made this explicit:

> In 1966, I adopted a perspective between anthropology and psycho-sociology of medicine. I never have self-identified as a 'Health Psychologist', continuing to work outside of disciplinary boundary constraints, but studied health questions moving first from psychology (and anthropology), through social psychology to sociology.
>
> (Herzlich, 2017: abstract)

Social representations work continues within critical health psychology and, if you want to know more Flick's (2000) paper on the topic is an excellent place to start. More generally, his more recent chapter on the approach is very useful (Flick and Foster, 2017).

The principles of critical health psychology

Critical health psychology adopts the broader and more contextualised definition of health as described in the previous section (Stainton Rogers, 1996). It is one that seeks to avoid stigmatising or scapegoating particular groups, and, rather, to promote human welfare. It uses a mix of methodological approaches, but much of its research uses qualitative methods and forms of analyses and interpretation designed to offer insight and understanding rather than the discovery of 'facts'. It too is transdisciplinary, seeking to transcend disciplinary boundaries and be open to innovation, such as arts-based research and alternative forms of communication such as *pecha kucha* at its conferences (there are lots of helpful demonstrations of pecha kucha on YouTube).

Aims

The aims of critical health psychology have been well-defined by the International Society for Critical Health Psychology (ISCHP), https://ischp.info/

- A pursuit of social justice in the topics studied and the approaches used.
- An active commitment to equity, transparency and inclusion in the way it is pursued.
- A truly international and multicultural spirit of collaboration and co-operation.
- An active avoidance of hierarchy and a determination to break down barriers that may exclude individuals and groups from full participation in its endeavours.

As you can see, it is very much a human psychology project, building on the ideas and approaches developed in this book.

Human welfare

The label 'welfare' is often seen rather narrowly as a matter of what goes on in 'welfare states' – the provision, by state governments, of various systems of support for its citizens in order to promote their wellbeing. Welfare services can be universal (such as education in most of the minority world and the UK National Health Service) but are more usually targeted to provide for specific people (such as those who have an inadequate income, nowhere suitable to live or are debilitated in some way by illness or infirmity). While welfare services are sometimes freely available to all, they are usually targeted in an incremental way depending on income. These welfare services include social care, health care, childcare, education, vocational training and leisure and sporting facilities.

What is human welfare?

However, in this chapter I am using the term '*human* welfare' to cover a broader philosophical perspective: one that brings together a range of positive concepts such as wellbeing, wellness, quality of life and human flourishing. The Greeks had their own word for it – *Eudaimonia*, its underlying ethics based on the virtue of 'living well' but meant in a *collective* sense, as it includes a responsibility to 'do good'. Human welfare, from this perspective, is what enables us to 'live well', in harmony with others and actively contributing to the common good. My concern here is not with a form of welfare that accepts that some people will only be able to 'make do', but about all people having the capacity to live meaningful, satisfying and comfortable lives. It is about them feeing secure and that they belong, that others care about them and are willing to care for them when they need it. It is living a life where you can achieve your potential, both in yourself and as part of your family and community. It is collective in its nature and very much to do with social connectedness.

It is crucial to recognise that this definition of human welfare (as with *Eudaimonia*) is *not* about living a life of luxury, indulgence and excess. Realistically, we are talking more about living in *lagom*, a Swedish word meaning something like 'in just the right sort of way'. The closest we get to it in English is in the proverb 'enough is as good as a feast', suggesting that people are happier when they have enough to be comfortable without being ostentatiously rich. Similar concepts are expressed in many languages across the world, including Thai and Javanese. In Russian and Slav languages it is a nuanced form of the term 'normal' and 'getting on fine'. This caveat is important, as seeking a life of *lagom* is a very different ambition from the goals promoted by neoliberalism, which are directed towards making profit by stimulating in people the desire for consuming 'high-end goods', that are 'better' and more 'luxurious' than others can afford; status symbols that mark you out as 'having arrived'. Indeed, this is probably not enough. Given our environmental crisis, we need to live much more frugally; 'living in the right sort of way' gets a lot tougher once we acknowledge just how damaging the lives we take for granted have become.

The social and community basis of human welfare

There is good evidence that when people have strong, positive relationships and are soundly connected within the community to which they belong they live longer and happier lives. A meta-analytic study by Holt-Lunstad, Smith and Layton (2010) which looked at 148 studies overall, found that strong social connections lifted people's life expectancy by up to 50%, with evidence that the stronger the interconnectedness, the more people gained from it. In research analyses like these, based on very large samples but using only questionnaire data, it can be hard to really understand what is going on – and very hard indeed to attribute causality. For instance, if you add high levels of compassion and empathy into the equation, the benefits appear to be even greater (Seppala, Rossomando and Doty, 2013). In other words, even if it seems perhaps too obvious to say it, people who live in close, supportive and caring families, friendship groups and tight-knit, caring communities tend to flourish in ways that people who live lonely and isolated lives, surrounded by hostile and risky communities, do not. It takes a lot more than medical services for people to be hale and healthy.

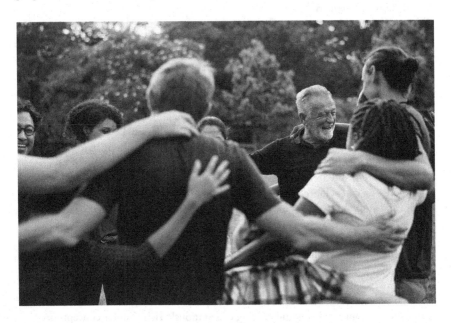

Photo: Shutterst

Living well

In a neoliberal world, it is not surprising that Sainsbury's, one of the UK's middle-market supermarkets, has jumped onto this bandwagon. Working with the National Centre for Social Research and Oxford Economics, they have come up with a Living Well Index (see Resources, p. 261), with which they seek to measure – and promote – people's wellbeing. Their initial survey in September 2017 was based on data collected from 8,000 British adults. They initially identified four key factors as strongly influencing 'living well' (according to their definition):

1   Getting enough sleep and waking up feeling refreshed.
2   Being satisfied with your sex life.
3   Feeling you have enough time to do the things you need to.
4   Generally eating your meals with others rather than eating alone.

A more recent report, based on a further survey, was published in May 2018. This one found that over the six months the Living Well score had fallen slightly but significantly, alongside a slight dip in people's feelings of wellbeing. They attributed this mostly to the impact of the severe winter of 2017 which kept people indoors and limited their social lives. But they also found that worries about money also appeared as a possible factor, especially for parents.

When they looked at the second expanded set of data in detail, overall they found that having mental health conditions badly undermined wellbeing. The report's authors concluded that: 'real social connections are essential to living well – and . . . digital interactions are no substitute' (10). Thus, while online contact appeared to have no impact on living well, actually getting together with family, neighbours and friends and eating together with others was much more important.

Reflection 10.3

Look at the 2018 report (see the Resources at the end of the chapter) and read it in full if you can. It gives a pretty good impression of what this kind of data analysis looks like, and what it can do. It is quite complicated and has its limitations, but make some notes on what you think are its key messages. Pay particular attention to the nuances available through the breakdown of the data according to things like age and whether people had children. Spend some time speculating about the limitations of using surveys. What more do you think we could learn by actually talking to people and observing them discuss 'living well' with each other?

Social connectedness

In Chapter 4, we looked at two other aspects of human relationships that are beneficial to human welfare, especially at times of trouble – social capital and community resilience. Here we will get into a bit more detail about them in terms of their impact on human welfare.

Social capital

According to Borgonovi (2010), social capital can benefit health in a number of ways. Communities with high social capital will often have people in them with knowledge about how to live a healthy life, who approve of such a lifestyle and support it. It is much easier to avoid smoking among people where it is seen as not 'cool' to smoke or feel strongly that children must be protected from cigarette smoke. Social groups where people help each other out and are supportive at times of trouble can do a great deal to reduce anxiety and distress that can undermine health, both directly and by reducing the temptation to turn to alcohol or drugs for solace. And, quite simply, it is a lot easier to fight cuts to services and lobby for a safer environment as part of an active community. Wilkinson and Pickett (2010) point out that in countries where there is a small difference between rich and poor, these features of social capital are much easier to achieve compared with countries where the gap is huge. Inequality tends to lead to a lack of social cohesion in communities and undermines good social relationships.

More concerned with human welfare than economics, the sociologist Susanne Martikke (2017) points out some of the problems with this term. She draws attention to the way it has been appropriated by politicians looking for cheap ways to 'solve' social problems – for the Labour Party (left wing) to combat ghettoisation and social exclusion; and for the Conservative Party (right wing) to provide a vision of a 'Big Society' where communities support each other by volunteering for charity work and the like. But then she gets into a more nuanced and detailed exploration of social capital, starting with the work of Pierre Bordieu, who, as she says, gets to the heart of the matter. He defines social capital as a matter of 'resources that are based on membership in a group' (Bourdieu, 1983: 191). Being connected into a network of friends, close family and people like the local rabbi, the person who runs the corner-shop and the nurse at the local surgery is a good start to 'living well'. But if, for example, you get on well with the local police chief, have a close friend who manages the food bank and an aunt who is a magistrate, then your capacity to garner support will be even better. Social capital does not just relate to the size of the networks that can offer support, more crucially, it depends on the ability of those in the network to gain access to resources.

Reflection 10.4

Spend some time creating a list of the people in your network. Don't bother with their names, just list them in terms of the resources to which they can provide access. Now consider what the network would be for somebody who is either more privileged or less privileged than you. Make a list of one or the other. Use your imagination to work out the sorts of people who could help them in times of trouble – both in times of crisis and when facing, say, chronic health problems or ongoing money troubles.

Mainly this activity is intended to bring home to you the way social capital is linked to privilege of different forms. It shows why Bourdieu's concept of habitus (see Chapter 3) helps us to better comprehend how social capital works. Martikke makes the point that, 'as habitus determines everything individuals and collectives do, it is also significant for the development of social capital' (Martikke, 2017: 8). What she is saying here is that our social standing is made obvious by the ways in which we present ourselves and live our lives through symbolic capital as an indication of our position in society. How we behave, gesture, hold ourselves and talk; what we eat and where we go for a drink or to exercise – these are all ways by which we are recognised as 'posh' or 'salt-of-the earth' or 'a bit common':

> Life-styles are thus the systematic products of habitus . . . sign systems that are socially qualified (as 'distinguished', 'vulgar' etc.). The dialectic of conditions and habitus is the basis of an alchemy which transforms the distribution of capital, the balance-sheet of a power relation, into a system of perceived differences, distinctive properties, that is, a distribution of symbolic capital.
>
> (Gieseking, 2014: 140)

Martikke makes it clear that social capital is not, in itself, a 'good thing'. It can be divisive and exclusionary. But for these in privileged positions it can be very much a basis for human welfare.

Community resilience

Look back at Chapter 4 if you need a reminder of what community resilience means and how it works. It is, in a way, a particular kind of social capital, one which enables communities to deal with harsh conditions and overcome disasters of various kinds. A good illustration of it is Louise Thornley and her colleagues' paper on lessons learned following the earthquakes that repeatedly devastated the city of Christchurch, New Zealand, in 2010–2011 (Thornley et al., 2015). These earthquakes were pretty well unique in recent history in their intensity and in the repeated damage they did to the large urban and suburban communities, as well as the central business district and the cathedral.

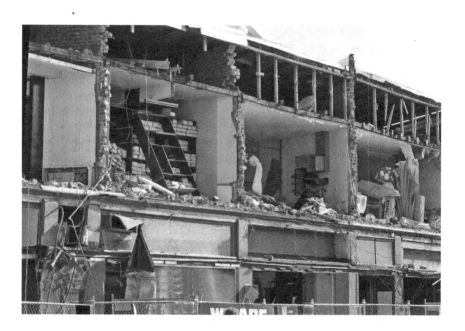

o the hospital
hurch following
quakes.
utterstock

Among the elements Thornley and her colleagues identified as important for recovery were those relating to individuals, particularly their pre-existing health/*whānau* and the survival skills they had developed previously from living in adversity. However, community connectedness was a major theme, mentioned by all six communities studied. Here is what one of the participants said:

> 'You need to have a sense of community before the disaster . . . because you do get that initial surge of 'community togetherness' in the immediate aftermath when the adrenalin is still pumping – but it can dissipate . . . once the going gets tough'.

> (Thornley et al., 2015: 24)

In Christchurch this included the use of texting and social media, which increased dramatically and was very useful in the aftermath of the quakes. Later on, getting together for ceremonies and memorial events helped to strengthen community connections, especially since many people had tended to stay at home and felt isolated because of the threat of further tremors. At the community infrastructure level, pre-existing community groups and projects (like time-banks) were crucial, as were local leaders who knew the community well and shared communication channels (such as community radio, websites, newsletters and email networks). Some communities had formal systems for organising volunteer labour, and new groups were also formed, such as the Student Volunteer Army. But in the context of a bi-cultural society, there were distinctly local strengths:

> A particularly strong example of pre-existing community infrastructure is that of Ngāi Tahu who, participants reported, was able to mobilise quickly because of [their] well-established tribal infrastructure based around marae. This was led by the tribal chair of Te Rūnanga o Ngāi Tahu and 18 Papatipu Rūnanga (local tribal council) leaders and was based on the cultural values and worldviews of the iwi. In the marae communities studied, Māori highlighted the key role of marae as hubs for providing emergency support and hospitality. The role of the marae is exemplified in the cultural construct of manaaki-tanga (hospitality and caring). Marae are well placed to care for large groups of people at a moment's notice. In ordinary times, they regularly offer support to Māori and other communities.
>
> (Thornley et al., 2015: 26–7)

Ok, this is a lot of language to get your head around. But try it! From the context you can guess quite a lot, but also use resources like www.maorilanguage.info/mao_defns.html to help. There is a lot of fascinating detail buried in those words.

Reflection 10.5

Compare the Christchurch example with the town of Jasper described in Chapter 4. Each community had its own strengths particular to its social and cultural composition, but I think you will agree that they differ in some interesting ways too. Reflect upon the implications for the welfare of the people involved.

Jasper was an unusual place in the US in that, before the 'lynching', it already had well-established community links across the black–white divide. This was particularly helpful in the context of the prejudices of much of the media and the attempts by particular groups and individuals to capitalise upon the catastrophe the town faced. Also it was a very specific and focused event, whereas the Christchurch earthquakes damaged up to 80% of the city-centre, with its impact being felt across a wide area and for a long time. But Christchurch faced little hostility – quite the reverse, in fact, with a groundswell of concern and empathy expressed across the world. Even so, I hope, like me, you find both communities inspirational, showing the strengths that can be found in sometimes surprising places. We can contrast these with the Grenfell

Tower fire in London in 2017, where the authorities failed the residents and their community so very badly. If you can, use an Internet search to explore what your government is doing – and recommending – to build resilience into the way it relates to its local communities.

The role of faith and religion

Dawn Foster, a journalist, writes of her experience suffering from a devastating epileptic fit. Her doctor asked her if she had made a will – it was that serious.

> I was sent home, and because I was lucky enough to have excellent friends, messages flooded in from people in London and farther afield offering to visit, shop for anything, I was only to ask. One group did away with such pragmatic codes: friends at my local church didn't ask but told me. I was to come for dinner; they were on the way to my house; we were all going to meet up in a few hours' time. We're a tightknit group – but the way church groups operate has always been different to the way my other groups of friends behave.
>
> (Foster, 2018: 5)

The point she is making in her article is that, for all the horrors that religious organisations are going through in relation to discoveries of historical abuse, for many members of faith groups, their religious community can provide a very special kind of support.

Reflection 10.6

Perform an Internet search to find out a bit more about the complex interface between religion and health – would you expect it to be simple? Make a few notes summarising the broad findings of the research that has been done.

The trouble is, in my view, that so much of this research is again based on quantitative data, which is very good at indicating correlation but has little value in aiding in understanding what is going on in any depth. For example, a study carried out in the predominantly Christian US links church attendance with a reduction in mortality (Gillum et al., 2008). Basically, people who regularly go to church tend to live that bit longer. However, there is no way to know whether this is a result of the act of going to church, the impact of having faith, the prohibition of religion towards indulgence such as alcohol or whatever else! Which is why, I believe, that human psychology should mainly use qualitative methods which get to the questions of 'why?' and 'what is going on?'

That having been said, I have included this section as it makes us aware that religious creeds are crucial to the worldviews adopted by large numbers of people worldwide (as I found in my research on discourses of health, see Chapter 9). In today's world, religion tends to get very bad press in that it is held to be responsible, in its extreme forms, for a great deal of human conflict. Foster's words remind us that religious creeds can also be very effective means to promote positive human values.

Promoting human welfare

In this section we will explore the ways in which state action can be taken to promote human welfare. We have already looked at the impact of social and community support. Now we will turn to what services can be formally provided at state level. Basically the question is – what does a 'good society' put in place to support the welfare of its citizens?

Reflection 10.7

What do you think is the most important service that government can provide to promote the human welfare of its citizens? What service most allows people to flourish and 'live well'?

Did you say medical care? Things like providing health centres, hospitals and ambulances; medicines like antibiotics and insulin; schemes to screen for conditions like cancer; or immunisation programmes? That's what many people think, but by now you may well suspect that this is not the case. Good medical care and treatment certainly makes an enormous difference to those of us who have access to them. But medical care on its own cannot operate effectively without certain pre-conditions being put in place. In this section we will look at three underlying state-based drivers that promote human welfare. Only when these are functioning well can a system for health care and medical treatment make a real difference across the population. The three drivers are:

- The public health measures a state puts in place;
- The actions the state takes for tackling inequality;
- Its health and safety law to protect the welfare and wellbeing of its citizens.

There is well-established evidence that, historically, the major impact on what we usually think of as human health and wellbeing has been from public health measures, most of which were established in the minority world beginning in the 18th century. Progress in public health provision included creating proper sanitation and decent housing, ensuring the availability of adequate and nutritious food (increased by the delivery of food that is fresh, made possible by the railways), enacting legislation limiting working hours, setting standards for health and safety at work and restricting the employment of children. What mattered was making all this available to the population as a whole and not just the rich and powerful.

Not convinced? Then look at the graph shown in Figure 10.1 as an example of what went on. It shows the reduction in cases of death from whooping cough and measles among children up to the age of 15, from 1850–1960. You can see that rates began to fall – and fall dramatically – well before the discovery of the organism that causes

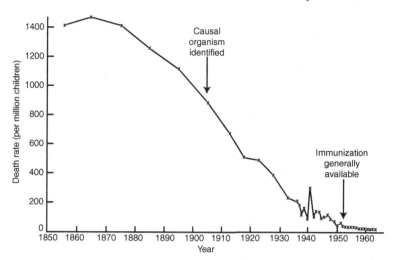

the disease in question, and even further ahead of the point at which pharmaceuticals and immunisation became freely available. Increasingly, lives were being saved because children were becoming less exposed to infection – they were living in less crowded and more sanitary conditions, getting more and better food, all of this making them more likely to survive relatively minor illnesses like whooping cough.

Thomas McKeown (1976) published a large number of such graphs for many infectious diseases, including dysentery, smallpox, scarlet fever and tuberculosis. In his highly perceptive book, he spelt out in detail the history of how humankind's health improved dramatically in the UK from around the mid-17th century when records began. Similar patterns undoubtedly occurred in other locations, but the UK is relatively unusual in how far back the data are formally recorded. Across the minority world, the impact of the same sorts of improvements in public health measures have also systematically reduced ill-health and premature death. Many counties, especially in Europe, have outstripped the UK in extending life expectancy, and, worryingly, recent data suggest that in the US and UK we are actually beginning to see a reduction in life expectancy, especially among those living in poverty.

There is now compelling and sustained evidence that, across the world today, lack of infrastructure (like good drains and proper housing) are the main causes of ill-health globally, and improvements like these should be fundamental to promoting human welfare worldwide. Tackling these is much more effective for the overall wellbeing of the majority of a country's population than building hospitals. However, there is also growing and compelling evidence that there are new dangers to human health building up – including environmental pollution, climate change and neoliberalism in the way it creates conditions where employment has become increasingly precarious and exploitative.

Poverty and health

Although it has been known for some considerable time that people living in poverty are in poorer health, in the UK it was the Black report, published in 1980, that really brought our attention the fundamental and far-reaching influence of poverty on health. The report had been commissioned by the UK Government, and if you look it up on the Internet, you should find an image of a battered copy of the original, only a few of which were produced. This itself speaks volumes! The report was 'sneaked out' covertly, away from public view, since its conclusions were so damning. A paper published later by Alistair McIntosh Grey (1982) provides an excellent summary, including of the attempts to suppress its findings – a very worthwhile read. A contemporary source, Health Scotland (2019) describes health inequalities like this:

> Health inequalities are the unjust and avoidable differences in people's health across the population and between specific population groups. Health inequalities go against the principles of social justice because they are avoidable. They do not occur randomly or by chance. They are socially determined by circumstances largely beyond an individual's control. These circumstances disadvantage people and limit their chance to live longer, healthier lives.

This stance illustrates the way that the UK's devolved governments (mainly Scotland and Wales) have tended to adopt policies based on social justice, in contrast to the adversity policy that has dominated the political agenda in England. The difference demonstrates the way social policy (including resource allocation) profoundly influences human wellbeing.

Reflection 10.8

Conduct an Internet search to explore the policy stance towards inequality taken by the government where you live. Look, in particular, at the underlying assumptions and principles on which it is based. List these and reflect upon the implications they have for your own welfare. Now do a similar exploration of a place where the situation is very different, and then consider the impact living there would have on you.

The Scottish approach is explicitly based on the principle of social justice – one that actively strives to reduce inequality because it is unfair. It is a collectivist approach, based on an assumption of universal human rights; it seeks to improve the health of *all* people. Contrast that with the 'safety net' approach adopted in many other countries, where 'welfare' is very much a 'boo word' – either seen as something to feel ashamed about, and/or dispensed in a condescending way, and for which recipients are expected to be grateful. Put it another way – health inequalities not only reflect the lack of material resources needed to support health, but the stigmatisation of a deficit identity (described earlier, Scott and Wilson, 2011), and all the distress that kind of labelling implies.

In their groundbreaking book, *The Spirit Level*, Richard Wilkinson and Kate Pickett (2010) argue that there is another, more collective, process at work here, where greater equality can be better for *everyone*. They cite extensive evidence to show that countries where there is a relatively small gap between the household income of the richest and the poorest (i.e. Japan and Scandinavia), its people have better overall health and there are fewer social problems than in countries where the gap is largest (i.e. the US, Portugal and the UK). More recently they have explored in more depth the psychological consequences of inequality – how 'inequality gets under the skin' and makes people feel anxious, insecure and lacking in self-worth; it undermines trust within communities, creates ghettos and 'no go' areas. Inequality, they argue, has a direct impact on health in terms of conditions like obesity and poor dental hygiene; it reduces educational attainment and exacerbates social problems such as crime (Wilkinson and Pickett, 2018). They conclude that humans are not 'naturally' competitive, and live most contentedly within societies that are based on fundamental principles of equality, sharing and reciprocity.

Another way to get a 'handle' on what goes on in situations like these is to watch some or all of the TV series *The Wire* (there were five seasons from 2002–2009). And if you're not from urban Baltimore, do use the subtitles function! Alternatively, you can watch some key sections on YouTube to get the general gist. A third option is to dip into Johnathan Abrahams' (2018) book *All the Pieces Matter: The Inside Story of the Wire*. The series offers a complex and subtle exploration of the impact of gross inequality in an urban setting, of how its problems are so very intractable and how much they reflect the very human qualities of the protagonists. It asks us to consider what actions can be taken and examines a whole range of consequences.

For me the series says something very important about what is wrong with popularism, and it says it very eloquently – every episode rams home the realisation that there are no simple and straightforward solutions to situations like these. Not simple either are the processes and conditions that lead to such situations in the first place. The series gives a fine-grained impression of how and why these conditions have become established as 'just how things are', and all the different components that work to maintain them and resist attempts to bring about change. All of these are highly complicated and intricately interconnected with each other in convoluted power-plays going on between various individuals, groups and whole communities, including the local residents, the homicide police and the US Justice Department. What better excuse could you have for binge-watching the whole series! It has certainly been used (even by Simon himself) to teach undergraduate classes in subjects varying from criminology to film theory.

Legislation
In this section we look at three key forms of law that are important for human welfare:

- Human rights
- Anti-discrimination
- Health and safety

Human rights law
The situation over human rights law worldwide and locally is complex and also open to change. It operates at a number of different levels.

Reflection 10.9

Conduct an Internet search to review the human rights laws that apply to you in the place where you live. Look first at the United Nations Convention on Human Rights (UNCHR), and find out which parts of it apply to you (Start by checking whether your country has signed up). Then look at any specific legislation more local to you. For example, if you live in France, you will have protections under the UNCHR, under EU law and under French law. Finally, find out if there are special provisions because of your situation – because you are a refugee or a migrant worker, for example. Do not spend too long on this as it is complicated – even lawyers cannot agree over many aspects of it. Just get a sense of what is 'out there' and how it might apply to you. When you have done that, reflect upon the principles behind the concept of 'human rights'. Make some notes if you have time. This would be a great activity to do as a group, with information-finding divided up as a task to be done first and then reflecting on what you have found out in a group discussion. It could also be done as a formal debate on, say, 'Human rights are the fundamental basis of human welfare'.

Human rights – as a concept – is very much about human welfare. It sets benchmarks for the way people should treat each other, both as individuals and in terms of the responsibilities of states, their obligations towards their citizens and the limits on their powers. The principles of human rights are collective in nature, quite different from more individualistic approaches – such as neoliberalism – that stress the importance of personal freedom and the rights of companies and institutions (such as the World Bank) to make decisions based on profit-making and fiscal 'prudence'. Human rights are often treated as 'problems', portrayed as impractical, unrealistic or involving too much bureaucracy; as limiting personal and commercial freedom and governmental sovereignty. Or, in many ways worse, human rights are ignored and marginalised – for example, by providing insufficient regulation and inadequate sanctions to ensure their implementation.

Anti-discrimination law

All this applies too to anti-discrimination law. At the time of writing, the key legislation in the UK is the Equality Act 2010 which makes it illegal to discriminate against a person because they have one of the 'protected characteristics' defined in the Act: age, disability, gender reassignment, marriage and civil partnership, race, religion or belief, sex, and sexual orientation. It is worth finding out what anti-discrimination law is in place where you live. In the UK the Act applies to employment, access to education, public services, private goods and services and premises (such as access to rental housing). For people with disabilities, for example, the Act places a duty on employers to remove the barriers they face because of their disability so they can do their job effectively and apply for jobs in the same way as someone who's not disabled.

Reflection 10.10

Conduct an Internet search to examine a different example of the 'protected characteristics' covered by this law. Find out about the duties accorded to such people, and reflect on the way in which this can contribute to human welfare. Look to see what resources are available (such as organisations providing advice) to such people and the mechanisms in place to make sure the duties are fulfilled. Then reflect on how much, in practice, they actually make a difference.

Health and safety law

Although often treated with derision, laws on 'health and safety' have dramatically improved human welfare in the countries where they have been introduced. The Industrial Revolution in England, for example, led to large numbers of very poor people from the countryside moving to towns and cities to find work – a trend that still continues and can be seen today pretty well worldwide. Although farm work had (and has) its dangers, working in factories, mines and mills was (and is) far more of a threat to human welfare, especially for children. In England's Industrial Revolution, children as young as 4 were employed in mills, as they were sufficiently small to get under the machinery.

In England this threat was first addressed by Sir Robert Peel, a factory owner himself, who responded to the popular outcry over the harm being done by the conditions under which children were forced to work. He introduced into parliament the Health and Morals of Apprentices Act 1802, commonly known as the Factory Act. It specified that factories:

- Must have sufficient ventilation and be kept clean.
- Limit the working hours of apprentices to no more than 12 hours a day (excluding time taken for breaks) and prohibit them from working between 9 pm and 6 am.
- Provide suitable clothing and sleeping accommodation to every apprentice.
- Educate them in reading, writing, arithmetic and the principles of the Christian religion.

This law only applied to certain children, but, particularly through activism among working people, in 1833 these controls were extended to all children working in factories and mills. However, it was the appointment of inspectors to enforce this law that gave it real impact. Starting with just four of them to inspect about 3,000 textile mills, gradually the numbers were built up and the legislation extended, for example, to providing guards over dangerous machinery. The influence here became more collective, as public opinion towards health and safety changed because of a rising consciousness of how employers exploited the people (including children) who worked for them.

This shift in popular opinion was stimulated by novelists such as Charles Dickens, and, in particular, by the development of Marxist theory by Frederic Engels, set out in his groundbreaking book *The Condition of the Working Class in England*, published in German in 1845 and in English in 1847. It was based on his personal observations and research in Manchester, as well as epidemiological data about the differences between the rural and urban poor. Karl Marx was deeply impressed by the book, and the two became lifelong friends, publishing many books and articles together, including the *Communist Manifesto* in 1848.

Reflection 10.11

As you can see, a range of influences drove the development of employment law in the UK – including Victorian philanthropy, activism among working people, a shift in the perception of what is and is not acceptable in society (such as sending children to work down the mines) and the introduction of ideologies such as Marxism. However, today, working conditions have significantly changed because of the increased use of ICT and practices like hot-desking, as well as the shift in what is acceptable under neoliberalism. Conduct an Internet search to get an impression of the situation of health and safety legislation as it operates today where you live. Look at both what the law requires and then at how well it is enforced. Then consider its impact upon human welfare where you are.

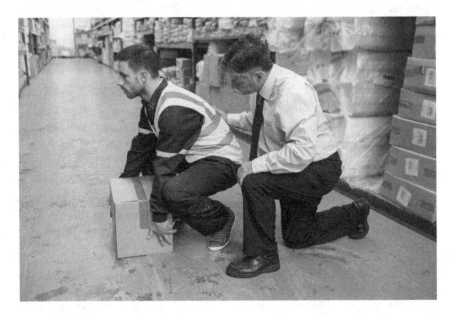

Training staff in
required by hea
safety legislati

In general, neoliberalism undermines workers' rights to work in conditions that protect their safety and wellbeing. For example, the casualisation of employment (such as 'contracting out' and zero-hours contracts) makes employment more precarious and income unpredictable, leading to lower wages and distress. Equally, the use of performance indicators and bonus incentives within a growing 'gig economy' limit the ability to protect health and safety, exacerbated by an increasing level of monitoring made possible by ICT. Workers can now be given wristbands or microchipped to in ways that keep a record of their location and hand movements.

> There are tech companies selling products that can take regular screenshots of employees' work, monitor keystrokes and web usage, and even photograph them at their desks using their computers' webcams. Working from home offers no protection, as all this can be done remotely. Software can monitor social media usage, analyse language or be installed on employees' phones to monitor encrypted apps such as WhatsApp. Employees can be fitted with badges that not only track their location, but also monitor their tone of voice, how often they speak in meetings and who they speak to and for how long.
>
> (Saner, 2018)

These practices are often defended, in part, as promoting workers' safety – but just how healthful is this level of surveillance? Already a handheld device is being used by Amazon for its warehouse staff that begins a countdown as soon as something is picked up in a quest to speed up response rates. James Bloodworth (2018) describes in painful detail just how anxiety-provoking and demoralising such systems can be, hounding workers constantly to increase their productivity, and threatening them if they don't – or can't – 'match up'. He describes how the whole regime of threatening disciplinary action, humiliating and unpaid security checks and sanctions for taking breaks made him feel 'less than human'.

Even in better-paid and more prestigious jobs, managers not only face the same kinds of performance management themselves, but are expected to collude with undermining the protections the law affords workers. Their performance assessments put them under pressure to limit health and safety compliance. In this way they are incentivised to avoid the assessments that are required, for instance, to make adjustments to ensure that screen-working is safe and to prevent it causing damage to workers. Managers are also under pressure not to allow sufficient time for health and safety inspections to be made. This strategy goes right to the top, with trades unions representatives who undertake this role today incrementally losing their capacity to undertake these responsibilities in their work-time (see Sherlock, 2017).

Is welfare 'health' by other means?

Throughout this chapter I have argued that people in the minority world (and rich people in the majority world) live in a world dominated by biomedicine. This is based on a worldview which values very highly the high-tech 'fixes' that medicine can provide for when our bodies fail to function properly, and often treats with disdain the very ordinary and mundane things like having a reliable sewage system, a more equal distribution of income and good community cohesion. Yet it is things like these that fundamentally enable people to 'live well'. Medicine is generally seen as really glamorous (more so if what you do is high-tech and involves expensive machines) in a way that fills the coffers of the charities that have become so good at tugging at our heart-strings, and feeds the profits of 'Big Pharma', not to mention insurance companies. Furthermore, so valued has 'good health' become that striving for it has become not only a preoccupation for many, but also an expectation of the 'good citizen'.

Please don't get me wrong. I am utterly grateful to the way my life has been saved several times by medical treatment and the ongoing care I get that literally keeps me alive. Furthermore, as I am convinced by the evidence, I also work hard to be as healthy as I can, especially as I age. I recognise the crucial expertise of medical knowledge, and, indeed, seek to contribute to it, currently by working for NICE (National Institute for Health and Care Excellence) in its Centre for Guidelines. Nevertheless, I believe we must not be so beguiled by the glamour of biomedicine that we overlook – and undervalue – the very many other things that contribute to promoting human welfare. I hope this chapter has made you think – and certainly more aware of what is a very complex (but often very inspirational) range of human endeavours that are seeking to make life better for much more of humanity than it does just now.

Resources

The ISCHP Website. **https://ischp.info/.** This website offers a great way to find out about psychologists who take a critical approach to human welfare and to keep up-to-date with what is 'moving and shaking' in this field.

Martikke's, S. (2018) *Overview of Social Capital.* **www.gmcvo.org.uk/system/files/social_capital_an_overview_0.pdf.** This is an excellent and accessible resource. It was prepared for the Greater Manchester Centre for Voluntary Organisations.

The Sainsbury's Living Well Index. **www.oxfordeconomics.com/recent-releases/the-sainsbury-s-living-well-index. www.about.sainsburys.co.uk/news/latest-news/ /22-05-18-living-well-index.** This survey offers some really interesting insights into what makes it possible for people to 'live well'. Well worth using it to keep up with any future developments.

Wilkinson, R. and Pickett, K. (2010) *The Spirit Level: Why Equality Is Better for Everyone.* **Penguin: London.** This book was a game-changer when it came out, making a convincing and systematic argument that inequality is very harmful to human welfare. Its use of comparative data is compelling. Despite its critics, the case being made is generally recognised as well-founded.

Wilkinson, R. and Pickett, K. (2018) *The Inner Level: How More Equal Societies Reduce Stress, Restore Sanity and Improve Everyone's Wellbeing.* **Penguin: London.** Their most recent book looks in more detail at the psychological impacts of inequality, especially on aspects like self-esteem and confidence.

The Wire TV Series. **https://thewire.fandom.com/wiki/David_Simo.** This is a great resource to explore the complex ways in which human welfare can be compromised and improved. Produced explicitly to examine life in urban US settings and see just how difficult it is to solve social problems.

Bibliography

Abrahams, J. (2018) *All the Pieces Matter: The Inside Story of the Wire*. No Exit Press: Harpenden.

Adorno, T. W., Frenkel-Brunswick, E., Levinson, D. J. and Sandford, R. N. (1950) *The Authoritarian Personality*. Harper: New York, NY.

Ahmed, S. (2014) *The Cultural Politics of Emotion*. Edinburgh University Press: Edinburgh.

Ahmed, S. (2017) *Living a Feminist Life.* Duke University Press: Durham, NC.

Ajzen, I. and Fishbein, M. (1972) Attitudes and Normative Beliefs as Factors Influencing Behavioural Intentions. *Journal of Personality and Social Psychology*, 21(1): 1–9.

Akhtar, M. (2016) *Positive Psychology for Overcoming Depression.* Watkins: London.

Aldridge, J. and Becker, S. (1993) Children Who Care. *Childright*, 97: 13–14.

Allport, G. W. (1935) Attitudes. In G. Murchison (ed) *Handbook of Social Psychology.* Clark University Press: Worchester, MA.

Arfken, M. (2017) Marxism as a Foundation for Critical Social Psychology. In B. Gough (ed) *The Palgrave Handbook of Critical Social Psychology*, 37–58. Palgrave: London.

Ashworth, P. (2003) The Phenomenology of the Lifeworld and Social Psychology. *Social Psychological Review*, 5(1): 18–34.

Atwood, M. (1985; 2017) *The Handmaid's Tale.* Penguin: London.

Audre Lorde, A. (1997) *Sister Outsider: Essays and Speeches.* Crossing Press: Berkeley, CA.

Augoustinos, M., Tuffin, K. and Every, D. (2005) New Racism, Meritocracy and Individualism: Constraining Affirmative Action in Education. *Discourse & Society*, 16(3): 315–340. https://doi.org/10.1177/0957926505051168

Augoustinos, M., Walker, I. and Donaghue, N. (2006) *Social Cognition: An Integrated Introduction*, 2nd Edition. Sage: New York, NY.

Bache, G. M. (1895) Reaction Time With Reference to Race. *Psychological Review*, 2: 475–486.

Baddley, A. (2013) *Essentials in Human Memory.* Psychology Press: London.

Bakhtin, M. (1968; 1984) *Rabelais and His World.* Indiana University Press: Bloomington, IN.

Barker, M. and Langdridge, D. (2008) II: Bisexuality: Working with a Silenced Sexuality. *Feminism & Psychology*, 18(3): 389–394. https://doi.org/10.1177/0959353508092093

Barker, M-J. (2018) *Rewriting the Rules: An Anti-Self-Help Guide to Love, Sex and Relationships.* Routledge: London.

Barthes, R. (1957; 1967) *Elements of Semiology.* Hill and Wang: New York, NY.

Bartlett, F. C. (1932) *Remembering.* Cambridge University Press: Cambridge.

Bauman, Z. (2005) *Liquid Life.* Polity Press: Oxford.

Beard, M. (2017) *Women & Power: A Manifesto.* Profile: London.

Beattie, G. (2004) *Visible Thought: The New Psychology of Body Language.* Routledge: London.

Becker, S. (2004) Carers. *Research Matters*, August Special Issue: 5–10.

Berger, J. (2008) *Ways of Seeing.* Penguin: London.

Blackman, L. and Walkerdine, V. (2001) *Mass Hysteria: Critical Psychology and Media Studies.* Palgrave: London.

Blaikie, N. (2010) *Designing Social Research*, 2nd Edition. Polity Press: Oxford.

Bloodworth, J. (2018) *Hired: Six Months Undercover in Low-Wage Britain.* Atlantic Books: London.

Bogonovi, F. (2010) A Life-Cycle Approach to the Analysis of the Relationship Between Social Capital and Health in Britain. *Social Science & Medicine*, 71(11): 1927–1934.

Böhme, H. (2014) *Fetishism and Culture: A Different Theory of Modernity.* De Gruyter: ProQuest Ebook Central. http://ebookcentral.proquest.com/lib/open/detail.action?docID=1317881

Bourdieu, P. (1977) *Outline of a Theory of Practice* (trans. R. Nice). Cambridge University Press: Cambridge.

Bourdieu, P. (1983) The Field of Cultural Production, or The Economic World Reversed. *Science Direct,* 12(4–5): 311–356.

Brah, A. (1996) *Cartographies of Diaspora.* Taylor and Francis: London.

Brandth, B. and Kvande, E. (2009) Norway: The Making of the Father's Quota. In S. Kamerman, and P. Moss (eds) *The Politics of Parental Leave Policies,* 191–206. Policy Press: Cambridge.

Braun, V. and Clarke, V. (2006) Using Thematic Analysis in Psychology. *Qualitative Research in Psychology,* 3: 77–101.

Braun, V. and Clarke, V. (2017) Thematic Analysis. In C. Willig and W. Stainton Rogers (eds) *The Sage Handbook of Qualitative Research in Psychology.* Sage: London.

Breckler, S. J. and Wiggins, E. C. (1989) Affect Versus Evaluation in the Structure of Attitudes. *Journal of Experimental Social Psychology,* 25: 253–271.

Brinkmann, S. (2017) *Stand Firm: Resisting the Self-Improvement Craze* (trans. T. McTurk). Polity Press: Oxford.

Brooks, J., Mccluskey, S., Turley, E. and King, N. (2015) The Utility of Template Analysis. *Qualitative Research in Psychology,* 12(2): 202–222.

Broverman, I., Vogel, S., Broverman, D., Clarkson, F. and Rosenkrantz, P. (1972) Sex-Role Stereotypes: A Current Appraisal. *Journal of Social Issues,* 28: 59–78.

Brown, S. (2012) Experiment: Abstract Experimentalism. In C. Lury and N. Wakefield (eds) *Inventive Methods: The Happening of the Social.* Routledge: Abingdon.

Brown, S. and Stenner, P. (2009) *Psychology Without Foundations: History, Philosophy and Psychosocial Theory.* Sage: London.

Brown, W. (2012) Neoliberalism and the End of Liberal Democracy. *Theory & Event,* 15(2). 10.1353/tae.2003.0020

Bruner, J. (1957) On Perceptual Readiness. *Psychological Review,* 64: 123–152.

Bulhan, H. A. (1985) *Frantz Fanon and the Psychology of Oppression.* Springer: Heidelberg, Germany.

Burkitt, I. (2002) Complex Emotions: Relations, Feelings and Images in Emotional Experience. *The Sociological Review,* 50(2): 151–167.

Burman, E. (2016) *Deconstructing Developmental Psychology,* 3rd Edition. Routledge: London.

Burr, V. (1998) *Psychology and Gender.* Routledge: London.

Butler, J. (1993) *Bodies That Matter: On the Discursive Limits of 'Sex'.* Routledge: New York, NY.

Butt, T. (1981) Economics is the Method; the Object Is to Change the Heart and Soul, *The Sunday Times,* 3rd May.

Byrne, B. (2006) In Search of a 'Good Mix', Class, Gender and Practices of Mothering. *Sociology,* 40(6): 1001–1017.

Caddick, N. (2018) How Sport and Exercise Helps Veterans Heal – and How It Can Do It Better. ISCHP Blog, January. http://ischp.info/2018/01/02/how-sport-and-exercise-helps-veterans-heal-and-how-it-can-do-it-better/

Campbell, B. (1980) A Feminist Sexual Politics: Now You See It, Now You Don't. *Feminist Review*, 5: 1–18.

Carnegie, D. (1937) *How to Win Friends and Influence People*. Simon and Shuster: New York, NY.

Cartwright, S. A. (1851) Report on the Diseases and Particularities of the Negro Race. *New Orleans Medical and Surgical Journal*, 69: 1–715.

Casas, C., Sadurni, M., Coenders, G. and Dannerbeck, A. (2010) *Quality-of-Life Research on Children and Adolescents*. Springer: Dordrecht, Netherlands.

Chabris, C. (1999) Prelude or Requiem for the 'Mozart Effect'? *Nature*, 400: 826.

Chamberlain, M. (1999) Brothers and Sisters, Uncles and Aunts: A Lateral Perspective on Caribbean Families. In E. Silva and C. Smart (eds) *The New Family*. Sage: London.

Chamberlain, K., McGuigan, K., Anstiss, D. and Marshall, K. (2018) A Change of View: Arts-Based Research and Psychology. *Qualitative Research in Psychology*, 15(2–3): 131–139.

Cherlin, A. J. and Furstenberg, F. F. (1992) *The New American Grandparent: A Place in the Family, a Life Apart*. Harvard University Press: Cambridge, MA.

Chinese Culture Connection. (1987) Chinese Values and the Search for Culture-Free Dimensions of Culture. *Journal of Cross-Cultural Psychology*, 18: 143–164.

Cho, H. (2012) Examining Gender Differences in the Nature and Context of Intimate Partner Violence. *Journal of Interpersonal Violence*, 21(13): 2665–2684.

Churchwell, S. (2018) End of the American Dream? The Dark History of 'America First', *Guardian*, 21st April, 2008.

Clarke, R. (2017) The NHS is not immune to sexual harassment: It happened to #metoo. *Guardian*, G2, 29th November.

Clough, P. T. and Halley, J. (2007) *The Affective Turn: Theorising the Social*. Duke University Press: Durham and London.

Cocozza, P. (2018) Sad summer's over? 18 ways to keep the health, humour and happiness of your holiday alive. *Guardian*, 3rd September.

Cohen, C. (1997) Punks, Bulldaggers, and Welfare Queens: The Radical Potential of Queer Politics? *GLQ: A Journal of Lesbian and Gay Studies*, 3: 437–485.

Coleman, J. S. (1916;1988) Social Capital in the Creation of Human Capital. *American Journal of Sociology*, 94: S95–S120. https://doi.org/10.1086/228943

Connoly, W. E. (2002) Film Technique and Micropolitics. *Theory & Event*, 6(1). John Hopkins University Press. 10.1353/tae.2002.0003

Crawford, R. (1980) Healthism and the Medicalization of Everyday Life. *International Journal of Health Services*, 10(3): 365–388.

Crawford, R. (1984) A Cultural Account of Health: Control, Release and the Social Body. In J. B. McKinlay (ed) *Issues in the Political Economy of Health Care*. Tavistock: London.

Crawford, R. (2006) Health Is a Meaningful Social Practice. *Health: An Interdisciplinary Journal for the Social Study of Health, Illness and Medicine*, 10(4): 401–420.

Cromby, J. (2015) *Feeling Bodies: Embodying Psychology*. Palgrave Macmillan: Basingstoke.

Curt, B. (1994) *Textuality and Tectonics: Troubling Social and Psychological Science*. Open University Press: Stony Stratford.

Damasio, A. R. (1994) *Descartes' Error: Emotion, Reason and the Human Brain*. Picador: London.

Davies, W. (2018) *Nervous States: How Feeling Took Over the World*. Jonathan Cape: London.

Day, C. and Nicholls, K. (2018) *"They don't think like us": Exploring attitudes of non-transgender students towards transgender people using discourse analysis.* Paper presented at the BPS Sexualities Conference, London.

Day, K., Rickett, B. and Woolhouse, M. (2017) Towards a Critical Social Psychology of Social Class. In B. Gough (ed) *The Palgrave Handbook of Critical Social Psychology*, 469–490. Palgrave Macmillan: London.

De Vogel, V., Stam, J., Bouman, H. A., Terterst, P. and Lamncel, M. (2015) Violent Women: A Multicentre Study Into Gender Differences in Forensic Psychiatric Patients. *Journal of Forensic Psychiatry and Psychology*, 27(2): 145–168.

Deleuze, G. and Guattari, F. (1977) *Anti-Oedipus: Capitalism and Schizophrenia*. University of Minnesota Press: Minneapolis, MN.

Deleuze, G. and Guattari, F. (1987) *A Thousand Plateaus* (trans. B. Massumi). University of Minnesota Press: Minneapolis, MN.

Deleuze, G. (1992) *Expressionism in Philosophy: Spinoza* (trans. M. Joughin). Zone: New York, NY.

Douglass, F. (1854) The Claims of the Negro Ethnologically Considered. In H. Brotz (ed) *Negro Social and Political Thought 1850–1920, Representative Texts*. Basic Books: New York, NY.

Douglas, S. J. and Michaels, M. (2004) *The Mommy Myth*. Free Press: New York, NY.

Du Gay, P., Evans, J. and Redman, P. (2000) *Identity: A Reader*. Sage: London.

Dunant, S. (1994) *The War of the Words: The Politically Correct Debate*. Virago: London.

Eagleton, T. (1981) *Walter Benjamin or Towards a Revolutionary Criticism*. Verso: London.

Eagly, A. H. and Chaiken, S. (1998) Attitude Structure and Function. In D. T. Gilbert, S. T. Fiske and G. Lindzey (eds) *The Handbook of Social Psychology*. McGraw-Hill: New York, NY.

Eatough, V. and Smith, J. (2017) Interpretative Phenomenological Analysis. In C. Willig and W. Stainton Rogers (eds) *The Sage Handbook of Qualitative Research in Psychology*. Sage: London.

Eddo-Lodge, R. (2018) *Why I'm No Longer Talking to White People About Race*. Bloomsbury: London.

Edwards, A. R. (1989) Sex/Gender, Sexism and Social Justice: Some Theoretical Considerations. *International Journal of the Sociology of Law*, 17(2): 165–184.

Edwards, R., Hadfield, L., Lucey, L. and Mauthner, M. (2006) *Sisters and Brothers: Sibling Identities and Relationships*. Routledge: London.

Ehrenreich, B. (2018) *Natural Causes: Life, Death and the Illusion of Control*. Granta: London.

Ekman, P. (1973; 2003) *Emotions Revealed*. Times Books: New York, NY.

Enloe, C. (2017) *The Big Push: Exposing and Challenging the Persistence of Patriarchy*. Myrad: Oxford.

Eysenk, H. J. (1971) *Race, Intelligence and Education*. Temple Smith: London.

Fanon, F. (1952;1986) *Black Skin, White Masks*. Pluto Press: London.

Fenton-O'Creevy, M. (2001) *Leadership in the New Organisation, Block 2*. Open University: Milton Keynes.

Ferrier, J. N. (2018) Beyond the Non/Monogamy System: Fluidity, Hybridity, and Transcendence in Intimate Relationships. *Psychology & Sexuality*, 9(1).

Fiedler, K. and Bless, H. (2001) Social Cognition. In M. Hewstone and W. Stroeber (eds) *Introduction to Social Psychology*, 3rd Edition. Blackwell: Oxford.

Finlay, L. (2014) Embodying Research. *Qualitative Research in Psychology*, 13(1): 4–18.

Finn, M. (2012) Monogamous Order and the Avoidance of Chaotic Excess. *Psychology & Sexuality*, 3(2): 123–136.

Fishbein, M. and Ajzen, I. (1975) *Belief, Attitude, Intention and Behaviour: An Introduction to Theory and Research*. Addison-Wesley: Reading, MA.

Fiske, S. T. and Taylor, S. E. (1991) *Social Cognition*, 2nd Edition. McGraw-Hill: New York, NY.

Fletcher, G. (2018) 'Instead of a scar, I had a piece of art': Women on their post-mastectomy tattoos. *Guardian*, 22nd September.

Flick, U. (2000) Qualitative Inquiries into Social Representations of Health. *Journal of Health Psychology*, 5(3): 309–318.

Flick, U. (2015) Qualitative Research as Social Transformation. In M. Murray (ed) *Critical Health Psychology*, 2nd Edition, pp. 182–199. Palgrave: London.

Flick, U. and Foster, J. (2017) Social Representations. In C. Willig and W. S. Rogers (eds) *The Handbook of Qualitative Research in Psychology*. Sage: London.

Floridi, L. (2014) *The 4th Revolution: How the Infosphere Is Reshaping Human Reality*. Oxford University Press: Oxford.

Fornäs, J. (1995) *Cultural Theory and Late Modernity*. Sage: London.

Foster, D. (2018) Why the Catholic church is still a force for good. *Guardian, Opinion*, 6th September.

Foucault, M. (1976) *The History of Sexuality (Volume 1)* (trans. R. Hurley). Pantheon Books: New York, NY.

Foucault, M. (1977; 1980) *Surveiller et punir: Naissance de la Prison*. Gamillard: Paris; *Discipline and Punish*. Penguin: Harmondsworth.

Foucault, M. (1978) *The History of Sexuality* (trans. R. Hurley). Penguin: Harmondsworth.

Foucault, M. (1988) *Politics, Philosophy, Culture: Interviews and Other Writings, 1977–1984* (ed. L. Kritzman). Routledge: London.

Freidan, B. (1963) *The Feminine Mystique*. Penguin: Harmondsworth.

Freire, P. (1972; 1995) *The Pedagogy of the Oppressed*. Penguin: Harmondsworth.

Freud, S. (1964) An Outline of Psychoanalysis. In *The Complete Psychological Works of Sigmund Freud* (Vol. XXIII), Standard Edition. Hogarth Press: London.

Friedson, E. (1970) *The Profession of Medicine: A Study of the Sociology of Applied Knowledge*. Dodd Mead: New York, NY.

Frosh, S. (2010) Psychoanalytic Perspectives on Identity: From Ego to Ethics. In M. Wetherell and C. Mohanty (eds) *Sage Handbook of Identities*, 29–46. Sage: London.

Frosh, S. and Saville Young, L. (2017) Psychoanalytic Approaches to Qualitative Psychology. In C. Willig and W. Stainton Rogers (eds) *The SAGE Handbook of Qualitative Research in Psychology*. Sage: London.

Furedi, F. (2005) *The Politics of Fear: Beyond left and Right*. Continuum: New York, NY.

Fusco, C. (2006) Inscribing Healthification: Governance, Risk, Surveillance and the Subjects and Spaces of Fitness and Health. *Health and Place*, 12(1): 55–78. https://doi.org/10.1016/j.healthplace.2004.10.003

Gabb, J., Klett-Davies, M., Fink, J. and Thomas, M. (2013) *Enduring Love? Couple Relationships in the 21st Century*. Open University Press: London.

Game, A. (1991) *Undoing the Social: Towards a Deconstructive Sociology*. Open University Press: Buckingham.

Geertz, C. (1975) On the Nature of Anthropological Understanding. *American Scientist*, 63: 47–53.

Georgi, A., Georgi, B. and Morley, J. (2017) The Descriptive Phenomenological Psychological Method. In C. Willig and W. S. Rogers (eds) *The Sage Handbook of Qualitative Research in Psychology*. Sage: London.

Gieseking, J. J. (2014) *The People, Place, and Space Reader*. Taylor and Francis: London.

Gill, R. and Kanai, A. (2018) Mediating Neoliberal Capitalism: Affect, Subjectivity and Inequality. *Journal of Communication*, 68(2): 318–326.

Gill, R. and Orgad, S. (2018) The Amazing Bounce-Backable Woman: Resilience and the Psychological Turn in Neoliberalism. *Sociology Research Online*, 23(2): 477–495.

Gilligan, C. (1982) *In a Different Voice: Psychological Theory and Women's Development*. Harvard University Press: Cambridge, MA.

Gillum, R., King, D., Obisesan, T. and Koenig, H. (2008) Frequency of Attendance at Religious Services and Mortality in a U.S. National Cohort. *Annals of Epidemiology*, 18(2): 124–129.

Gil-Rivas, V. and Kilmer, R. P. (2016) Building Community Capacity and Fostering Disaster Resilience. *Journal of Clinical Psychology*, 72(12): 1318–1332.

Ging, D. (2017) Alphas, Betas, and Incels: Theorizing the Masculinities of the Manosphere. *Men and Masculinities*. https://journals.sagepub.com/doi/abs/10.1177/1097184X17706401

Glazzard, J. (2018) *The experiences of Trans young people in schools: Barriers to and facilitators of inclusion*. Paper Presented at the Gender Conference, Leeds Beckett University, 6th March.

Glick, P. and Fiske, S. T. (2001) An Ambivalent Alliance: Hostile and Benevolent Sexism as Complementary Justifications for Gender Inequality. *American Psychologist*, 56: 109–118. Goffman, E. (1959) *Stigma: Notes on the Management of Spoiled Identity*. Prentice Hall: Englewood Cliffs, CA.

Goffman, E. (1955) On Face-Work: An Analysis of Ritual Elements in Social Interaction. *Psychiatry*, 18: 213–231.

Goffman, E. (1959) *The Presentation of Self in Everyday Life*. Doubleday: New York.

Goffman, E. (1963) *Behaviour in Public Places*. Free Press: New York, NY.

Goffman, E. (1967) *Interaction Ritual: Essays on Face-to-face Behaviour*. Garden City, NY: Anchor.

Goodley, D., Lawthom, R. and Cole, K. R. (2014) Posthuman Disability Studies. *Subjectivity*, 7(4): 342–361.

Gough, B. (2017) *The Palgrave Handbook of Critical Social Psychology*. Palgrave Macmillan: London.

Gough, B. and Edwards, D. (1998) The Beer Talking: A Carry out and the Reproduction of Masculinities. *The Sociological Review*, 46(3): 409–455.

Greenhalgh, T. (2017) Adjuvant Chemotherapy: An Autoethnography. *Subjectivity*, 10(4): 340–357.

Greenhalgh, T. and O'Riordan, L. (2018) *The Complete Guide to Breast Cancer*. Penguin: London.

Hall, E. T. (1966) *The Silent Language*. Doubleday: New York, NY.

Haraway, D. (1984) Primatology Is Politics by Other Means. In R. Blier (ed) *Feminist Approaches to Science*. Pergamon: London.

Haraway, D. (2004) Situated Knowledges: The Science Question in Feminism and the Privileges of Partial Perspective. In E. Y. Lincoln (ed) *Turning Points in Qualitative Research: Tying Knots in a Handkerchief*. Alta Mira Press: Walnut Creek, CA.

Harvey, D. (2006) *Spaces of Global Capitalism*. Verso: London.

Health Scotland (2019) What are health inequalities. http://www.healthscotland. scot/health-inequalities/what-are-health-inequalities

Heider, F. (1953) *The Psychology of Interpersonal Relations*. Wiley: New York, NY.

Heidigger, M. (1927; 2010) *Being and Time: A Revised Edition of the Stambaugh Translation* (SUNY series in Contemporary Continental Philosophy). State University of New York Press: Albany, NY.

Heilbrun, K., DeMatteo, D., Marczyk, G. and Goldstein, A. (2008) Standards of Practice and Care in Forensic Mental Health Assessment: Legal, Professional, and Principles-Based Consideration. *Psychology, Public Policy, and Law*, 14(1): 1–26.

Henderson, A., Harmon, S. and Newma, H. (2016) The Price Mothers Pay, Even When They Are Not Buying It: Mental Health Consequences of Idealized Motherhood. *Sex Roles*, 74(11–12): 512–526.

Henriques, J., Hollway, W., Venn, C. and Walkerdine, V. (1984) *Changing the Subject: Psychology, Social Regulation and Subjectivity*. Routledge: London.

Herriot, P. (1974) *Attributes of Memory*. Methuen: London.

Herrnstein, C. and Murray, R. (1994) *The Bell Curve: Intelligence and Class Structure in American Life*. The Free Press: New York, NY.

Herzlich, C. (1974) *Health and Illness*. Academic Press: London.

Herzlich, C. (2017) A Journey in the Field of Health: From Social Psychology to Multi-Disciplinarity. *Journal of Health Psychology*, 23(3): 386–396.

Hill, D. (2000) Feminism in the 21st Century. *Guardian*, 11th December.

Hobbes, T. (1998) *On the Citizen* (ed. & trans. Richard Tuck and Michael Silverthorne). Cambridge University Press: Cambridge.

Hochschild, A. (1983) *The Managed Heart*. University of California Press: Berkeley, CA.

Hochschild, A. and Ehrenreich, B. (2004) *Global Woman: Nannies, Maids and Sex Workers*. Macmillan: London.

Hoff, E. (2013) Interpreting the Early Language Trajectories of Children From Low-SES and Language Minority Homes: Implications for Closing Achievement Gaps. *Developmental Psychology*, 49(1): 4–14. http://dx.doi.org/10.1037/a0027238

Hofstede, G. (1983) Dimensions of National Cultures in Fifty Countries and Three Regions. In J. Deregowski, S. Dziurawiec and R. Annis (eds) *Explications in Cross-Cultural Psychology*. Swets and Zeitlinger: Lisse.

Hogg, M. A. and Vaughan, G. M. (1998) *Social Psychology*. Prentice-Hall: Englewood Cliffs, NJ.

Hogg, M. A. and Vaughan, G. M. (2017) *Social Psychology: An Introduction*. Pearson: London.

Hollway, W. (1989) Gender Difference and the Production of Subjectivity. In J. Henriques, W. Hollway, C. Curwen, C. Venn and V. Walkerdine (eds) *Changing the Subject: Psychology, Social Regulation and Subjectivity*. Routledge: London.

Hollway, W. (2010) Relationality: The Intersubjective Foundations of Identity. In M. Wetherell and C. Mohanty (eds) *Sage Handbook of Identities*, 216–232. Sage: London.

Holt-Lunstad, J., Smith, T. B. and Layton, J. B. (2010) Social Relationships and Mortality Risk: A Meta-analytic Review. *PLOS Medicine*, 7(7). https://doi.org/10.1371/journal.pmed.1000316

Hook, D. (2004) Critical Psychology: The Basic Co-Ordinates. In D. Hook, A. Collins, P. Kiguwa and N. Mkhize (eds) *Critical Psychology*. University of Cape Town Press: Cape Town, South Africa.

Hostetler, A. J. (2009) Single by Choice? Assessing and Understanding Voluntary Singlehood Among Mature Gay Men. *Journal of Homosexuality*, 56(4): 499–531.

Hrdy, S. B. (1999) *Mother Nature: Maternal Instincts and How They Shape the Human Species*. Ballantine: New York, NY.

Humberstone, B. (2011) Embodiment and Social and Environmental Action in Nature-Based Sport: Spiritual Spaces. *Leisure Studies*, 30(4): 495–512.

Illouz, E. (2007) *Cold Intimacies: The Making of Emotional Capitalism*. Polity Press: Oxford.

Illouz, E. (2008) *Saving the Modern Soul: Therapy, Emotions and the Culture of Self-Help*. University of California Press: Berkeley, CA.

Jaensch, E. R. (1939) Der Hünerhof als Forschungs- und Aufklärungsmittel in menschlichen Rassenfragen. *Zeitschrift für Tierpsychologie*, 2: 223–258.

James, W. (1907) *Psychology*. Macmillan: London.

Janoff-Bulman, R. and Frieze, I. H. (1987) The Role of Gender in Reactions to Gender Victimization. In R. C. Barnett, L. Beiner and G. K. Baruch (eds) *Gender and Stress*. Free Press: New York, NY.

Jensen, A. R. (1969) How Much Can We Boost IQ and Scholastic Achievement? *Harvard Educational Review*, 39: 1–123.

Johansen-Berg, H. and Duzel, E. (2016) Effects of Physical and Cognitive Activity on Brain Structure and Function. *Neurolimage*, 131: 1–238.

Johnston, D. D. and Swanson, D. H. (2007) Cognitive Acrobatics in the Construction of Worker – Mother Identity. *Sex Roles*, 57: 447–459.

Jones, E. E. and Davis, K. E. (1965) A Theory of Correspondent Inferences: From Acts to Dispositions. In L. Berkovitz (ed) *Advances in Experimental Social Psychology*, Vol. 2. Academic Press: New York, NY.

Jones, L. and McDaid, H. (eds) (2017) *Nasty Women: A Collection of Essays and Accounts on What It Is to Be a Woman in the 21st Century*. 404 Ink: Edinburgh.

Jorgensen, C. (2003) Frederick Douglass and the Early Social Psychology of Racial Oppression. *Race and Society*, 6: 3–20.

Jourard, S. M. (1966) An Exploratory Study of Body Accessibility. *British Journal of Social and Clinical Psychology*, 5: 221–231.

Kahneman, D. (2003) A Perspective on Judgement and Choice. *American Psychologist*, 58: 697–720.

Kahneman, D. (2011) *Thinking Fast and Slow*. Penguin: London.

Kaniasty, K. and Norris, F. H. (2004) Social Support in the Aftermath of Disasters, Catastrophes, and Acts of Terrorism: Altruistic, Overwhelmed, Uncertain, Antagonistic, and Patriotic Communities. In R. J. Ursano, A. E. Norwood and C. S. Fullerton (eds) *Bioterrorism: Psychological and Public Health Interventions*, 200–229. Cambridge University Press: Cambridge.

Kawachi, I., Subramanian, S. V. and Kim, D. (2008) Social Capital and Health: A Decade of Progress and Beyond. In I. Kawachi, S. V. Subramanian and D. Kim (eds) *Social Capital and Health*, 1–28. Springer: New York, NY.

Kelley, H. H. (1967) Attribution Theory in Social Psychology. In D. Levine (ed) *Nebraska Symposium on Motivation*, Vol. 15.

Kevles, D. J. (1995) *In the Name of Eugenics: Genetics and the Uses of Human Heredity*. Harvard University Press: Cambridge, MA.

Khaled, R., Biddel, R., Noble, J., Barr, P. and Fischer., H. (2006) *Persuasive interaction for collectivist cultures*. Paper given at the Seventh Australasian User Interface Conference (AUIC 2006) Hobart, Australia.

Kim, J. M. (2011) Is 'the Missy' the New Femininity? In R. Gill and C. Scharff (eds) *New Femininities: Postfeminism, Neoliberalism and Subjectivity*. Palgrave: London.

Kimhi, S. and Shamai, M. (2004) Community resilience and the impact of stress: Adult response to Israel's withdrawal from Lebanon. *Journal of Community Psychology*, 32(4): 439–451.

Kitzinger, C. and Frith, H. (1999) Just Say No? The Use of Conversational Analysis in Developing a Feminist Perspective on Sexual Refusal. *Discourse and Society*, 10(3): 293–316.

Kline, W. (2002) *Building a Better Race: Gender, Sexuality, and Eugenics From the Turn of the Century to the Baby Boom*. University of California Press: Berkeley, CA.

Kohlberg, L. (1984) *The Psychology of Moral Development: The Nature and Validity of Moral Stages* (Essays on Moral Development, Volume 2). Harper & Row: New York, NY.

Kondo, D. (1990) *Crafting Selves: Power, Gender and Discourses of Identity in a Japanese Workplace*. University of Chicago Press: Chicago.

Lahti, A. (2018) Bisexual Desires for More Than One Gender as a Challenge to Normative Relationship Ideals. *Psychology & Sexuality*, 9(2): 132–147.

Lalljee, M. (2000) The Interpreting Self: A Social Constructionist Perspective. In R. Stevens (ed) *Understanding the Self*. Sage: London.

Lambert, C. (2015) *Shadow Work: The Unpaid, Unseen Jobs That Fill Your Day*. Counterpoint: Berkeley, CA.

Langridge, D. (2007) *Phenomenological Psychology: Theory, Research and Method*. Pearson: Harlow.

Langer, S. (1967) *Mind: An Essay on Human Feeling (Volume 1)*. The Johns Hopkins University Press: Baltimore, MD.

Langer, S. (1972) *Mind: An Essay on Human Feeling (Volume 2)*. The Johns Hopkins University Press: Baltimore, MD.

Langer, S. (1982) *Mind: An Essay on Human Feeling (Volume 3)*. The Johns Hopkins University Press: Baltimore, MD.

Latané, B. and Darley, J. M. (1968) Group Inhibition of Bystander Intervention in Emergencies: Diffusion of Responsibility. *Journal of Personality and Social Psychology*, 8(4): 377–383.

Latané, B. and Darley, J. M. (1976) Help in Crisis: Bystander Response to an Emergency. In J. W. Thibout and J. T. Spence (eds) *Contemporary Topics in Social Psychology*, 309–332. General Learning Press: Morristown, NJ.

Latour, B. (2004) How to Talk About the Body? The Normative Dimension of Science Studies. *Body & Society*, 10(2–3): 205–229. https://doi.org/10.1177/1357034X04042943

Latour, B. (2005) *Reassembling the Social: An Introduction to Actor-Network Theory*. Oxford University Press: Oxford.

Latshaw, B. A. and Hale, S. I. (2016) 'The Domestic Handoff': Stay-at-Home Fathers' Time-Use in Female Breadwinner Families. *Journal of Family Studies*, 22: 97–120.

Lazarus, R. S. (1991) *Emotion and Adaptation*. Oxford University Press: Oxford.

Lenoble, R. (1943) *Essai sur la notion de l'experience (Essay on the Concept of the Experience)*. Vrin: Paris.

Levinson, D. J., with Darrow, C. N, Klein, E. B. and Levinson, M. (1978) *Seasons of a Man's Life*. Random House: New York, NY.

Lewis, G. (2009) Birthing Racial Difference: Conversations With My Mother and Others. *Studies in the Maternal*, 1(1).

Lindesmith, A. R., Strauss, A. L. and Denzin, N. K. (1999) *Social Psychology*, 8th Edition. Sage: London.

Littler, J. (2017) Meritocracy: The great delusion that ingrains inequality. *Guardian, Opinion*, 20th March.

Locke, A., Lawthom, R. and Lyons, A. (2018) Social Media Platforms as Complex and Contradictory Spaces for Feminisms: Visibility, Opportunity, Power, Resistance and Activism. *Feminism & Psychology*, 28(1): 3–10.

Locke, A. and Yarwood, G. (2017) Exploring the Depths of Gender, Parenting and 'Work': Critical Discursive Psychology and the 'Missing Voices' of Involved Fatherhood. *Community, Work & Family*, 20(1): 4–18.

Lorimer, H. (2005) Cultural Geography: The Busyness of Being 'More-Than-Representational'. *Progress in Human Geography*, 29(1): 83–94. https://doi.org/10.1191/0309132505ph531pr

Lowe, I. (2009) *A Big Fix: Radical Solutions for Australia's Environmental Crisis*, 2nd Edition. Black Inc.: Melbourne, Australia.

Lucey, H. (2007) Families. In W. Hollway, H. Lucey and A. Pheonix (eds) *Social Psychology Matters*. Open University Press: London.

Lukes, S. (2005) *Power: A Radical View*, 2nd Edition. Palgrave Macmillan: Basingstoke.

Luria, A. R. (1968) *The Mind of a Mnemonist* (trans. L. Solototaroff). Harvard University Press: Cambridge, MA.

MacDonald, M. (2013) Women Prisoners, Mental Health, Violence and Abuse. *International Journal of Law and Psychiatry*, 36(3–4): 293–303.

Machiavelli, N. (2017) *The Prince*. Penguin Classics: London.

Madill, A., Jordan, A. and Shirley, C. (2000) Objectivity and Reliability in Qualitative Analysis: Realist, Contextualist and Radical Constructionist Epistemologies. *British Journal of Psychology*, 91: 1–20.

Malpert, A.V., Suiter, S.V., Kivell, N. M., Perkins, D.D., Bess, Evans, S. D., Hanlin, C.E., Conway, P., Mccown, D. and Prilleltensky, I. (2017) , in C. Willig and W. Stainton Rogers (Eds.) The Sage Handbook of Qualitative Research in Psychology. Sage: London.

Mangan, L. (2013) *Hopscotch and Handbags: The Truth About Being a Girl*. Hachette: London.

Manstead, A. S. R. and Semin, G. (1980) Social Facilitation Effects: More Enhancement of Dominant Responses? *British Journal of Social and Clinical Psychology*, 19: 119–136.

Marlowe, L. (2018) Eva Illouz: Sex, power and the behaviour of men. *Irish Times*, 14th March.

Marsh, P., Rosser, E. and Harré, R. (1974) *The Rules of Disorder*. Routledge and Kegan Paul: London.

Martikke, S. (2017) *Overview of Social Capital*, written for the Greater Manchester Centre for Voluntary Organisations. www.gmcvo.org.uk/system/files/social_capital_an_overview_0.pdf

Martin, C. L. and Halverson, C. F. (1981) A Schematic Processing Model of Sex Stereotyping in Children. *Child Development*, 52(4): 1119–1134.

Mason, J. and Davies, K. (2009) Coming to Our Senses? A Critical Approach to Sensory Methodology. *Qualitative Research*, 9(5): 587–603.

Mason, P. (2018) A new politics of emotion is needed to beat the far right. *Guardian, Journal*, 26th November.

Massey, D. (2004) Geographies of Responsibility. *Geografiska Annaler: Series B, Human Geography*, 86(1): 5–18.

Massumi, B. (1996) Becoming-Deleuzian. *Environment and Planning D: Society and Space*, 14(4): 395–406. https://doi.org/10.1068/d140395McDougall, W. (1919) *An Introduction to Social Psychology*. Methuen: London.

McIntosh Grey, A. (1982) Inequalities in Health: The Black Report: A Summary and Comment. *International Journal of Health Services*, 12(3): 349–380

McKeown, T. (1976) *The Role of Medicine: Dream, Mirage or Nemesis?* The Nuffield Trust: London.

McRuer, R. (2006) *Crip Theory: Cultural Signs of Queerness and Disability*. New York University Press: New York, NY.

Merleau-Ponty, M. (1964; 2012) *The Phenomenology of Perception* (trans. D. A. Landes). Routledge: New York, NY.

Mielewczyk, M. and Willig, C. (2007) Old Clothes and an Older Look: The Case for a Radical Makeover in Health. *Theory & Psychology*, 17(6): 811–837.

Miller, G. A., Galanter, E. and Pribram, K. H. (1960) *Plans and the Structure of Behavior*. Henry Holt: New York, NY.

Millward-Hopkins, J. (2017) Easiest to Get By Searching for 'Neoliberal Psychology'. *openDemocracy*. https://www.opendemocracy.net/en/transformation/neoliberal-psychology/

Mol, A. (2008) *The Logic of Care: Health and the Problem of Patient Choice*. Routledge: London.

Monbiot, G. (2018a) We won't save the Earth with a better kind of disposable coffee cup. *Guardian*, 6th September.

Monbiot, G. (2018b) Electric food – The new sci-fi diet that could save our planet. *Guardian*, 31st October.

Monbiot, G. (2019) The Fear That Lies Behind Aggressive Masculinity. *Guardian*, 16th January.

Moscovici, S. (1961) *La Psychanalyse, Son Image, Son Public*, PUF. First Published in English in 1985 and then in 2008: *Psychoanalysis: Its Image, Its Public*. Polity Press: Oxford.

Moscovici, S. (1985) Society and Theory in Social Psychology. In J. Israel and H. Tajfel (eds) *The Context of Social Psychology: A Critical Assessment*. Academic Press: New York, NY.

Moscovici, S. and Hewstone, M. (1983) Social Representations and Social Explanations: From the 'Mature' to the 'Amateur' Scientist. In M. Hewstone (ed) *Attribution Theory: Social and Functional Explanations*. Blackwell: Oxford.

Moore, S. (2019) It takes more than a T-shirt to be a feminist. *Guardian,* 30th May.

Mrazek, P. B. and Mrazek, D. A. (1981) The Effects of Child Abuse: Methodological Considerations. In P. B. Mrazek and C. H. Kempe (eds) *Sexually Abused Children and Their Families*, 235–246. Pergamon: New York, NY.

Mudde, C. and Kaltwasser, C. R. (2017) *Populism: A Very Short Introduction.* Oxford University Press: Oxford.

Mulkay, M. (1991) *Sociology of Science: A Sociological Pilgrimage.* Open University Press: Milton Keynes.

Mulvey, L. (1975) Visual Pleasure and Narrative Cinema. *Screen*, 16(3): 6–18.

Murray, D. A. B. (2003) Who Is Takatāpui? Māori Language, Sexuality and Identity in Aotearoa/New Zealand. *Anthropologica*, 45(2): 233–244. www.jstor.org/stable/25606143

Nagata, D., Yang, W. and Tsai-Chae, A. (2010) Chinese American Grandmothering: A Qualitative Exploration. *Asian American Journal of Psychology*, 1(2): 151–161.

Nagle, A. (2017) *Kill All Normies: The On-line Culture Wars From Tumblr and 4chan to the Alt-Right and Trump.* Zero Books: Winchester.

Neisser, U. (1967) *Cognitive Psychology.* Prentice-Hall: Englewood Cliffs, NJ.

Newman, H. (2016) The Price Mothers Pay, Even When They Are Not Buying It: Mental Health Consequences of Idealized Motherhood. *Sex Roles*, 74(11–12): 512–526.

Ngozi Adichie, C. (2014) I decided to call myself a Happy Feminist. *Guardian*, 17th October.

Nisbett, R. E. and Ross, L. (1980) *Human Inference: Strategies and Shortcomings of Social Judgement.* Prentice Hall: Englewood Cliffs, NJ.

Norberg, J. (2016) *Progress: Ten Reasons to Look Forward to the Future.* Oneworld: London.

Norris, F. E., Stevens, S. P., Pfefferbaum, B., Wyche, K. F. and Pfefferbaum, R. (2008) Community Resilience as a Metaphor, Theory, Set of Capacities, and Strategy for Disaster Readiness. *American Journal of Community Psychology*, 41: 127–150.

O'Dell, L. (1997) Child Sexual Abuse and the Academic Construction of Symptomatologies. *Feminism & Psychology*, 7(3): 334–339. https://doi.org/10.1177/0959353597073006

O'Dell, L., Crafter, S., De Abreu, G. and Cline, T. (2010) Constructing 'Normal Childhoods': Young People Talk About Young Carers. *Disability and Society*, 25(6): 643–655.

Oliver, M. (1990) *Understanding Disability: From Theory to Practice.* Macmillan Education: Basingstoke.

Oliver, M. and Barnes, C. (2012) *The New Politics of Disablement*, 2nd Edition. Palgrave Macmillan: Basingstoke.

Orr, N. and Phoenix, C. (2015) Photographing Physical Activity: Using Visual Methods to 'Grasp at' the Sensual Experiences of the Ageing Body. *Qualitative Research*, 15(4): 454–472.

Orwell, G. (2004) *Nineteen Eighty-Four.* Penguin Classics: London.

O'Sullivan, S. (2018) *It's All in Your Head: Stories From the Frontline of Psychosomatic Illness.* Chatto and Windus: London.

Paton, D. and Johnston, D. (2017) *Disaster Resilience*, 2nd Edition. Charles C Thomas: Springfield, IL.

Parker, I. (1989) *The Crisis in Modern Social Psychology, and How to End It.* Routledge: London.

Parsons, T. (1951) *The Social System*. The Free Press: Glencoe, IL.

Peirce, C. S. (1940) Abduction and Induction. In J. Bulchder (ed) *The Philosophy of Peirce: Selected Writings*. London: Routledge and Keegan Paul. (Republished in 1955 as *Philosophical Writings of Pierce*. Dover: New York, NY.)

Perry, G. (2017) *The Descent of Man*. Penguin: London.

Perry, G. (2018) *The Lost Boys: Inside Muzafer Sherif's Robbers Cave Experiment*. Scribe Publications: Victoria, Australia.

Peterson, C. M., Mathews, A., Copps-Smith, E. and Connard, L. A. (2017) Suicidality, Self-Harm, and Body Dissatisfaction in Transgender Adolescents and Emerging Adults With Gender Dysphoria. *Suicide and Self-Threatening Behaviour*, 47(4): 75–482.

Phoenix, C. and Orr, N. (2014) Pleasure: A Forgotten Dimension of Activity in Older Age. *Social Science & Medicine*, 115: 94–102.

Pinker, S. (2014) Daniel Kahneman changed the way we think about thinking: But what do other thinkers think of him? *Observer*, 16th February.

Potkay, A. (2007) *The Story of Joy: From the Bible to Late Romanticism*. Cambridge University Press: Cambridge.

Potter, J. (2017) Discursive Psychology and Discourse Analysis. In *The Routledge Handbook of Discourse Analysis*, 130–145. Routledge: London.

Potter, J. and Wetherell, M. (1987) *Discourse and Social Psychology: Beyond Attitudes and Behaviour*. Sage: London.

Powell, D. (2018) Marketing 'Childhood Obesity' and 'Health'. *International Society of Critical Health Psychology blog*. https://ischp.info/2018/07/31/marketing-childhood-obesity-and-health/

Press, I. (1980) Problems in the Definition and Classification of Medical Systems. *Social Science and Medicine*, 14b: 45–57.

Putnam, N. D. (2001) *Bowling Alone: The Collapse and Revival of American Community*. Simon and Shuster: New York, NY.

Rachman, S. (2013) *Anxiety*. Psychology Press: London.

Radley, A. (2000) Health Psychology, Embodiment and the Question of Vulnerability. *Journal of Health Psychology*, 5(3): 297–304.

Raisbrough, J. (2018) *The troubles of age and ageing: An optimist's account*. Keynote lecture given at the Psychology of Women and Equalities conference, Cumberland Lodge, July.

Rambukkana, N. (2015) *Fraught intimacies: Non/monogamy in the Public Sphere*. The University of British Columbia: Vancouver, Canada.

Randal, M. (2013) Through the Eyes of Ex-Foster Children: Placement Success and the Characteristics of Good Foster Carers. *Social Work in Action*, 25(1). https://doi.org/10.1080/09503153.2013.775236

Raskin, P. (2006) *The great transition today: Report from the future*. GTI Paper Series. Tellis Institute: Boston, MA. www.tellus.org/tellus/publication/the-great-transition-today-a-report-from-the-future

Reynolds, J. and Taylor, S. (2004) Narrating Singleness: Life Stories and Deficit Identities. *Narrative Inquiry*, 15(2): 297–215.

Richards, G. (1997) 'Race', Racism and Psychology: Towards a Reflexive History: Routledge: London.

Ricoeur, P. (1955) The Model of the Text: Meaningful Actions Considered as Texts. *Social Research*, 38: 530–547.

Ricoeur, P. (1970) *Freud and Philosophy: An Essay in Interpretation* (trans. D. Savage). Yale University Press: New Haven, CT.

Riggs, D. and Peel, E. (2016) *Critical Kinship Studies*. Palgrave Macmillan: London.

Riggs, D. and Treharne, G. (2017) Queer Theory. In B. Gough (ed) *The Palgrave Handbook of Critical Social Psychology*. Palgrave Macmillan: London.

Riley, S. (2010) Constructions of Equality and Discrimination in Professional Men's Talk. *British Journal of Psychology*, 41(3): 443–461.

Riley, S. and Evans, A. (2017) Gender. In B. Gough (ed) *The Palgrave Handbook of Critical Social Psychology*, 37–58. Palgrave Macmillan: London.

Robbins, T. W. and Costa, R. M. (2017) Habits. *Current Biology*, 27(22).

Rohleder, P. and Flowers, P. (2018) Towards a Psychology of Sexual Health. *Journal of Health Psychology*, 23(2): 143–144.

Rokeach, M. (1973) *The Nature of Human Values*. Free Press: New York, NY.

Rokeach, M. (1976) The Nature of Human Values and Value Systems. In E. P. Hollander and R. G. Hunt (eds) *Current Perspectives in Social Psychology*, 4th Edition. Oxford University Press: New York, NY.

Rose, N. (1979) The Psychological Complex: Mental Measurement and Social Administration. *Ideology and Consciousness*, 5: 5–68.

Rose, N. (1999) *Governing the Soul: The Shaping of the Private Self*, 2nd Edition. Routledge: London.

Ryan, F. (2017) We still get turned away from buses: We still have nowhere to live. *Guardian*, 15th November.

Saini, A. (2017) *Inferior: How Science Got Women Wrong – and the New Research That's Rewriting the Story*. Fourth Estate: London.

Saner, E. (2018) Employers are monitoring computers, toilet breaks – even emotions. Is your boss watching you? *Guardian*, 14th May.

Santiago-Delefosse, M. and del Rio Carral, M. (2018) The Rapid Expansion of (Mainstream) Health Psychology in France: Historical Foundations. *Journal of Health Psychology*, 23(3): 372–385.

Saussure, F. de (1974) *Course in General Linguistics* (ed. J. Culler; trans. W. Baskin). Fontana: London.

Scase, R. (1999) *Britain Towards 2010*. Economic Research Council: Swindon.

Scott, A. and Wilson, L. (2011) Valued Identities and Deficit Identities: Wellness Recovery Action Planning and Self-Management in Mental Health. *Nursing Inquiry*, 18: 40–49.

Sedgewick, P. (1982) *Psychopolitics*. Pluto: London.

Segal, L. (2017) *Radical Happiness: Moments of Collective Joy*. Verso: London.

Seppala, E., Rossomando, T. and Doty, J. R. (2013) Social Connection and Compassion: Important Predictors of Health and Well-Being. *Social Research: An International Quarterly*, 80(2): 411–430.Sheers, O. (2018) *To Provide All People: A Poem in the Voice of the NHS*. Faber: London.

Shaxson, N. (2018) *The Finance Curse: How Global Finance Is Making Us All Poorer*. The Bodley Head: London.

Sherlock, P. (2017) *Statutory time off for trade union health and safety representatives to undertake 'Safety Representative Functions'*. Report to the University of Salford Council Health and Safety Committee.

Shotter, J. (1981) Telling and Reporting: Prospective and Retrospective Self-Ascriptions. In C. Antaki (ed) *The Psychology of Ordinary Explanations of Behaviour*. Academic Press: London.

Shotter, J. (1993) *Conversational Realities: Constructing Life Through Language*. Sage: London.

Silk, M. L. and Andrews, D. L. (2006) The Fittest City in America. *Journal of Sport and Social Issues*, 30(3): 315–327. https://doi.org/10.1177/0193723506290677

Skeggs, B. (2004) *Class, Self and Culture*. Routledge: London.

Smith, E. R. and Mackie, D. M. (2000) *Social Psychology*. Taylor and Francis: Philadelphia, PA.

Spiegel, A. (2008) *Two families grapple with sons' gender preferences*. National Public Radio. www.npr.org/templates/sory/story.php?storyId=90247842

Stainton Rogers, R. and Stainton Rogers, W. (1992) *Stories of Childhood*. Harvester Wheatsheaf: London.

Stainton Rogers, R., Stenner, P., Gleeson, K. and Stainton Rogers, W. (1995) *Social Psychology: A Critical Agenda*. Polity Press: Cambridge.

Stainton Rogers, W. (1991) *Explaining Health and Illness: An Exploration of Diversity*. Harvester Wheatsheaf: Hemel Hempstead.

Stainton Rogers, W. (1996) Critical Approaches to Health Psychology. *Journal of Health Psychology*, 1(1): 65–77.

Stainton Rogers, W. (2011) *Social Psychology*. Open University: Maidenhead.

Stainton Rogers, W. (2015) Promoting Better Childhoods: Constructions of Child Concern. In M. J. Kehiley (ed) *An Introduction to Childhood Studies*, 3rd Edition. Open University Press: Maidenhead.

Stainton Rogers, W. and Stainton Rogers, R. (2001) *The Psychology of Gender and Sexuality*. Open University Press: Stony Stratford.

Stainton Rogers, W., Stainton Rogers, R., Vyrost, J. and Lovás, L. (2006) Worlds Apart: Young People's Aspirations in a Changing Europe. In J. Roche, S. Tucker, R. Thompson and R. Flynn (eds) *Youth in Society*, 19–27. Sage: London.

Steffen, W., Rockström, J., Richardson, K., Lenton, T., Folke, C., Liverman, D., . . . Hans Schellnhuber, J. (2018) Trajectories of the Earth System in the Anthropocene. *Proceedings of the National Academy of Science of the United States of America*, 115(33): 8252–8259.

Stenner, P. (2017) *Liminality and Experience: A Transdisciplinary Approach to the Psychosocial*. Palgrave Macmillan: London.

Stephenson, W. (1935) Technique of Factor Analysis. *Nature*, 136: 297.

Stephenson, W. (1953) *The Study of Behaviour: Q Technique and Its Methodology*. University of Chicago Press: Chicago, IL.

Stephenson, W. (1986) Protoconcursus: The Concourse Theory of Communication. *Operant Subjectivity*, 9(2): 30–72.

Stoppard, M. (2013) Agony Aunt Feature, *The Daily Mirror*, UK, 17th June.

Strawson, G. (2011) Thinking fast and slow by Daniel Kahneman: Review. *Guardian*, 13th December.

Sugarman, J. (2015) Neoliberalism and Psychological Ethics. *Journal of Theoretical and Philosophical Psychology*, 35(2): 103–116. http://dx.doi.org/10.1037/a0038960

Talapade Mohanty, C. (2010) Social Justice and the Politics of Identity. In Wetherell, M. and Talpade Mohanty, C. (eds), *The Sage Handbook of Identities*. Sage: London.

Taussig, M. (1980) Reification and Consciousness of the Patient. *Social Science and Medicine*, 14b: 3–13.

Teo, T. (2018) *Outline of Theoretical Psychology: Critical Investigations*. Palgrave Macmillan: London.

Terman, L. M. (1916) *The Measurement of Intelligence*. Houghton Mifflin: Boston, MA.

Thompson, L., Rickett, B. and Day, K. (2018) Feminist Relational Discourse Analysis: Putting the Personal in the Political in Feminist Research. *Qualitative Research in Psychology*, 15(1): 93–115.

Thornley, L., Ball, J., Signal, L., Lawson-Te Aho, K. and Rawson, E. (2015) Building Community Resilience: Learning From the Canterbury Earthquakes. *Kotuitui: New Zealand Journal of Social Sciences Online*, 10(1): 23–35. DOI: 10.1080/1177083X.2014.934846

Thorup, K. (2016) The dangerous 'zombie identities' of those left behind by global capitalism. *OpenDemocracy*, 4th December. www.opendemocracy.net/author/kristian-thorup

Tiffin, J., Knight, F. B. and Josey, C. C. (1940) *The Psychology of Normal People*. Heath: Boston, MA.

Tremain, R. (2016) *The Gustav Sonata*. Vintage: London.

Turley, E. L., King, N. and Monro, S. (2018) 'You Want to Be Swept up In It All': Illuminating the Erotic in BDSM. *Psychology & Sexuality*, 9(2): 148–160.

Turner, J. C. (1991) *Social Influence*. Pacific Grove, CA: Brooks/Cole.

Tyler, I. (2011) Pregnant Beauty: Maternal Femininities Under Neoliberalism. In R. Gill and C. Scharff (eds) *New Femininities: Postfeminism, Neoliberalism and Subjectivity*. Palgrave: London.

Underdown, A. (2002) 'I'm Growing up Too Fast': Messages From Young Carers. *Children and Society*, 16: 57–60.

Ussher, J. M. (1989) *The Psychology of the Female Body*. Routledge: London.

van Manen, M. (1990) *Researching Lived Experience: Human Science for an Action Sensitive Pedagogy*. State University of New York Press: New York, NY.

Venäläinen, S. (2018) A Poem About Studying Women as Perpetrators of Violence That Is Not. *Qualitative Research in Psychology*, 15(2–3): 188–191.

Vickers, J. (1982) Memoirs of an ontological exile: the methodological rebellions of feminist research, in A. Miles and G. Finn (eds) *Feminism in Canada: From Pressure to Politics*. Montreal: Black Rose.

Wachtel, A. and Scott, B. (1991) The Impact of Child Sexual Abuse in Developmental Perspective. In C. R. Bagley and R. J. Thomlinson (eds) *Child Sexual Abuse: Critical Perspectives on Prevention, Intervention and Treatment*. Wall and Emerson: Toronto.

Wacquant, L. (2005) Carnal Connections: On Embodiment, Apprenticeship, and Membership. *Qualitative Sociology*, 28(4): 445–474.

Walkerdine, V. (2007) *Children, Gender, Video Games: Towards a Relational Approach to Multimedia*. Palgrave Macmillan: Basingstoke.

Walkerdine, V. (2010) Communal Beingness and Affect: An Exploration of Trauma in an Ex-Industrial Community. *Body & Society*, 16(1): 91–116. 10.1177/1357034X09354127

Waller, J. (2008) *A Time to Dance, a Time to Die: The Extraordinary Story of the Dancing Plague of 1518*. Icon Books: Cambridge.

Warner, M. (2000) *The Trouble With Normal: Sex, Politics and the Ethics of Queer Life*. Free Press: New York, NY.

Watts, J. (2018) World is finally waking up to climate change, says 'hothouse Earth' author. *Guardian*, 19th August.

Watts, S. and Stenner, P. (2005) Doing Q Methodology: Theory, Method and Interpretation. *Qualitative Research in Psychology*, 2(1): 67–69.

Weiwei, A. (2018) The refugee crisis isn't about refugees. It's about us. *Guardian, Opinion,* 2nd February.

Wetherell, M. (2010) The Field of Identity Studies. In M. Wetherell and C. Talapade Mohanty (eds) *The Sage Handbook of Identities,* 3–26. Sage: London.

Wetherell, M. (2012) *Affect and Emotion: A New Social Science Understanding.* Sage: London.

Wetherell, M. (2013) Affect and Discourse – What's the Problem? *Subjectivity,* 6(4): 349–368.

Wetherell, M. and Maybin, J. (2000) The Distributed Self: A Social Constructionist Perspective. In R. Stevens (ed) *Understanding the Self.* Sage: London.

Wetherell, M. and Talpade Mohanty, C. (2010) *The Sage Handbook of Identities.* Sage: London.

Wicke, T. and Cohen Silver, R. (2009) A Community Responds to Collective Trauma: An Ecological Analysis of the James Byrd Murder in Jasper, Texas. *American Journal of Community Psychology,* 44: 233–248.

Wiggins, S. and Potter, J. (2017) Discursive Psychology. In C. Willig and W. Stainton Rogers (eds) *The Sage Handbook of Qualitative Research in Psychology.* Sage: London.

Wilbraham, L. (2004) Discursive Practice: Analysing as Loveliness Text on Sex Communications for Parents. In D. Hook, A. Collins, P. Kiguwa and N. Mkhize (eds) *Critical Psychology.* University of Cape Town Press: Cape Town, South Africa.

Wilkinson, R. and Pickett, K. (2010) *The Spirit Level: Why Equality Is Better for Everyone.* Penguin: London.

Wilkinson, R. and Pickett, K. (2018) *The Inner Level: How More Equal Societies Reduce Stress, Restore Sanity and Improve Everyone's Wellbeing.* Penguin: London.

Wilkinson, S. (1991) Feminism & Psychology: From Critique to Reconstruction. *Feminism & Psychology,* 1(1). https://doi.org/10.1177/0959353591011001

Williams, F. (2004) *Rethinking Families.* Calouste Gulbenkian Foundation: London.

Williams, R. (1977) *Marxism and Literature.* Oxford University Press: Oxford.

Williamson, L. M., Buston, K. and Sweeting, H. (2009) Young Women and Limits to the Normalisation of Condom Use: A Qualitative Study. *AIDS Care,* 21(5): 561–566.

Willig, C. and Stainton Rogers, W. (2017) *The Sage Handbook of Qualitative Research in Psychology,* 2nd Edition. Sage: London.

Wood, H. (2009) *Talking With Television: Women, Talk Shows and Modern Self-Reflexivity.* University of Illinois Press: Urbana and Chicago.

Yeung, W-J. (2013) Asian Fatherhood. *Journal of Family Issues,* 34(2): 143–160.

Young, M. (1958; 1972) *The Rise of the Meritocracy.* Routledge: London.

Young, M. (2001) Down with meritocracy. *Guardian, Politics,* 29th June.

Younge, G. and Barr, C. (2017) How Scotland reduced knife deaths among young people. *Guardian,* 3rd December.

Zucker, K. J. and Bradley, S. J. (1995) *Gender Identity Disorder and Psychosexual Problems in Children and Adolescents.* Guilford Press: New York, NY.

6

DEALING WITH SOCIAL EXCLUSION

An analysis of psychological strategies

Susanna Timeo, Paolo Riva, and Maria Paola Paladino

Social exclusion has been defined as the experience of being kept apart from others physically (e.g., social isolation) or emotionally (e.g., being ignored or told one is not wanted; Riva & Eck, 2016). Social exclusion has many facets. It can be used by individuals or groups to punish a rule violation, or with malicious intentions to hurt the victim (see Rudert & Greifeneder, 2019). These various forms of social exclusion have in common their ability to hurt a given target. Williams (2009) compares ostracism to a flame that instantaneously hurts the skin, no matter what the circumstances are. The pain of social exclusion has been likened to the experience of physical pain (Eisenberger, & Lieberman, 2004). Exclusion triggers negative emotions, threatens basic psychological needs such as self-esteem and belonging, and can itself foster aggression (see Williams, Hales & Michels, 2019). Most relevant, however, is how people respond to the negative outcomes caused by social exclusion. Individuals can either choose to cope with it in functional ways, thus ultimately increasing their chances for social inclusion, or in dysfunctional ways: promoting a vicious cycle of exclusion, maladaptive responses, further instances of exclusion, and social isolation. Accordingly, in recent years, researchers have started to devote attention to the psychological and behavioral strategies that might help individuals to cope with this unpleasant situation (Eck & Riva, 2016; Riva, 2016). The purpose of this chapter is twofold. On one side, we will review and systematize research on psychological strategies that have demonstrated some efficacy against social exclusion. This will help us to depict a general state of the art and to point out gaps in the literature. On the other side, we will suggest the use of other strategies, which have been tested in other domains of psychological wellbeing and critically discuss their effectiveness against exclusion.

The starting point to any evaluation of strategies for coping with exclusion is to acknowledge the negative effects of this experience on the individual's wellbeing.

Exclusion threatens the individual's basic psychological needs (Williams, 2009) and impacts people's personal wellbeing (Niu et al., 2016, see Williams et al., 2019). Williams (2009) points out that at least four needs are involved: the need to belong, the need for self-esteem, the need to have control, and the need for a meaningful existence. The need to belong refers to an impulsive desire to be connected with others and to feel part of a social group. Self-esteem is the need to have a positive vision of oneself. Control refers to the sense of being in charge of one's own life as well as being able to dominate its circumstances. Finally, the need for a meaningful existence refers to the need to feel that one's own life has value and purpose. In this perspective, exclusion threatens the self in its core aspects.

In his Temporal Need-Threat model, Williams (2009) identifies three stages to observe the effect of ostracism: reflexive, reflective and resignation (see Williams et al., 2019). The reflexive stage occurs right after the ostracism episode and includes increased negative emotions (i.e., anger, sadness, anxiety), and decreased satisfaction of fundamental psychological needs. The reflective stage involves efforts to cope with ostracism and includes the attribution of meaning and motivation to the event, along with the fortification of depleted needs (i.e., attempts to become more socially attractive). According to Williams, this is the only stage where coping strategies may have an impact on the person's feelings and recovery can be observed. Finally, the resignation stage occurs after a prolonged experience of ostracism and consists in the inability to react or fortify needs. This stage may lead to depression and alienation. In this perspective, exclusion will always hurt people at the very beginning, and this is also considered adaptive since detecting even subtle signs of exclusion might be vital for the individual's fit into the society. In this view, coping strategies will never eliminate the sting of exclusion. Instead, their role should be to help people manage the negative feelings and threatened needs connected with exclusion and to accelerate the recovery process. Moreover, coping strategies should also temper the individual's possible negative behavioral reactions (i.e., isolation or aggression, see Williams et al., 2019; Täuber, 2019) which may be detrimental for future successful interactions.

In this chapter, we will depict a multifaceted array of strategies. After looking at those that had already been tested, we identified two main classes. The first class—which we named *Changing Perspective*—comprises approaches that lessen the perceived threats of exclusion, for instance, by acquiring a different perspective on the situation or the self. Accordingly, these strategies include positive reappraisal, acceptance, self-distancing, distraction, and focused attention (see Orvell & Kross, 2019). Some of these approaches (e.g., positive reappraisal) imply changing how the exclusionary event is perceived, whereas others (e.g., distraction) involve shifting the attention away from the event. However, all these strategies can help people to avoid ruminating on negative events and move on more quickly from unpleasant situations. Therefore, they can reduce the impact of daily forms of exclusion and rejection.

Other strategies, rather than mitigating the effects of social exclusion (e.g., by directing the attention away from the exclusionary event), focus on managing the effects of exclusion once they have occurred. As previously described, social exclusion threatens four individual psychological needs. The most commonly studied strategies in the field of exclusion involve the recovery of the threatened needs by directly working to raise their level of satisfaction. Specific strategies proved to contrast the negative effects on belonging, self-esteem, control, and meaningful existence. We have therefore grouped them together in the class *Restoring the Threatened Needs*. In the following sections, we will review strategies included in these two main classes.

Changing perspective

In this broad class are listed all the strategies that can reduce the impact of social exclusion. The main idea behind these strategies is that not only does the objective experience of exclusion hurt people, but also that their personal interpretation and reaction to it is affected (see Greifeneder & Rudert, 2019). In a sense, shifting the perspective of exclusion into a relative, more positive and rational view could help victims minimize its negative effects. Therefore, these strategies are mostly based on a cognitive reinterpretation of events or on averting attention from them.

Acceptance

Acceptance is a core element of mindfulness-based intervention (Germer, 2005) where the painful situation is not avoided, and the negative feelings are embraced. This process involves the conscious and not evaluative acceptance of negative feelings and thoughts. This is also a core element of a promising cognitive-based therapy, namely Acceptance and Commitment Therapy (Hayes, Luoma, Bond, Masuda, & Lillis, 2006). Based on this approach, experiential avoidance is a harmful behavior which consists of running away from negative (or negatively framed) situations. By doing so, people are constantly looking for negative situations to avoid and the focus on negative events is amplified. Acceptance-based therapy helps people consciously embrace negative feelings instead of escaping or reducing them. The acceptance of temporary negative events may help people to focus more on their broader values, thus increasing goal-oriented behavior. In this direction, recent work has shown that people who are more psychologically flexible perceived lower stress following ostracism (Waldeck, Tyndall, Riva, & Chmiel, 2017).

To date, an acceptance-based intervention has never been applied to the context of social exclusion. In one such study, however, have tested the acceptance strategy to cope against stressful experiences. In one such study, the acceptance-oriented strategy promoted heart-rate habituation and recovery over an evaluative strategy (Low, Stanton, & Bower, 2008). Moreover, acceptance-enhanced expressive writing has shown favorable results in preventing low to mild symptoms of depression (Baum, & Rude, 2013), alongside a wide range of psychological benefits for adolescents (Holder-Spriggs, 2015). Learning to accept negative events and the feelings connected with them might be a promising strategy to cope against social exclusion. In effect, if people learn to accept the negative social interactions that they might encounter, they may not charge those episodes with anxiety. This in turn may lead to an easier recovery from those situations.

Positive reappraisal

Positive reappraisal is a classical strategy of emotion regulation and takes place when a person tries to create positive meaning to a negative situation in terms of personal growth to decrease its emotional impact (Gross, 1998). Some studies have tested positive reappraisal in the context of social exclusion, finding promising results (Poon & Chen, 2016; Sethi, Moulds, & Richardson, 2013). Poon and Chen (2016) primed participants with beliefs that ostracism was either detrimental (loss frame) or beneficial (gain frame) for people's relationships. The gain frame eliminated people's inclination to act aggressively toward their perpetrator. In the same direction, Chen and colleagues (Chen, DeWall, Poon & Chen, 2012) manipulated people's beliefs on relationships. In the destiny belief condition, people were told that interpersonal relationships are usually either going to work or not regardless of their efforts. In the growth belief condition, people were told that although some relationships are troubled, they can be improved through effort and hard work. In this framework, people were encouraged to interpret exclusion as an event that could be overcome and may even help with their own personal growth (positive reappraisal). In effect, in the growth belief condition, participants showed less aggressiveness toward the perpetrator when they were excluded.

Self-distancing

Self-distancing is a strategy used to detach from the present situation and has been proven to be adaptive when facing negative experiences (Kross, Ayduk, & Mischel, 2005; Orvell & Kross, 2019). When self-distancing, people face the negative situation with less emotional arousal and can reconstruct it, giving it meaning and closure. To our knowledge, there are no studies specifically using self-distancing manipulation to cope with social exclusion. However, a recent study has shown that people with a more abstract (i.e., more detached) and less concrete thinking style reported less threat to belonging when excluded (Pfundmair, Lermer, Frey & Aydin, 2015). Moreover, participants primed with an abstract thinking style reported higher levels of belonging. In any case, abstract thinking only has a positive effect when it helps people put the situation into a broader framework, thereby reappraising the single event. In this regard, Rude and colleagues (2011) differentiated the abstract–evaluative (i.e., "Why do you think this happened?") from the abstract–contextual style (i.e., "How do you think you will view this event in 1–2 years?") and found that the latter led to less rumination and fewer depressive symptoms following rejection than the first and control conditions. The concrete–experiential condition (i.e., "As you recall the event, what physical sensations do you notice?") performed equally well.

Distancing can be reached by taking an external perspective on the event. It is important, however, not to evoke the presence of an observer, as this might bring feelings of shame and anxiety, and worsen the impact of social exclusion. Lau and colleagues (Lau, Moulds, & Richardson, 2009) found that, when instructing people to use an observer perspective instead of a self-focused recall, these people recovered more slowly from ostracism. Altogether, these findings suggest that self-distancing might be an interesting strategy to use for social exclusion, although it may bring some insidious side effects (i.e., evaluation-related stress).

Distraction

Distraction is a common reaction to negative situations and consists of turning attention away from unpleasant thoughts. Distraction has often been contrasted with rumination, which consists of constantly thinking of negative situations and feelings (Garnefski, Teerds, Kraaij, Legerstee, & van den Kommer, 2004). Whereas rumination as a coping strategy has been linked to internalizing problems (Garnefski et al., 2004), distraction has turned out to be a better coping strategy against negative events (Nolen-Hoeksema, Morrow, & Fredrickson, 1993). Distraction has also been used with success in controlling physical pain (Damme, Crombez, Wever, & Goubert, 2008). In the field of social exclusion, distraction has produced promising results. Studies have found distraction after exclusion to produce less distress than rumination (Wesselmann, Ren, Swim, & Williams, 2013) and to have similar effects to prayer and self-affirmation strategies (Hales et al., 2016).

It has been argued that distraction is only a temporary, short-term solution (Linehan, 1993). However, in the context of social exclusion, distraction is an easy coping strategy to implement just after the negative event and may work better for isolated and sporadic exclusion than for prolonged exclusion. It is highly likely that more conscious coping or problem-solving strategies, used in combination with distraction, are necessary to cope with negative events. In a one-year longitudinal study, it was found that when in high-stress job situations, frequent use of problem-solving and distraction lead to less stress and better job performance (Shimazu & Schaufeli, 2007).

Focused attention

Focused attention is one ingredient of mindfulness intervention and consists of conscious awareness of the present moment without any judgment or attachment to the experience (Germer, 2005). Although it may be counterintuitive to think that focusing on the present moment can help distract from a negative situation, the basis of focused attention is that the experience is always flowing from one moment to the next. By focusing attention on the present experience, the person can quickly leave the exclusion episode behind and move on to the next event.

Moreover, mindfulness is based on the pure observation of the scene from a detached point of view. The experience is described but not valued. In this sense, focused attention is connected with both non-judgmental distancing and accept-ance of the situation as it is. Past research has shown mindfulness meditation to be more effective than just distraction in reducing dysphoric mood (Broderick, 2005). In the context of social exclusion, one study (Molet, Macquet, Lefebvre, & Williams, 2013) showed that ostracized participants who were trained with focused attention intervention felt the same need-threat as that of ostracized par-ticipants without the intervention. However, those in the focused attention con-dition recovered more quickly. Moreover, a recent study also showed the efficacy of focused attention in reducing the propensity to commit ostracism (Ramsey & Jones, 2015). Focused attention could be a promising strategy against exclusion, even though it requires more effort than just pure distraction.

Summary

The strategies reviewed in this macro section aim to facilitate the cognitive elaboration of the situation by accepting or reappraising it, or by shifting peo-ple's attention away from it (e.g., self-distancing, distraction, focused attention). They all constitute potentially effective bumpers against the well-known nega-tive effects of social exclusion, helping victims to protect themselves from con-sequences that would otherwise make them highly vulnerable. These strategies are spontaneously used, but they can also be taught for prevention (before any negative event), or suggested after the exclusion has occurred. From this perspec-tive, even though exclusion will always be interpreted as hurtful, the range of strategies for changing perspective should help affected people reconstruct the exclusionary experience in a less negative way.

Restoring the threatened needs

Social exclusion constitutes a direct threat to the self. In effect, social exclusion threatens at least four fundamental needs: self-esteem, belonging, control, and meaningful existence (Williams, 2009). From this perspective, one possibility is to cope with exclusionary experiences by trying to satisfy one or more of these threatened needs. Strategies that facilitate the recovery of need-satisfaction include self-affirmation; reminding oneself of existing social bonds and social surrogates, as well as control, power, or the denigration of the excluding person.

Reaffirming belonging

Amongst other negative effects, social exclusion particularly threatens the indi-vidual's need to belong (DeWall, & Richman, 2011). When people are excluded they are left alone, which makes them think they are not liked by others (see Claypool & Bernstein, 2019). However, an experience of exclusion from one group or person does not necessarily mean that the target will be excluded by all human beings. Focusing on other existing positive social relationships is a strategy to overcome the experience of ostracism. Thinking of a friend or family member makes excluded people behave less aggressively (Twenge et al., 2007) and fulfill some need-satisfaction (McConnell, Brown, Shoda, Stayton, & Martin, 2011). Even thinking of one's own pet is sufficient to restore people's need (McConnell et al., 2011). Moreover, belonging to a majority group seems to protect against need-threat, but only for individuals who have a high need to belong (Eck, Schoel, & Greifeneder, 2016). Finally, even when people activate the group construct by themselves, it facilitates recovery from threats of exclusion (Knowles, & Gardner, 2008). Training people to remind themselves of their social bonds could be an easy, ready-to-use strategy to implement. Thinking of other relationships could also be a way to detach from the specificity of the present exclusionary event and evaluate it in a more relative rather than an absolute way.

Social surrogates act in the same way as reminders of social bonds, although they are only a substitute for real human relationships. This strategy consists of making people think of someone (i.e., famous people, fictional characters) or something (e.g., nature or God) they like and evokes a sense of connectedness with human or non-human entities. In this sense, the use of social surrogates might be an effective short-term strategy, simulating the sense of belonging and acceptance, although with less intensity than in a real social bond. Research on social exclusion has uncovered different types of social surrogates, like parasocial attachment to TV characters (Derrick, Gabriel, & Hugenberg, 2009), comfort food (Troisi & Gabriel, 2011), connectedness to nature (Poon, Teng, Wong, & Chen, 2016), and religion (Hales et al., 2016). These surrogates have been shown to protect self-esteem (Derrick et al., 2009), the sense of belonging (Troisi & Gabriel, 2011) and to decrease intentions of aggression (Poon et al., 2016).

Reaffirming self-esteem

There are several strategies which might serve the ultimate goal of satisfying the fundamental need of perceiving oneself as a valuable person threatened by social exclusion.

Self-affirmation is a strategy that reminds people of their values and positive aspects (Steele, 1988). Within the context of social exclusion, self-affirmation may be a strategy to raise self-esteem. Accordingly, recent studies showed some promising results. Self-affirmation seems to improve need-satisfaction (Hales, Wesselmann, & Williams, 2016) and the executive control of excluded participants (Burson, Crocker, & Mischkowski, 2012). Moreover, even though exclusion threatens social relationships when given a chance to affirm a social or an intellectual area of life, excluded people still prefer to talk about the importance of social values (Knowles, Lucas, Molden, Gardner, & Dean, 2010). This result may be taken as proof of the importance of relationships to human beings.

However, the mechanism by which self-affirmation works is still under debate. Some researchers argue that instead of just raising self-esteem, the recall of personal values produces a big-picture focus (Wakslak & Trope, 2009). Focusing on values would make people think of the most important aspects of their lives, thus enlarging their horizon of priorities compared to an exclusionary experience. Self-affirmation helps people put the negative event or threat into a broader perspective and focus on long-term values, thus minimizing the detrimental effects of a single instance of social disconnection.

Derogation is another self-defensive strategy that attempts to diminish the partner's value in a relationship (Murray et al., 2002). This allows people to distance themselves from the source of social threat, restoring their self-esteem and self-value by depicting the perpetrator as less worthy (MacDonald & Leary, 2005). This strategy is especially used when ostracism is due to a moralizing issue (see Täuber, 2019). Bourgeois and Leary (2001) showed that rejected participants rated their perpetrators less positively and thought they knew them less well than their included counterparts. Most importantly, derogating their perpetrator helped participants to maintain positive affect after rejection. However, derogation as a defensive strategy seems to be used more by people with low self-esteem and has been linked with high levels of stress-phase cortisol (Ford & Collins, 2010). This strategy seems to be more of an impulsive reaction to a personal threat, probably related to anger or anxiety, which may protect the victim's self-esteem while fostering interpersonal hostility.

Reaffirming control or power

Social exclusion or rejection also threatens the need for control. In their meta-analysis, Gerber and Wheeler (2009) found a correlation between loss of control and an increase in aggression, showing that when control is threatened, people tend to act antisocially. Moreover, in the victim–offender relationship, studies have demonstrated that a higher sense of power facilitates victims' forgiveness (Côté et al., 2011; Karremans, & Smith, 2010). In the context of social exclusion, different studies have shown that being in a powerful position buffers the negative effects of exclusion (Kuehn, Chen, & Gordon, 2015; Schoel, Eck, & Greifeneder, 2014). Furthermore, monetary compensation (Lelieveld, Moor, Crone, Karremans, & van Beest, 2013) or reminders of money as a symbol of socio-economic power (Zhou, Vohs, & Baumeister, 2009) have also been shown to have positive effects against exclusion. Finally, a recent study showed that just thinking about being physically invulnerable could be a sufficient buffer against the negative effects of exclusion (Huang, Ackerman, & Bargh, 2013).

Reaffirming a meaningful existence

The last need that is threatened by social exclusion is the sense of having a meaningful existence. Especially when prolonged over time, exclusion makes people feel as if they are invisible and do not deserve the attention of others. From this perspective, restoring one of the other needs (i.e., self-esteem or control) will also improve the sense that one is living a meaningful existence. Alternatively, some studies showed that mere acknowledgment of the person's presence may be sufficient to improve the sense of meaning (Rudert, Hales, Greifeneder, & Williams, 2017; Wesselmann, Cardoso, Slater, & Williams, 2012). As Rudert and collaborators (2017) showed, even negative attention is better than no attention. From this perspective, being ignored and ostracized seems to be the ultimate punishment, and might even be worse than receiving hostile attention.

Summary

All the strategies listed in this section aim at reaffirming at least one of the four threatened needs. Social exclusion is one threat to the self, which comes from the social environment surrounding the person. As other social threats (i.e., identity or self-threat), it may undermine people's self-esteem and perception of self-worth (Branscombe, Ellemers, Spears, & Doosje, 1999). These strategies try to compensate for each threat by restoring its correlated need. Thus, the *social bonds* and *social surrogates* strategies may help people to protect their sense of belonging by finding comfort and reassurance in their real (or imagined) social networks. The *self-affirmation* and *denigration of the perpetrator* strategies can be used by victims to protect their personal value and self-view by enhancing positive qualities. The *control/power* strategy may help people to heighten their sense of control by enhancing their perceived power. Overall, these strategies may also help people maintain their sense of meaningful existence by restoring positive qualities and agency to the individual. However, even *mere acknowledgment* of the person may be sufficient in restoring this last fundamental need. In general, it seems that these strategies may follow a hydraulic mechanism based on the oscillation of need-satisfaction. From this perspective, every time an episode of exclusion lowers need-satisfaction, using a specific strategy should help restore it to the previous level. In this sense, the use of a strategy should be implemented each time an episode of exclusion occurs.

However, one aspect still unclear is whether the use of a specific strategy would influence only one specific need or whether there would be a beneficial effect for all four needs. Previous studies have found that one strategy was able to raise the satisfaction of more than one need (Hales et al., 2016; McConnell et al., 2011). These strategies are addressing not just one but several needs at the same time. From this perspective, self-affirmation may work not only on self-esteem but also on increasing people's sense of control. An alternative hypothesis is that the four needs are related to one another. In this sense, working on self-esteem may also help people to increase their sense of a meaningful existence or their sense of control over events. However, more research is needed to assess these different explanations.

Discussion

In this review, we examined different coping strategies that have shown promising effects on the recovery from social exclusion or other self-threats. These strategies have been clustered into two categories. The first category includes strategies that help people to cognitively change their perspective toward exclusion or distance themselves from the event. They include accepting the exclusion episode without judgment (acceptance), looking at it from a broader perspective (distancing), framing it in a more positive light (positive reappraisal), shifting attention from the negative event to something more positive (distraction), or focusing on the present moment (focused attention). The second category includes strategies that help people reaffirm their threatened needs. These strategies include those which restore the need to belong, such as focusing on real or imagined positive social relationships (reminders of social bonds and social surrogates), strategies to restore self-esteem by focusing on one's positive aspects (self-affirmation), or decreasing the perpetrator's value (derogation of the other) and strategies that restore the victim's power or control. The second group of strategies is the most studied, and they try to directly heal a specific area that has been threatened. In a way, they address the consequences of the exclusion rather than the exclusion process itself. With a hydraulic metaphor, we could see the self as a bowl full of water, which represents need-satisfaction. While the water stays at a certain level, the system is balanced. The exclusion threat could be seen as a pin that punches a hole in the bowl so that some water starts to pour out, and the level of water inside the bowl gets lower. The system detects a problem. The strategies to recover need-satisfaction could be seen as pouring some water back into the bowl, so as to reach the previous level. With this metaphor, we can see that we would never reduce the water flowing out (need-threat), or reinforce the sides of the bowl (reduce the threat of exclusion). Moreover, it is interesting to observe that until need-satisfaction is back to a balanced level, more social connections will not produce beneficial effects, while only a reduction of need-satisfaction will be detected as problematic (see also sociometer theory, Leary & Baumeister, 2000). In this respect, inclusion will not result in a buffer against future exclusion.

The strategies which change perspective are meant, in the long-term, to change people's perspective on the threatening situation, and maybe also on the self. In this metaphor, they might help to make the self less vulnerable to social exclusion by either reinforcing the bowl's sides (i.e., positive reappraisal), or by simply embracing the fact that the bowl might not always be full (i.e., acceptance). In effect, a recent study has shown that people with a higher psychological flexibility (i.e. staying in the present moment without defence as fully human beings) are less vulnerable to social exclusion (Waldeck et al., 2017). Although exclusion will hurt at the very beginning, the long-term practice of these strategies may help make exclusion less emotionally painful.

A different discussion should be made for distraction. In this sense, it is not clear whether this strategy may stop need-threat by disengaging attention from the hurtful event (in the metaphor, moving the bowl far from the pin of exclusion). In this sense, although the immediate damage is avoided, no change has occurred in the self. In the metaphor, if another pin arrives, the bowl would be just as vulnerable, and so it would need to be moved again and again. Alternatively, distracting strategies might work as the strategies to restore need-satisfaction do: by filling the self with other pleasant experiences or feelings (i.e., filling the bowl with new water). Furthermore, the efficacy of this strategy may depend on the value of the relationship between the perpetrator and the victim (Richman & Leary, 2009), in that it may work well in a context with low relational value. For example, when a person is excluded by strangers in a new situation (a common background for the experimental manipulation of exclusion), distraction may be one of the best coping strategies they have in order to move on from the unpleasant event and erase any negative feelings associated with it. On the contrary, when a person is excluded by close friends, distraction may be more difficult to implement and may bring less effective results.

Altogether, these strategies may work on different aspects of the exclusion process, thus bringing more or less durable positive effects. However, the mechanisms behind these strategies are still to be investigated, and future research should help us to unravel these questions.

Strategies administered by others

Although this review has focused its attention on strategies that can be used by victims of social exclusion, it is important to point out that the people around victims can play an important role in their recovery. One example is represented by social norms. Some researchers (Rudert & Greifeneder, 2016) have in fact argued that social exclusion is a hurtful experience which is cognitively mediated. This means that exclusion needs to be interpreted as a negative event. For example, if a person is excluded but s/he does not recognize the exclusion, then the event would not hurt her/him. Moreover, researchers have argued that exclusion hurts people because our society has an expectation for inclusion, which qualifies exclusion as a negative experience. In some experiments, it has been shown that changing the expectation of inclusion diminished people's need-threat, negative mood, and intention to act aggressively toward their perpetrators (Greifeneder & Rudert, 2019; see also Rudert & Greifeneder, 2016; Schoel, et al., 2014). Another study conducted with children from one individualistic and one collectivistic economic culture showed that collectivistic children estimated ostracism to be less painful, punishing the ostracizer less harshly than individualistic children (Uskul & Over, 2017). From this perspective, working on the social norms of a given culture may loosen the anxiety connected with an exclusionary status.

The validation of emotion represents another strategy. This strategy has been used in therapy for chronic physical pain and consists of communicating an understanding of the patient's feelings (Edmond & Keefe, 2015). In this type of strategy, the caregiver supports the complaints of the patient, thus communicating that his/her experience is trustworthy and legitimate. In the context of social exclusion, just the simple acknowledgment of the victim's feelings may help them to feel legitimate in their experience and thus prevent self-blame. In a recent experiment, we have tested the validation strategy with a group of university students ($n=109$, M_{age} = 19.63 years, SD = .90 years, 21 Males). At the beginning of the study, participants' self-compassion, self-pity, and self-esteem levels were assessed. Afterward, participants played the Cyberball task, a manipulation of ostracism (Williams, Cheung, & Choi 2000). Participants were either included or excluded. As a cover story, participants were also told that the game session was being supervised by a member of staff, whose role it was to give technical support if needed. At the end of the game, participants received a message from the bogus staff member. In the control condition, the message included standard information about the duration of the session and the number of throws. In the validation condition, the message made an explicit reference to the exclusion situation. The staff member validated the perspective of the participant by saying that it was not a pleasant situation, and that other people had already been excluded in the past, and that their reaction was negative. After this, participants' need-satisfaction and emotions were assessed in the reflexive and reflective stages. Receiving a validation had positive effects on the emotional experience, especially for those participants who were low in self-compassion. In a way, it seems that a validating communication style could have helped the recovery of participants who were generally more critical toward themselves, and who might have blamed themselves for having been excluded. These preliminary results highlight the potential assistance that people surrounding the victim of exclusion might have to offer. In effect, exclusion is a social phenomenon that deprives the individual of social relationships. When surrounding people offer acceptance and support to the victim of exclusion, this could result in need restoration. Sometimes, when people feel they do not possess the instruments to cope with negative events, the best solution would be to look for external help. In a way, a strategy for the victims may even be considered to strategically turn to individuals that may offer them support. Finally, it is plausible that these strategies may be beneficial to some sub-populations, which may be more sensitive to the exclusion threat (i.e., low self-compassionate people in our research).

Conclusion

Despite the fact that much research has been carried out on the effects of exclusion, only a few studies have focused on the coping strategies that may buffer its negative outcomes and foster recovery (Riva, 2016). In this chapter, we revised the self-administered coping strategies that have shown some promising results in the field of social exclusion, or in closer research areas. We have proposed a clustering of these strategies based on the specific aspects of the exclusion process that they address. The strategies to change perspective aim at diminishing the negative impact of exclusion. In this sense, they try to prevent the negative feelings associated with need-threat by cognitively reappraising the situation. The strategies to restore need-satisfaction aim at repairing the damage caused by exclusion. They try to replenish the need fulfillment which has been lowered by the exclusionary situation. Although all these strategies have been proposed to promote recovery from exclusion, the exact effects of the approaches and the processes by which they work are still unclear. In this sense, more research is needed to better account for the underlying mechanism of these strategies. Moreover, research has focused almost entirely on self-administered strategies, although surrounding people may play an important role in the victim's recovery from a negative state. Because of the social relevance and the possible application of this topic, we hope that future studies will investigate in more depth the most effective strategies to teach people to cope with social exclusion.

References

Baum, E. S., & Rude, S. S. (2013). Acceptance-enhanced expressive writing prevents symptoms in participants with low initial depression. *Cognitive Therapy and Research*, *37*, 35–42. doi:10.1007/s10608-012-9435-x

Bourgeois, K. S., & Leary, M. R. (2001). Coping with rejection: Derogating those who choose us last. *Motivation and Emotion*, *25*, 101–111. doi:10.1023/A:1010661825137

Branscombe, N. R., Ellemers, N., Spears, R., & Doosje, B. (1999). The context and content of social identity threat. In N. Ellemers, R. Spears, & B. Doosje (Eds.), *Social identity: Context, commitment, content* (pp. 35–58). Oxford, UK: Blackwell Science.

Broderick, P. C. (2005). Mindfulness and coping with dysphoric mood: Contrasts with rumination and distraction. *Cognitive Therapy and Research*, *29*, 501–510. doi:10.1007/s10608-005-3888-0

Burson, A., Crocker, J., & Mischkowski, D. (2012). Two types of value-affirmation: Implications for self-control following social exclusion. *Social Psychological and Personality Science*, *3*, 510–516. doi:10.1177/1948550611427773

Chen, Z., DeWall, C. N., Poon, K. T., & Chen, E. W. (2012). When destiny hurts: Implicit theories of relationships moderate aggressive responses to ostracism. *Journal of Experimental Social Psychology*, *48*, 1029–1036. doi:10.1016/j.jesp.2012.04.002

Claypool, H. M., & Bernstein, M. J. (2019). Exclusion and its impact on social information processing. In S. C. Rudert, R. Greifeneder, & K. D. Williams (Eds.), *Current directions in ostracism, social exclusion, and rejection research*. London: Routledge.

Côté, S., Kraus, M. W., Cheng, B. H., Oveis, C., van der Löwe, I., Lian, H., & Keltner, D. (2011). Social power facilitates the effect of prosocial orientation on empathic accuracy. *Journal of Personality and Social Psychology*, *101*, 217–232. doi:10.1037/a0023171

Damme, S., Crombez, G., Wever, K. N., & Goubert, L. (2008). Is distraction less effective when pain is threatening? An experimental investigation with the cold pressor task. *European Journal of Pain*, *12*, 60–67. doi:10.1016/j.ejpain.2007.03.001

Derrick, J. L., Gabriel, S., & Hugenberg, K. (2009). Social surrogacy: How favored television programs provide the experience of belonging. *Journal of Experimental Social Psychology*, *45*, 352–362. doi:10.1016/j.jesp.2008.12.003

DeWall, C. N., & Richman, S. B. (2011). Social exclusion and the desire to reconnect. *Social and Personality Psychology Compass*, *5*, 919–932. doi:10.1111/j.1751-9004.2011.00383.x

Eck, J., & Riva, P. (2016). Bridging the gap between different psychological approaches to understanding and reducing the impact of social exclusion. In P. Riva & J. Eck (Eds.), *Social exclusion: Psychological approaches to understanding and reducing its impact* (pp. 199–225). Basel, Switzerland: Springer International Publishing.

Eck, J., Schoel, C., & Greifeneder, R. (2016). Belonging to a majority reduces the immediate need threat from ostracism in individuals with a high need to belong. *European Journal of Social Psychology*, *47*, 273–288. doi:10.1002/ejsp.2233

Edmond, S. N., & Keefe, F. J. (2015). Validating pain communication: Current state of the science. *Pain*, *156*, 215–219. doi:10.1097/01.j.pain.0000460301.18207.c2

Eisenberger, N. I., & Lieberman, M. D. (2004). Why rejection hurts: A common neural alarm system for physical and social pain. *Trends in Cognitive Sciences*, *8*, 294–300. doi:10.1016/j.tics.2004.05.010

Ford, M. B., & Collins, N. L. (2010). Self-esteem moderates neuroendocrine and psychological responses to interpersonal rejection. *Journal of Personality and Social Psychology*, *98*, 405–419. doi:10.1037/a0017345

Garnefski, N., Teerds, J., Kraaij, V., Legerstee, J., & van den Kommer, T. (2004). Cognitive emotion regulation strategies and depressive symptoms: Differences between males and females. *Personality and Individual Differences*, *36*, 267–276. doi:10.1016/S0191-8869(03)00083-7

Gerber, J., & Wheeler, L. (2009). On being rejected: A meta-analysis of experimental research on rejection. *Perspectives on Psychological Science*, *4*, 468–488. doi:10.1111/j.1745-6924.2009.01158.x

Germer, C. K. (2005). Teaching mindfulness in therapy. In C. K. Germer, R. D. Siegel, & P. R. Fulton (Eds.), *Mindfulness and psychotherapy* (Vol.1, pp. 113–129). New York, NY: Guilford Press.

Greifeneder, R., & Rudert, S. C. (2019). About flames and boogeymen: Social norms affect individuals' construal of social exclusion. In S. C. Rudert, R. Greifeneder, & K. D. Williams (Eds.), *Current directions in ostracism, social exclusion, and rejection research*. London: Routledge.

Gross, J. J. (1998). The emerging field of emotion regulation: An integrative review. *Review of General Psychology*, *2*, 271–299. doi:10.1037/1089-2680.2.3.271

Hales, A. H., Wesselmann, E. D., & Williams, K. D. (2016). Prayer, self-affirmation, and distraction improve recovery from short-term ostracism. *Journal of Experimental Social Psychology*, *64*, 8–20. doi:10.1016/j.jesp.2016.01.002

Hayes, S. C., Luoma, J. B., Bond, F. W., Masuda, A., & Lillis, J. (2006). Acceptance and commitment therapy: Model, processes and outcomes. *Behaviour Research and Therapy*, *44*, 1–25. doi:10.1016/j.brat.2005.06.006

Holder Spriggs, J. (2015). *Expressive writing interventions for children and young people: A systematic review and exploration of the literature* (Doctoral thesis, University of Southampton, Southampton, UK). Retrieved from https://eprints.soton.ac.uk/389518/

Huang, J. Y., Ackerman, J. M., & Bargh, J. A. (2013). Superman to the rescue: Simulating physical invulnerability attenuates exclusion-related interpersonal biases. *Journal of Experimental Social Psychology*, *49*, 349–354. doi:10.1016/j.jesp.2012.12.007

Karremans, J. C., & Smith, P. K. (2010). Having the power to forgive: When the experience of power increases interpersonal forgiveness. *Personality and Social Psychology Bulletin*, *36*, 1010–1023. doi:10.1177/0146167210376761

Knowles, M. L., & Gardner, W. L. (2008). Benefits of membership: The activation and amplification of group identities in response to social rejection. *Personality and Social Psychology Bulletin*, *34*, 1200–1213. doi:10.1177/0146167208320062

Knowles, M. L., Lucas, G. M., Molden, D. C., Gardner, W. L., & Dean, K. K. (2010). There's no substitute for belonging: Self-affirmation following social and nonsocial threats. *Personality and Social Psychology Bulletin, 36*, 173–186. doi:10.1177/0146167209346860

Kross, E., Ayduk, O., & Mischel, W. (2005). When asking "why" does not hurt distinguishing rumination from reflective processing of negative emotions. *Psychological Science, 16*, 709–715. doi:10.1111/j.1467-9280.2005.01600.x

Kuehn, M. M., Chen, S., & Gordon, A. M. (2015). Having a thicker skin: Social power buffers the negative effects of social rejection. *Social Psychological and Personality Science, 6*, 701–709. doi:10.1177/1948550615580170

Lau, G., Moulds, M. L., & Richardson, R. (2009). Ostracism: How much it hurts depends on how you remember it. *Emotion, 9*, 430–434. doi:10.1037/a0015350

Leary, M. R., & Baumeister, R. F. (2000). The nature and function of self-esteem: Sociometer theory. In M. P. Zanna (Ed.), *Advances in experimental social psychology* (Vol. 32, pp. 1–62). San Diego, CA: Academic Press.

Lelieveld, G., Moor, B., Crone, E. A., Karremans, J. C., & van Beest, I. (2013). A penny for your pain? The financial compensation of social pain after exclusion. *Social Psychological and Personality Science, 4*, 206–214. doi:10.1177/1948550612446661

Linehan, M. (1993). *Skills training manual for treating borderline personality disorder.* New York, NY: Guilford Press.

Low, C. A., Stanton, A. L., & Bower, J. E. (2008). Effects of acceptance-oriented versus evaluative emotional processing on heart rate recovery and habituation. *Emotion, 8*, 419–424. doi:10.1037/1528-3542.8.3.419

MacDonald, G., & Leary, M. R. (2005). Why does social exclusion hurt? The relationship between social and physical pain. *Psychological Bulletin, 131*, 202–223. doi:10.1037/0033-2909.131.2.202

McConnell, A. R., Brown, C. M., Shoda, T. M., Stayton, L. E., & Martin, C. E. (2011). Friends with benefits: On the positive consequences of pet ownership. *Journal of Personality and Social Psychology, 101*, 1239–1252. doi:10.1037/a0024506

Molet, M., Macquet, B., Lefebvre, O., & Williams, K. D. (2013). A focused attention intervention for coping with ostracism. *Consciousness and Cognition, 22*, 1262–1270. doi:10.1016/j.concog.2013.08.010

Murray, S. L., Rose, P., Bellavia, G. M., Holmes, J. G., & Kusche, A. G. (2002). When rejection stings: How self-esteem constrains relationship-enhancement processes. *Journal of Personality and Social Psychology, 83*, 556–573. doi:10.1037/0022–3514.83.3.556

Niu, G. F., Sun, X. J., Tian, Y., Fan, C. Y., & Zhou, Z. K. (2016). Resilience moderates the relationship between ostracism and depression among Chinese adolescents. *Personality and Individual Differences, 99*, 77–80. doi:10.1016/j.paid.2016.04.059

Nolen-Hoeksema, S., Morrow, J., & Fredrickson, B. L. (1993). Response styles and the duration of episodes of depressed mood. *Journal of Abnormal Psychology, 102*, 20–28. doi:10.1037/0021-843X.102.1.20

Orvell, A., & Kross, E. (2019). How self-talk promotes self-regulation: Implications for coping with emotional pain. In S. C. Rudert, R. Greifeneder, & K. D. Williams (Eds.), *Current directions in ostracism, social exclusion, and rejection research.* London: Routledge.

Pfundmair, M., Lermer, E., Frey, D., & Aydin, N. (2015). Construal level and social exclusion: Concrete thinking impedes recovery from social exclusion. *The Journal of Social Psychology, 155*, 338–355. doi:10.1080/00224545.2015.1015475

Poon, K. T., & Chen, Z. (2016). Assuring a sense of growth: A cognitive strategy to weaken the effect of cyber-ostracism on aggression. *Computers in Human Behavior, 57*, 31–37. doi:10.1016/j.chb.2015.12.032

Poon, K. T., Teng, F., Wong, W. Y., & Chen, Z. (2016). When nature heals: Nature exposure moderates the relationship between ostracism and aggression. *Journal of Environmental Psychology, 48*, 159–168. doi:10.1016/j.chb.2015.12.032

Ramsey, A. T., & Jones, E. E. (2015). Minding the interpersonal gap: Mindfulness-based interventions in the prevention of ostracism. *Consciousness and Cognition, 31*, 24–34. doi:10.1016/j.concog.2014.10.003

Richman, L., & Leary, M. R. (2009). Reactions to discrimination, stigmatization, ostracism, and other forms of interpersonal rejection: A multimotive model. *Psychological Review, 116*, 365–383. doi:10.1037/a0015250

Riva, P. (2016). Emotion regulation following social exclusion: Psychological and behavioral strategies. In P. Riva, & J. Eck (Eds.), *Social exclusion: Psychological approaches to understanding and reducing its impact* (pp. 199–225). Cham, Switzerland: Springer International Publishing.

Riva P, & Eck J. (2016). *Social exclusion: Psychological approaches to understanding and reducing its impact*. Basel, Switzerland: Springer International Publishing.

Rude, S. S., Mazzetti, F. A., Pal, H., & Stauble, M. R. (2011). Social rejection: How best to think about it? *Cognitive Therapy and Research, 35*, 209–216. doi:10.1007/s10608-010-9296-0

Rudert, S. C., & Greifeneder, R. (2016). When it's okay that I don't play: Social norms and the situated construal of social exclusion. *Personality and Social Psychology Bulletin, 42*, 955–969. doi:10.1177/0146167216649606

Rudert, S. C., & Greifeneder, R. (2019). Observing ostracism: How observers interpret and respond to ostracism situations. In S. C. Rudert, R. Greifeneder, & K. D. Williams (Eds.), *Current directions in ostracism, social exclusion, and rejection research*. London: Routledge.

Rudert, S. C., Hales, A. H., Greifeneder, R., & Williams, K. D. (2017). When silence is not golden: Why acknowledgment matters even when being excluded. *Personality and Social Psychology Bulletin, 43*, 678–692. doi:10.1177/0146167217695554

Schoel, C., Eck, J., & Greifeneder, R. (2014). A matter of vertical position: Consequences of ostracism differ for those above versus below its perpetrators. *Social Psychological and Personality Science, 5*, 149–157. doi:10.1177/1948550613488953

Sethi, N., Moulds, M. L., & Richardson, R. (2013). The role of focus of attention and reappraisal in prolonging the negative effects of ostracism. *Group Dynamics: Theory, Research, and Practice, 17*, 110–123. doi:10.1037/a0032436

Shimazu, A., & Schaufeli, W. B. (2007). Does distraction facilitate problem-focused coping with job stress? A 1 year longitudinal study. *Journal of Behavioral Medicine, 30*, 423–434. doi:10.1007/s10865-007-9109-4

Steele, C. M. (1988). The psychology of self-affirmation: Sustaining the integrity of the self. In L. Berkowitz (Ed.), *Advances in experimental social psychology* (Vol. 21, pp. 261–302). San Diego, CA: Academic Press.

Täuber, S. (2019). Moralization as legitimization for ostracism: Effects on intergroup dynamics social cohesion. In S. C. Rudert, R. Greifeneder, & K. D. Williams (Eds.), *Current directions in ostracism, social exclusion, and rejection research*. London: Routledge.

Troisi, J. D., & Gabriel, S. (2011). Chicken soup really is good for the soul: "Comfort food" fulfills the need to belong. *Psychological Science, 22*, 747–753. doi:10.1177/0956797611407931

Twenge, J. M., Zhang, L., Catanese, K. R., Dolan-Pascoe, B., Lyche, L. F., & Baumeister, R. F. (2007). Replenishing connectedness: Reminders of social activity reduce aggression after social exclusion. *The British Journal of Social Psychology, 46*, 205–224. doi:10.1348/014466605X90793

Uskul, A., & Over, H. (2017). Culture, social interdependence, and ostracism. *Current Directions in Psychological Science, 26*, 371–376. doi:10.1177/0963721417699300

Wakslak, C. J., & Trope, Y. (2009). Cognitive consequences of affirming the self: The relationship between self-affirmation and object construal. *Journal of Experimental Social Psychology, 45*, 927–932. doi:10.1016/j.jesp.2009.05.002

Waldeck, D., Tyndall, I., Riva, P., & Chmiel, N. (2017). How do we cope with ostracism? Psychological flexibility moderates the relationship between everyday ostracism experiences and psychological distress. *Journal of Contextual Behavioral Science, 6*, 425–432. doi:10.1016/j.jcbs.2017.09.001

Wesselmann, E. D., Cardoso, F. D., Slater, S., & Williams, K. D. (2012). To be looked at as though air: Civil attention matters. *Psychological Science, 23*, 166–168. doi:10.1177/0956797611427921

Wesselmann, E. D., Ren, D., Swim, E., & Williams, K. D. (2013). Rumination hinders recovery from ostracism. *International Journal of Developmental Science, 7*, 33–39. doi:10.3233/DEV-1312115

Williams, K. D. (2009). Ostracism: A temporal need-threat model. In M. P. Zanna (Ed.), *Advances in experimental social psychology* (Vol. 41, pp. 275–314). San Diego, CA: Elsevier Academic Press.

Williams, K. D., Cheung, C. K., & Choi, W. (2000). Cyberostracism: Effects of being ignored over the Internet. *Journal of Personality and Social Psychology, 79*, 748–762. doi:10.1037/0022-3514.79.5.748

Williams, K. D., Hales, A. H., & Michels, C. (2019). Social ostracism as a factor motivating interest in extreme groups. In S. C. Rudert, R. Greifeneder, & K. D. Williams (Eds.), *Current directions in ostracism, social exclusion, and rejection research*. London: Routledge.

Zhou, X., Vohs, K. D., & Baumeister, R. F. (2009). The symbolic power of money: Reminders of money after social distress and physical pain. *Psychological Science, 20*, 700–706. doi:10.1111/j.1467-9280.2009.02353.x

Chapter 7

Social accountability and action orientation

Strengthening the policy-making capacity of psychologists

Elizabeth Lira Kornfeld

Introduction

This chapter describes psychology's contribution to the recognition and reparation of victims of human rights violations committed in Chile during the military regime (1973–1990). Under the dictatorship, Chilean human rights organisations provided psychological care to victims and their families, documented the consequences of torture, forced disappearance and summary executions on individuals and families, and proposed methods of clinical intervention for victims and their relatives. The chapter describes the contribution of psychology to the recognition and reparation of victims in therapeutic, social and political relations in the reparation public policies after dictatorship.[1]

Salvador Allende had been elected president of Chile in 1970, heading the Popular Unity government which proposed a transition to socialism within the existing legal framework. Soon afterwards, Chilean society became divided by opposing views on what constituted the common good and social utopia. The Popular Unity government was overthrown in the context of the Cold War, influenced by national and international interests, followed by installation of a military dictatorship (1973–1990). The very day of the coup, harsh persecution was unleashed against government employees and supporters as well as community and political leaders. In the following weeks and months thousands of people were arrested, brutalised, tortured and murdered. Human rights violations were justified as necessary in order to save the country from the "Marxist menace".

The military coup conspirators declared the country to be in a state of siege and suspended constitutional guarantees. The situation became critical. Within a few days, several ecumenical entities were created to provide legal and social assistance (information, advice, food, shelter, sometimes money, depending on the victim's needs). One was the Committee for Peace in Chile (COPACHI). When this organisation was disbanded under pressure from the military government, in 1976, the Santiago Archdiocese's *Vicaría de la Solidaridad* assumed and expanded COPACHI's work. Moral (and political) resistance to human rights violations found expression in acts of solidarity with victims through legal defence and documented the repressive policies through cases filed in court. These organisations created an array of medical, psychological and social assistance programmes in support of victims.

At first, a network of volunteers and, later, specialised teams offered medical and psychological care. In late 1977 FASIC (Social Aid Foundation of Christian Churches) opened a medical psychiatric programme to provide specialised care to former political prisoners, torture victims and their families. From 1977 to 1985 the programme assisted 4,174 persons in personalised, family and group therapy processes (Weinstein, Lira, & Rojas, 1987, p. 17). In 1987, part of the team formed ILAS (Latin American Institute for Mental Health and Human Rights). In 1980 the Corporation for the Defence of People's Rights (CODEPU) opened its doors, prioritising care for victims of torture. CODEPU's mental health team worked on treatment of the tortured person and his or her family (unit DIT-T), documenting cases to research and denounce human rights violations during the dictatorship. Another mental health-based organisation, CINTRAS, was created in 1985. By the time the dictatorship drew to an end, six mental health teams existed within the various human rights organisations.

Political repression and psychotherapy under dictatorship

From the beginning, hundreds of people turned to the nascent human rights organisations for support in the aftermath of torture. Personalised care sought to bring relief to feelings of insecurity and disorientation that arose when faced with extremely violent situations. Torture was committed against thousands of detainees after September 11, 1973. Beatings, application of electric current and other forms of torture, sexual abuse and rape were the most common methods exercised against human beings held in conditions of extreme powerlessness and vulnerability (Comisión Nacional de Prisión Política y Tortura, 2004, pp. 223–257). In addition, the military government "disappeared" (detained and murdered) many people, denying that they had ever taken prisoners and any knowledge of their whereabouts (Chilean National Commission on Truth and Reconciliation, 1993).

Torture was exercised by Chileans, the majority members of the Armed Forces or police, on behalf of the state and the nation – the same state and the same nation of the prisoners. The torturer would then "forget" the prisoner's name and would categorically deny ever having mistreated and tortured anyone in every judicial process until now. The detainee could corroborate that the hatred was not personal, but rather the projection of political hatreds, that transformed the prisoner into a dangerous enemy, thus justifying the use of violence "to save the nation".

The deliberate subjection to pain, that sought to destroy a person, break down resistance and obtain information about political activities might last for days or months. Such practices paralysed the victims, eroding trust in other human beings, and provoked fear in the broader population, thereby consolidating control of the dictatorship. Each person attempted to endure extreme suffering looking for some meaning in their beliefs, values and political convictions. But torture nearly always is traumatic, and its effects are manifested through anguish, grief, afflictions and illness. In numerous cases, deep depression was generated by multiple losses, associated with feelings of frustration, powerlessness and fear. Upon release from prison, many former prisoners experienced great difficulty in resuming their lives.

Such situations affected not only the former prisoner but the whole family and children in particular. In situations related to the kidnapping and disappearance of a family member symptoms are similar to any other traumatic experience. The cases under treatment were classified by psychologists, psychiatrists and social workers by the specific repressive situation (former political prisoner, relative of a forcibly disappeared person, relative of victims of political execution, people coming from exile). The "situational" diagnosis emphasised the traumatic situation, seeking to make sense of the symptoms. The general diagnosis applied was that of "traumatic political experience". This expression referred to the nature of the harm, as well as individual and familiar consequences.

Most human rights mental health professional teams offered individual, family, group psychotherapy and occupational therapy. Most of them also provided physical and psychiatric health care. The purpose of the various different therapeutic interventions was:

> to repair the repercussions and traumatic side effects of violence related to torture and political repression of the individual who was harmed ... [We attempt] to restore the individual's relation to reality, restoring his/her story, ability to relate to other people and things, the ability to project into the future, by reaching a better understanding of oneself and one's own resources, by expanding his/her conscience concerning the experience.
>
> (Lira & Weinstein, 1984, p. 13)

Torture

Psychologists and other mental health workers were not prepared professionally to treat torture victims. In searching for work methods to help people manage the effects of experiences that for many were cataclysmic, the FASIC team employed *testimony* as a therapeutic tool inspired by old social sciences methodology (Lewis, 1962). In 1978, the team began documenting personal testimonies which were compiled in the form of texts that registered particularly extreme and brutal situations of torture. The text belonged to the author. The testimony was done, in part, for purposes of denunciation of torture in the legal arena (criminal courts and international instances), almost always without success, but leaving a public record of the criminal complaints that, many years later, have led to successful prosecutions (Lira & Loveman, 2005). Some victims used them to substantiate the complaints of torture presented at the time before the tribunals. Sometimes the victim's organisations sent the testimonies to support requests for solidarity with political prisoners and their families.

The patient and the therapist agreed on the purpose of the registry work. The narrative was tape-recorded, transcribed, reviewed and edited with the patient (Cienfuegos & Monelli, 1983). Each story was situated in a timeline of the person's life, the traumatic experience and the present (the moment of the consultation). Testimony resulted from a process, a material expression of a stage of work that meant reliving, working through and thinking about the life lived, not just the traumatic experiences inflicted by repression. Therapists observed that torture altered the functions of the self as disintegrating, prosecutorial and self-destructive fantasies emerged. We observed that the narrative developed by patients in the clinical setting made it easier to progressively recover and order the fragments of a disintegrated experience. It allowed patients to name terrifying, silenced and humiliating situations and we noted that people felt better after relating what had happened to them, although this improvement was transitory. The testimony operated as a catharsis, relieved anguish and enabled an initial emotional elaboration. Victims needed to vindicate their dignity, and their truth. They had been convicted for their statements under torture and tried without due process guarantees. The therapeutic space was constituted by a relationship based on the recognition of their dignity and their rights. However, family conflicts aggravated by the lack of employment and permanent persecution constituted an adverse context. For this reason, the achievements were often transitory. That was to be reckoned with.

Most men and women suffered sexual abuse as a form of torture (Cienfuegos & Ramírez, 2017, p. 127). The communication of these experiences was painful and almost always very difficult to report and denounce. Some men who suffered sexual torture filmed their testimony for denunciation purposes (Fliman, 1979). The complaint relieved the patients emotionally and morally. Their statements reaffirmed their experience, denied by the authorities and unknown to society. Some patients valued the recording of their testimony as a form of reliable documentation of their experience that would persist over time. CODEPU published a book on the heart-breaking experiences of surviving victims arrested shortly after the military coup. The testimonies were also collected by specialists who provided them with support and medical care between 1973 and 1974 (Rojas, Barceló & Reszczynski, 1991). Testimonies have remained over time as a subjective and political record of human rights violations.

The National Commission of Political Imprisonment and Torture (2003–2005)

The Valech Commission submitted its report in November of 2004. At the end of May 2005, 28,459 persons were recognised as victims of political imprisonment and torture from a total number of 34,690 detentions. Ninety-four per cent indicated that they were victims of torture. Among these individuals, 1,244 were under the age of 18 and 176 were under the age of 13; 12.72%, which is the equivalent of 3,621 persons, were women. The Report acknowledged the psychological contributions on the consequences of torture on its report (see Chapter 8). The Commission stated that torture had been a traumatic experience for victims, affecting their sense of personal dignity and integrity, overwhelmed by the self-perception of having abruptly changed into a different person due to having been stripped of all that comprised their previous life, identity, loyalties and values (CNPPT, 2005, pp. 583–612). The reparations measures established by law considered the physical and psychological needs of the victims.

Forced disappearances

The rupture of the life project, the death of loved ones, persecution, detention and torture, the numerous associated losses (housing, employment, income, social relationships) were part of the events experienced by thousands of people, who sought to face their difficulties and normalise daily life in a very adverse context. But there was a group of people who had no chance of returning to normality. They were faced with the forcible disappearance of a relative after detention at home, at work or on the street without witnesses. Most disappearances occurred between the years

1973 and 1977. The detained person did not reappear despite the writs of *habeas corpus* presented in his/her name by human rights lawyers (Vicaría de la Solidaridad, 1979). The disappeared detainees were militants of the persecuted political parties, community leaders, human rights advocates, labelled as *enemies of the nation* and kidnapped by agents of the state. In some cases, the detention, transfer, interrogation and disappearance of prisoners crossed national borders. Neighbouring countries conspired to form joint repressive policy operations, known as Operation Condor (Dinges, 2004).

The practice of forced disappearance installed the ghost of death that remained in its threatening ambiguity in the minds of people tied to the disappeared person. In spite of the authorities' denial of their responsibility for the detention, the relatives latched on to the hope of finding their loved ones alive. They filed countless legal actions, followed any number of leads, presented denunciations before international organisations and courts (United Nations, Organization of American States, International Labour Organization, among others). Legal recourses were inoperative, and authorities not only denied any relationship with the detained person but also constructed public interpretations to displace the responsibility of the disappearances to the victim's own decision or to their political organisations, declaring that they had gone "underground".

Families lived the absence of the "disappeared" as a forced and involuntary separation, which, when prolonged beyond the usual deadlines, nurtured anxiety and the fear that family members had been murdered. Over the years, the hope of finding them alive began to fade. Relatives, mainly women, organised themselves to keep up the search and demands upon the government and the judiciary to know the whereabouts and final destiny of their loved ones. Sometimes, but not always, the families, and especially the mothers, managed to create, with many difficulties, an adequate protective environment for the children. But economic difficulties led to families living in the home of parents, grandparents or relatives, requiring complex adaptations in daily living. It was an affective context besieged by a threatening reality, which could upset the family structure, which had been sustained and reorganised with immense difficulties while facing the disappearance of loved ones. Forced disappearances were a common practice with the same pattern and consequences in the Southern Cone, mainly in Argentina (Rojas, 2009).

According to the observations of the psychologists, in almost in all the families, after the father's arrest, the children experienced the impact of this catastrophe in many ways, depending on their age. Some presented regressive behaviours; others functioned out of control, reacting against every authority (at home, at school); others behaved in an over-adapted way, or in the role of a parent. Initial records showed that most of the children of disappeared persons who consulted presented anguish, sleep disorders, "nightmares in which they woke up crying in the middle of the night", stuttering, exaggerated search for affection, feeling of loneliness, flights of fantasy and others (Cerda & Lagos, 2017, pp. 181–183). Providing adequate clinical care was very complicated: how to care for those children who were orphans, but no one declared their orphanhood and took responsibility for it? How to deal with those women who were almost certainly already widows, but who in their daily struggle demanded that the government took responsibility and acknowledged the murder of their partner in order to assume their widowhood, but who, at the same time, still hoped for the husband to appear alive? Acknowledging death would have made it possible in some way to mourn the loss, but this declaration was the responsibility of the authorities. The situation has lasted for decades. Psychotherapy has been a complex process of accompaniment of a human being living each day with the hope of finding her/his "disappeared" alive and fearing to find him/her dead. The girls and boys who grew up in families traumatised by forced disappearance have reported (and denounced) decades later the sufferings and traumatic experiences that affected them.

Extrajudicial executions

More than 2,000 persons were executed/assassinated in the first months of military government. Many of them died under torture. Some were executed after sham trials by military court martial without ordinary due process – even the minimal protections offered by the Code of Military Justice. In some cases, the bodies of the executed were not delivered to family members for proper burial. The "executions" and deaths in supposed confrontations with the military and police were reported in local and national newspapers. In a small number of cases criminal complaints were filed but were usually heard by military courts and dismissed or rejected. Impunity was the rule.

Some family members of the executed persons consulted after 1979 in FASIC. Practically all the children attended by the mental health teams had witnessed violence exercised against their parents or other members of their families. They asked for psychological care, mainly for children.

> One had to connect all the feelings that the situation produced – pain, anger, sorrow, powerlessness – to other manifestations the child did not explain, such as poor attention span, difficulties in school learning, certain intense fears that overcame him/her. We could help the child cry and experience mourning. ... The deaths of these people have historic and social meaning, therefore, the task of reparation for these deaths pertains to society. As long as these children are not told by their families, and, moreover, by society the value of their parents' lives and death, reparation will be incomplete.
>
> (Cerda & Lagos, 2017, p. 195)

Soledad's case illustrates the consequences of her father's execution, the tragedy of her family, encapsulated in a traumatic oblivion that suffocated her childhood.[2] A creative therapeutic intervention contributed to recovery of her feelings and memories of her painful past. Soledad consulted during 1981, when she was visiting Chile for seven months. She had been living in exile since the execution of her father in 1973. When the family arrived at the country of exile, in March of 1974, her mother told her that her father had been executed. She grew up hurt and damaged, did not recover from the loss, rather hardly remembers it, developed with anger and sadness, was disturbed and sick. At the age of 15 she had great conflicts with her mother, used drugs and decided to return to Chile:

I feel empty ... I am unravelled inside ..., something is missing ..., I am permanently unsatisfied ..., I feel disunited with the things I have inside ..., sometimes I feel that I am going to go crazy ... I don't understand at all.

(Weinstein, 1984, pp. 37–38)

The psychotherapist decided to work with the emotional dissociation that Soledad presented. She experienced anguish, unable to remember what had happened to her before she learned that her father had been executed. All efforts to remember had been in vain. A therapeutic technique was then resorted to that would be essential for her; she was asked to invent, to create those seven months of her life that she lacked, those that go from the *coup d'état* to her departure into exile. The resulting written material was designated "The Void" and was analysed together with Soledad (Weinstein, 1984, p. 42). In that text she wrote in a fragmented way about memories and emotions:

There was something of love, but too much anguish, more anguish than I could bear ... the terrible anguish of my mother pressed me a lot;

Well, then I was running, I was running, I wanted to get out. I wanted to kill. I wanted to liberate the world. There were noises of war, people of war ... The days were cloudy, blind, without rain or light. I was running, ... I want to cry, I want to go out, I want to love, I want to merge the past with the present, I am afraid of the future, in it are lost loved ones.

... I've got everything blank; I don't remember. Only the days were sunny after all ... So that's how I stayed, meditating on life and death. Dying – living. I'm tired, I can't write any more.

(Weinstein, 1984, p. 48)

The psychotherapist wrote that Soledad returned to Chile to re-connect with her father and her roots and to recover her identity. Psychotherapy was for her the instance from which, with affection and companionship, she undertook the process of revealing the meanings of her confused and painful history. That emptiness that drowned her had been filled with tears, sorrow, joy, rage, in short, diverse emotions on which she could sustain herself to continue growing (Weinstein, 1984, p. 50). However, these moments of recovery were still unstable. The prognosis for Soledad was uncertain. This case, like many others, demonstrates that these patients have required professional support until they are able to sustain themselves independently – and that could require many years.

Other situations

Mental health teams also provided a variety of counselling and therapy services to different groups. In 1978 group sessions were held for former political prisoners whose prison sentences were commuted to exile. At the same time a programme was initiated for individuals and families returning from exile. These institutional experiences of psychosocial and therapeutic work, especially with teenagers and children returning to Chile from exile and carried out in FASIC, were documented and published in 1986 (Castillo, 1986; Salamovich & Domínguez, 1986; Weinstein, 1986).

National protests began in 1983 and were violently repressed, giving rise to great numbers of people seeking medical and psychological care. In response, therapists formed groups with people who had been arrested during the daylong protests held from 1983 to 1986, mainly adolescents and young people. On-site workshops were organised with support from volunteer professionals, primarily the Psychologists Guild (Colegio de Psicólogos de Chile), to offer emotional support after the mass raids of working-class neighbourhoods and deaths during protests. Such workshops were held in Catholic church parishes with communities that had been deeply affected by violence (Weinstein et al., 1987, p. 87). After 1984 this type of intervention for working through mourning processes with affected communities and families became quite common (Lira, Weinstein, & Kovalskys, 1987, p. 341).

Such situations led to a return to the issue of fear, comprising a facet of the mental health work that expanded increasingly (Lira, Weinstein, & Salamovich, 1986). Fear and silence reigned for many years. Public silence accompanied private horror and the suffering of torture and death. Fear was constructed through personal experiences. It was reinforced in the narratives of terror, in the lack of information, in the imagination, in the silence of the night, intensified under curfew (that lasted until 1988), in human beings silenced by censorship and by self-censorship. Fear swelled from the perception that the power to kill was unchecked by law and that it was limitless. Various activities were carried out to confront fear in social organisations and communities. The first step was to recognise and speak about fear as a personal and collective experience lived in family, neighbourhoods, schools and social organisations. Groups were organised to work through threats and intimidation against regime opponents and human rights organisations, which intensified from 1985 to 1989. A study on fear under dictatorship was developed by psychologists from 1987 to 1990. The study worked actively with leaders of more than 100 groups to prevent the emotional and practical consequences of fear, considering the importance of people participation before plebiscite (1988) and general elections (1989) to put an end to the dictatorship through constitutional rules (Lira & Castillo, 1991).

Lessons from this experience

An important synthesis of the initial lessons gleaned by mental health teams emerged during a meeting held in April 1980, which discussed the intervention models that had been implemented as well as the relation between political crisis, repressive violence and psychological damage. Professional experiences outside Chile, particularly in France and Belgium, with Latin American exiles were presented (Colectivo Chileno de Trabajo Psicosocial, 1982). In 1983, FASIC's team of psychologists was accorded the Premio Nacional Colegio de Psicólogos (Psychologists Professional Guild's national award) as recognition of its pioneering work on behalf of victims of political repression (Discurso, 1983).

Later writings regarding political repression and mental health services expanded and deepened the initial, somewhat improvisational, approaches. All of them stressed the need to characterise the experiences of the consultants and to describe the different intervention modalities implemented in order to understand how, in spite of their limitations, positive results were achieved. Most of the patients had suffered one loss after another: loss of rights, loss of a job, loss of physical integrity, loss of peace and stability of the family and the loss of the capacity to determine one's life course.

The traumatic experience of the victim is at the core of the therapeutic process. This process, when possible, starts in a professional mental health care context to build a therapeutic bond. The bond with this type of patient is characterised as a "committed bond" (Lira & Weinstein, 1984, pp. 12–13). It implies an *ethically non-neutral attitude* towards the patient's suffering. This kind of therapeutic bond helps to facilitate, and to re-establish, the patient's capacity to trust others, to establish a genuine relationship based on truth and to accept love, hate, sadness, loss, helplessness and desperation, not only in the context of this therapeutic bond, but as part of other relationships between human beings – re-establishing the capacity to trust, by building a true "human relationship sustained by comprehension and solidarity" (Pollarolo & Morales, 1984, p. 190).

However, confronting such trauma requires the differentiation of each repressive situation affecting individuals and families. The terrifying experiences the patient had endured were, to a great extent, irreparable. The therapeutic treatment of victims who have suffered such losses moves towards their acceptance of the fact that parts of their own identities and their social world have been destroyed. But, since the losses are real, only acceptance, mourning and, integration of the losses into their experience and activities can lead to the necessary transformation and reconstruction of their lives. The victims came to realise that individual therapeutic intervention was not enough: they needed to know that their society, as a whole, acknowledged what had happened to them. Individual reparation and social reparation were complementary.

This approach underlined the importance of the acknowledgement of the victims by society, and the therapeutic value of public recognition of the human rights violations and access to justice (Lira, 2016, p. 205). This role was assumed, to a certain extent, by the truth commissions, with the national government confirming and validating legally and symbolically the experiences endured by victims of repression during the dictatorship.

At the end of the dictatorship psychologists were concerned with the process of recognition of victims as a requisite of social peace and political reconciliation.

Political transition to democracy

Public policies regarding recognition and reparation of victims of human rights violations evolved gradually from 1990 until the present. In 1990, newly elected President Patricio Aylwin began to adopt several measures, including the creation of the National Commission for Truth and Reconciliation, 1990–1991 (known as the Rettig Commission) and several reparation policies in order to recognise and redress the victims of human rights violations under the dictatorship. Some psychologists from human rights organisations collaborated in drafting the recommendations of the Commission regarding provision of health services to victims. The Commission recommended the creation of a special health programme for them: "Such a program should seek technical cooperation from non-governmental health organisations, particularly those that have provided health care to this population and have accumulated valuable experience over all these years" (Chilean National Commission on Truth and Reconciliation, 1993, p. 1068). In 1991 the Program of Reparation and Comprehensive Health Care for Victims of Human Rights Violations, known as PRAIS, was implemented, and this offers both physical and mental health care to surviving victims.

In 2003 the Commission on Political Imprisonment and Torture (known as Valech Commission) was created by President Ricardo Lagos to "determine ... the individuals that suffered detention and torture for political reasons, as a result of acts of government agents or persons at their service" (CNPPT, 2005). In 2010, the government opened a new period for application for victims' recognition in the Advisory Commission for the Recognition of Disappeared Detainees, Victims of Extrajudicial Executions and Victims of Political Imprisonment and Torture (2010–2011). In all these instances, 41,513 persons were officially recognised as victims of human rights violations.

The Valech Commission's report described the medical, psychosocial and psychological consequences of torture and stated that:

> The psychosocial impact of torture cannot be gauged by an inventory of effects that comprise an anatomy of pain. The aggression victims suffered is not limited to them personally or to their closest circle; it affects and has implications for the entire society. The effects of human rights violations profoundly changed historic models of civic and citizen participation, and trust between people. ... Politics as a legitimate occupation became associated with death and losses. ... Medical and psychological diagnosis cannot adequately explain the unfathomable consequences of torture. ... The perception of this adverse and frustrating situation accentuated as a result of societal disinterest, incredulity, and denial regarding the existence of human rights violations.
>
> (CNPPT, 2005, p. 606)

Reparation policies included the right to rehabilitation in the PRAIS programme. PRAIS recognised as beneficiaries (direct family members, that is to say, fathers, mothers, children, siblings and grandchildren) the relatives of forced disappearances and those executed for political reasons, exiles who returned to the country, former political prisoners and victims of torture and people dismissed from their employment for political reasons (Domínguez, Poffald, Valdivia, & Gómez, 1994). PRAIS initiated its activities in 1991 as a programme of the Ministry of Health and was established by law 19,980 as a reparation programme in 2004.

In 2019, PRAIS was comprised of 29 public health teams with networks that covered the needs of more than 740,000 registered beneficiaries, including all the victims recognised by the state and their relatives. Medical doctors, psychologists and other professionals provide specialised health and mental health care. In addition to direct care, over time other activities were added at the request of the victims and according to the possibilities offered by the teams, including participation with the associations of victims in education and human rights activities. The PRAIS teams also participate in memory and justice initiatives, such as activities at sites of memory (the Museum of Memory, former centres of torture, monuments around the country, including the national cemetery in Santiago, among others), ceremonies of commemoration, psychosocial support during denunciation of victimisers, monitoring criminal judicial processes against victimisers, participation in the process of exhumation, identification and burial of victims who have remained disappeared for decades and whose remains, or partial remains, have been found. All of these activities have been considered part of the policy of reparation. It is important to note that the work of PRAIS has been possible thanks to the professionals working in each of the teams who have built the programme, by creating, in practice, concrete modalities of assistance, accompaniment and treatment according to the consultant's and families' needs.

Final reflections

A retrospective view enables us to see to what extent Chile's post-1990 public policies of acknowledgement and reparation of victims were based on the work, experience and documentation compiled by professional staff of human rights organisations, in most cases the same ones that had provided assistance during the dictatorship to people affected by political repression (Bernasconi, Ruiz, & Lira, 2018).

The work of the psychologists since its inception had as its main objective to recognise and care for the victims. The therapeutic process involved recognising personal resources and strengths and rescuing what could be repaired even though the losses were irreparable. These therapeutic processes have taught us that the improvement of the victims has not depended solely on the processes of psychic working through. Given that their suffering originated in political and social conditions, the public recognition of the facts that affected them, material and symbolic reparation policies, as well as the judicial convictions of the perpetrators, have contributed to many victims feeling "repaired", experiencing significant improvements in their mental health. But we have also learned that for many victims nothing will be enough to repair the physical and psychological injuries they have suffered. These relationships between political and personal processes, sometimes evident, sometimes disguised or deeply buried in victims and family members, have implications that greatly exceed the impact of clinical interventions.

Reparation as a social, psychological and political process cannot ignore the fact that most of the damages and losses that give the right to be recognised and repaired are, paradoxically, irreparable. For this reason, a reparation policy must ensure preventive measures in the sphere of the institutions involved in the violations of human rights and in the socio-cultural sphere, to ensure educational measures and civic memory that give full respect for the human rights of all and the non-repetition of these violations in a new conflict.

Questions

1. Are we talking about victims or survivors? What is the meaning of referring to individuals and families as victims in cases of human rights violations?
2. As regards the limits of psychotherapy in cases of enforced disappearance, how are we to conceptualise mourning and grief in cases where there is no information about the final destination and whereabouts of the remains of a victim of enforced disappearance?

3. What is the role of judicial processes (condemnation of those responsible, recognition of the events that occurred, recognition of the victims and their compensation) in relation to the mental health of the victims, when these results are produced 40 years after the events?

4. With regard to the individual and family consequences of the summary execution of a family member in the immediate present and over the years: how are we to conceptualise mourning and grief, and how should we accompany its processing in the context of a dictatorship?

5. Discuss the registration of the memory and truth of victims as a resource for the truth and collective memory of society and its role in the construction of democratic coexistence after the violence of political repression.

Notes

1 This chapter is based on documentation gathered for the project "Political Memory Technologies: Contemporary Uses and Appropriations of Devices for Recording Human Rights Violations Perpetrated by the Civil-Military Dictatorship in Chile" (Conicyt PIA-SOC18005). Memory and Human Rights Programme, Alberto Hurtado University.

2 Soledad is a pseudonym. The case was anonymised. She gave permission for publication to her therapist in 1984. Soledad died a few years ago.

References

Bernasconi, O., Ruiz, M., & Lira, E. (2018). What defines the victims of human rights violations? The case of the Comité Pro Paz and Vicaría de la Solidaridad in Chile (1973–1992). In V. Druliolle & R. Brett (Eds.), *The politics of victimhood in post-conflict societies. Comparative and analytical perspectives* (pp. 101–131). Cham: Palgrave Macmillan.

Castillo, M. I. (1986). La identidad en adolescentes retornados: una experiencia grupal (The identity of returning adolescents: A group experience). In *Exilio 1986–1978* (pp. 35–45). Santiago: FASIC/Amerinda Ediciones.

Cerda, M., & Lagos, E. (2017). Los niños y las experiencias de pérdida en el marco de la represión política chilena. In Lira, E. (ed.) Colectivo *Chileno de Trabajo Psicosocial Lecturas de Psicología y Política. Crisis Política y Daño Psicológico* (Children and experiences of loss in the framework of Chilean political repression. In Chilean collective of psychosocial work, readings of psychology and politics. Political crisis and psychological distress) (pp. 179–191). Santiago: Reedición Ediciones, Universidad Alberto Hurtado.

Chilean National Commission on Truth and Reconciliation. (1993). *Report of the Chilean National Commission on Truth and Reconciliation*. University of Notre Dame Press.

Cienfuegos, A. J., & Monelli, C. (1983). The testimony of political repression as a therapeutic instrument. *American Journal of Orthopsychiatry*, 53(1), 43–51.

Cienfuegos, A. J., & Ramírez, M. J. (2017). Daño Psicológico de la represión política en el individuo, en Colectivo chileno de trabajo psicosocial *Lecturas de Psicología y Política. Crisis Política y Daño Psicológico*. (The individual psychological distress of political repression in Chilean collective of psychosocial work readings of psychology and politics. Political crisis and psychological damage). (pp. 126–135). Santiago: Reedición Ediciones Universidad Alberto Hurtado.

CNPPT. (2005). (Informe de la Comisión Nacional Sobre la Prisión Política y Tortura) Report of the Valech commission 2005 available at http://www.memoriachilena.gob.cl/602/w3-art icle-85804.html

Colectivo Chileno de Trabajo Psicosocial. (1982). *Lecturas de Psicología y Política. Crisis Política y Daño Psicológico* (Readings of psychology and politics. political crisis and psychological damage). Santiago: 2 tomos.

Comisión Nacional sobre Prisión Política y Tortura. (2004) *Informe de la Comisión Nacional sobre Prisión Política y Tortura* (Report of the National Commission on Political Detention and Torture). Santiago. Retrieved from https://bibliotecadigital.indh.cl/handle/123456789/455

Dinges, J. (2004). *The Condor years: How Pinochet and his allies brought terrorism to three continents*. New York: The New Press.

Discurso de agradecimiento al premio Colegio de Psicólogos de Chile (Speech of thanks to the Chilean college of psychologists award) (1983). La verdad reparadora Revista *Mensaje ("The restorative truth" Message Magazine)*. 326, 29–31.

Domínguez, R., Poffald, L., Valdivia, G., & Gómez, E. (1994). *Salud y Derechos Humanos. Una experiencia desde el sistema público de salud chileno*, (Health and human rights. An experience from the Chilean public health system). Santiago: Ministerio de Salud.

Fliman, H. (1979). *Chile testimonio 1 (Chile testimony 1)*. (video 52 min). Archivo Museo de la Memoria. Retrieved from http://archivomuseodelamemoria.cl/index.php/186783;isad

Lewis, O. (1962). *The children of Sanchez – The autobiography of a Mexican family*. London: Secker & Warburg.

Lira, E. (2016). Reflections on rehabilitation as a form of reparation in Chile after Pinochet's dictatorship. *International Human Rights Law Review*, 5(2), 1–23.

Lira, E., & Castillo, M. I. (1991). *Psicología de la amenaza política y del miedo* (The psychology of political threat and fear). Santiago: Ediciones Ilas- Cesoc.

Lira, E., & Loveman, B. (2005). *Políticas de reparación. (Politics of reparation). Chile: 1990–2004*. Santiago: LOM/DIBAM and Universidad Alberto Hurtado.

Lira, E., & Weinstein, E. (1984). *Psicoterapia y represión política (Psychotherapy and political repression)*. México D.F: Editorial Siglo XXI.

Lira, E., Weinstein, E., & Kovalskys, J. (1987). Subjetividad y represión política: Intervenciones psicoterapéuticas (Subjectivity and political repression: Psychotherapeutic interventions). In M. Montero & I. Martín Baró (Eds.), *Psicología política latinoamericana* (pp. 317–346). Caracas: Ed. Panapo.

Lira, E., Weinstein, E., & Salamovich, S. (1986). El miedo. Un enfoque psicosocial (The fear. A psychosocial approach). *Revista Chilena De Psicología*, 8(1), 51–56.

Pollarolo, F., & Morales, E. (1984). Claustrofobia, paralización y participación: psicoterapia de un militante politico (Claustrophobia, paralysis and participation: Psychotherapy of a political militant). In E. Lira & E. Weinstein (Eds.), *Psicoterapia y represión política* (pp. 180–192). México: Siglo XXI.

Rojas, P. (2009). *La Interminable ausencia, Estudio médico, psicológico y politico de la desaparición forzada de personas* (The endless absence, medical, psychological and political study of the forced disappearance of people). Santiago: LOM.

Rojas, P., Barceló, P., & Reszczynski, K. (1991). *Tortura y resistencia en Chile (Torture and resistance in Chile)*. Santiago: Emisión.

Salamovich, S., & Domínguez, R. (1986). Proceso psicológico de desexilio: una respuesta psicoterapéutica (The psychological process of desexiliation: a psychotherapeutic response). En *Exilio 1986–1978* (pp. 47–60). Santiago: FASIC/Amerinda Ediciones.

Vicaría de la Solidaridad, Arzobispado de Santiago. (1979). *Dónde están* (Where are they). Santiago: 7 tomos.

Weinstein, E. (1984). "Soledad y vacío: un caso de psicoterapia con un familiar de ejecutado" (Loneliness and emptiness: A case of psychotherapy with a relative an executed individual). In E. Lira & E. Weinstein (Eds.), *Psicoterapia y represión política* (pp. 38–50). México: Siglo XXI.

Weinstein, E. (1986). Algunas orientaciones acerca de la Psicoterapia con retornados del exilio (Some guidelines for Psychotherapy with returnees from exile). In *Exilio 1986–1978* (pp. 63–80). Santiago: FASIC/Amerinda Ediciones.

Weinstein, E., Lira, E., & Rojas, M. E. (1987). *Trauma, duelo y reparación. Una experiencia de trabajo en Chile psicosocial* (Trauma, bereavement and reparation. A psychosocial work experience in Chile). Santiago: FASIC/Interamericana.

Printed in the United States
By Bookmasters